PROGRESS IN BRAIN RESEARCH

VOLUME 32

PITUITARY, ADRENAL AND THE BRAIN

PROGRESS IN BRAIN RESEARCH

PROGRESS IN BRAIN RESEARCH
VOLUME 32

PITUITARY, ADRENAL
AND THE BRAIN

EDITED BY

D. DE WIED

AND

J. A. W. M. WEIJNEN

Rudolf Magnus Institute for Pharmacology,
University of Utrecht, Medical Faculty
Vondellaan 6, Utrecht, The Netherlands

ELSEVIER PUBLISHING COMPANY
AMSTERDAM / LONDON / NEW YORK
1970

ELSEVIER PUBLISHING COMPANY
335 JAN VAN GALENSTRAAT,
P.O. BOX 211, AMSTERDAM, THE NETHERLANDS

ELSEVIER PUBLISHING CO. LTD.
BARKING, ESSEX, ENGLAND

AMERICAN ELSEVIER PUBLISHING COMPANY, INC.
52 VANDERBILT AVENUE, NEW YORK, N.Y. 10017

This volume contains the Proceedings of an International Conference on

THE PITUITARY–ADRENAL AXIS AND THE NERVOUS SYSTEM

*The Conference was organized by the Rudolf Magnus Institute for Pharmacology,
University of Utrecht, and held at Vierhouten,
The Netherlands, 22–24 July, 1969*

LIBRARY OF CONGRESS CATALOG CARD NUMBER 70–110965

STANDARD BOOK NUMBER: 444-40854-1

PRINTED IN THE NETHERLANDS

List of Contributors

A. N. BHATTACHARYA, Department of Physiology, School of Medicine, University of Pittsburgh, Pittsburgh, Penn., U.S.A.

B. BOHUS, Institute of Physiology, University Medical School, Rákóczi út 80, Pécs, Hungary.

P. K. BRIDGES, Department of Psychological Medicine, Royal Free Hospital, London, W.C.1, England.

R. A. CLEGHORN, Department of Psychiatry, Allan Memorial Institute, McGill University, 1025 Pine Avenue West, Montreal 112, Province Quebec, Canada.

A. J. COPPEN, M.R.C. Neuropsychiatric Research Unit Carshalton, and West Park Hospital, Epsom, Surrey, England.

H. CORRODI, Biochemical Laboratory, AB Hässle, Fack, 402 20 Göteborg, Sweden.

N. DAFNY, Department of Neurology, Hadassah University Hospital, Jerusalem, Israel.

J. DELACOUR, Centre d'Etudes de Physiologie Nerveuse, Département de Psychophysiologie du Comportement, 4, Avenue Gordon-Bennet, Paris 16 ème, France.

D. A. DENTON, Howard Florey Laboratories of Experimental Physiology, Department of Physiology, University of Melbourne, Parkville, Victoria 3052, Australia.

D. DE WIED, Rudolf Magnus Institute for Pharmacology, University of Utrecht, Medical Faculty, Vondellaan 6, Utrecht, The Netherlands.

E. ENDRÖCZI, Institute of Physiology, University Medical School, Rákóczi út 80, Pécs, Hungary.

T. FEKETE, Institute of Physiology, University Medical School, Rákóczi út 80, Pécs, Hungary.

S. FELDMAN, Department of Neurology, Hadassah University Hospital, Jerusalem, Israel.

J. FRANKEL, Paediatric Metabolic and Endocrine Service and Rogoff-Wellcome Medical Research Institute, Division of Paediatrics, Beilinson Hospital, Tel Aviv University Medical School (and Psychology Department, Bar-Ilan University), Israel.

C. FRANKLIN, Department of Physiology, Health Sciences Centre, The University of Western Ontario, London, Ontario, Canada.

K. FUXE, Department of Histology, Karolinska Institutet, 104 01 Stockholm 60, Sweden.

W. H. GISPEN, Rudolf Magnus Institute for Pharmacology, University of Utrecht, Medical Faculty, Vondellaan 6, Utrecht, The Netherlands.

E. GLASSMAN, Department of Biochemistry and the Neurobiology Curriculum, University of North Carolina, Chapel Hill, N. C., U.S.A.

M. M. HALL, Department of Pharmacology, Ohio State University College of Medicine, Columbus, Ohio, U.S.A.

G. W. HARRIS, University of Oxford, Department of Human Anatomy, South Parks Road, Oxford, England.

R. I. HENKIN, Section of Neuroendocrinology, Experimental Therapeutics Branch, National Heart Institute, National Institutes of Health, Bethesda, Md20014, U.S.A.

J. R. HODGES, Department of Pharmacology, Royal Free Hospital School of Medicine, 8, Hunter Street, London W.C.I., England.

T. HÖKFELT, Department of Histology, Karolinska Institutet, 104 01 Stockholm 60, Sweden.

M. T. JONES, Sherrington School of Physiology, St. Thomas' Hospital, London S.E.I., England.

G. JONSSON, Department of Histology, Karolinska Institutet, 104 01 Stockholm 60, Sweden.

M. KARP, Paediatric Metabolic and Endocrine Service and Rogoff-Wellcome Medical Research Institute, Division of Paediatrics, Beilinson Hospital, Tel Aviv University Medical School, Israel.

R. KLEIN, Pediatric Clinical Center, Boston City Hospital, Boston, Mass. 02118, U.S.A.

L. KORÁNYI, Institute of Physiology, University Medical School, Rákóczi út 80, Pécs, Hungary.

W. A. KRIVOY, National Institute of Mental Health, Addiction Research Center, P.O. Box 2000, Lexington, Ky., U.S.A.

S. LANDE, Section of Dermatology, Department of Medicine, Yale University School of Medicine, New Haven, Conn., U.S.A.

Z. LARON, Paediatric Metabolic and Endocrine Service and Rogoff-Wellcome Medical Research Institute, Division of Paediatrics, Beilinson Hospital, Tel Aviv University Medical School, Israel.

D. LEAK, McGregor Clinic and St. Joseph's Hospital, Hamilton, Ontario, Canada.

S. LEVINE, Stanford University School of Medicine, Department of Psychiatry, Stanford, Calif. 94305, U.S.A.

K. LISSÁK, Institute of Physiology, University Medical School, Rákóczi út 80, Pécs, Hungary.

B. H. MARKS, Department of Pharmacology, Ohio State University College of Medicine, 1645 Neil Avenue, Columbus, Ohio 43210, U.S.A.

L. MARTINI, Institute of Pharmacology, University of Milan, 32, Via Vanvitelli, 20129, Milano, Italy

B. S. MCEWEN, Rockefeller University, 66th and York Avenue, New York, N.Y. 10021, U.S.A.

K. MILKOVIĆ, Institute of General Biology, Medical Faculty, University of Zagreb, Yugoslavia.

S. MILKOVIĆ, Laboratory for Experimental Medicine, General Hospital "Dr. Mladen Stojanović", Vinogradska c. 29, Zagreb, Yugoslavia.

I. A. MIRSKY, Laboratory of Clinical Sciences, University of Pittsburgh School of Medicine, 3811 O'Hara Street, Pittsburgh, Penn. 15213, U.S.A.

J. MONEY, Department of Psychiatry and Behavioral Sciences and Department of Pediatrics, The Johns Hopkins Hospital, Baltimore, Md. 21205, U.S.A.

M. MOTTA, Institute of Pharmacology, University of Milan, 32, Via Vanvitelli, 20129, Milano, Italy

A. H. MULDER, Rudolf Magnus Institute for Pharmacology, University of Utrecht, Medical Faculty, Vondellaan 6, Utrecht, The Netherlands.

J. F. NELSON, Howard Florey Laboratories of Experimental Physiology, Department of Physiology, University of Melbourne, Parkville, Victoria 3052, Australia.

J. PAUNOVIĆ, Institute of General Biology, Medical Faculty, University of Zagreb, Yugoslavia.

A. PERTZELAN, Paediatric Metabolic and Endocrine Service and Rogoff-Wellcome Medical Research Institute, Division of Paediatrics, Beilinson Hospital, Tel Aviv University Medical School, Israel.

F. PIVA, Institute of Pharmacology, University of Milan, 32, Via Vanvitelli, 20129, Milano, Italy.

E. J. SACHAR, Montefiore Hospital and Medical Center, 111 East 210th Street, Bronx, N.Y. 10467, U.S.A.

J. P. SCHADÉ, Netherlands Central Institute for Brain Research, IJdijk 28, Amsterdam-O, The Netherlands.

P. SCHOTMAN, Laboratory for Physiological Chemistry, Medical Faculty, University of Utrecht, Vondellaan 24a, Utrecht, The Netherlands.

I. SENČAR, Laboratory for Experimental Medicine, General Hospital "Dr. Mladen Stojanović", Vinogradska c. 29, Zagreb, Yugoslavia.

J. L. SLANGEN, Rudolf Magnus Institute for Pharmacology, University of Utrecht, Medical Faculty, Vondellaan 6, Utrecht, The Netherlands.

P. G. SMELIK, Department of Pharmacology, Free University, P.O. Box 7161, Amsterdam, The Netherlands.

F. A. STEINER, Department of Experimental Medicine, F. Hoffmann-La Roche & Co. Ltd., Basel, and Institute for Brain Research, University of Zurich, Switzerland.

J. A. F. STEVENSON, Department of Physiology, The University of Western Ontario, London, Ontario, Canada.

A. M. L. VAN DELFT, Rudolf Magnus Institute for Pharmacology, University of Utrecht, Medical Faculty, Vondellaan 6, Utrecht, The Netherlands.

TJ. B. VAN WIMERSMA GREIDANUS, Rudolf Magnus Institute for Pharmacology, University of Utrecht, Medical Faculty, Vondellaan 6, Utrecht, The Netherlands.

J. A. W. M. WEIJNEN, Rudolf Magnus Institute for Pharmacology, University of Utrecht, Medical Faculty, Vondellaan 6, Utrecht, The Netherlands.

J. M. WEISS, Rockefeller University, 66th and York Avenue, New York, 10021, N.Y., U.S.A.

J. E. WILSON, Department of Biochemistry and the Neurobiology Curriculum, University of North Carolina, Chapel Hill, N. C., U.S.A.

A. WITTER, Rudolf Magnus Institute for Pharmacology, University of Utrecht, Medical Faculty, Vondellaan 6, Utrecht, The Netherlands.

PROGRESS IN BRAIN RESEARCH

Preface

For several years we have felt that it would be appropriate to organize a meeting on the pituitary–adrenal axis and the nervous system. The present expansion of research in this area called for a survey of the field in order to gain insight into the significance of the interaction between the pituitary–adrenal axis and the brain and to set new goals for future research.

It was intended to examine the subject of the conference from different angles. The meeting started with a discussion on the influence of the nervous system on pituitary–adrenal activity, a topic which has been extensively studied during the last two decades. Subsequently, the action of the pituitary–adrenal axis on the nervous system was discussed, an area which has been recently expanding. The third aspect of the meeting was the relationship between the pituitary–adrenal system and animal behavior, which is an important topic in our own research. The conference ended with studies on the interaction between pituitary–adrenal system hormones and human behavior.

During the meeting, a magnificent accomplishment was made when the first human being set foot on the moon. This spectacular technological achievement hopefully is indicative of the speed with which knowledge on the living organism will be attained in the near future. One would wish that the achievements in this area of research would parallel the progress made in sounding the universe during the last decade. May this conference have contributed to the understanding of the organ essential for all our accomplishments: The Brain.

I am grateful to all who contributed to the success of the conference, to the chairmen Professors R. A. Cleghorn, G. W. Harris, K. Lissák and I. A. Mirsky, and to the speakers and the discussants who were so kind to accept my invitation to participate in the meeting. I would also like to mention the valuable assistance of the secretarial staff with special reference to Miss T. A. Baas, the technical staff, and in particular the organizing committee consisting of Drs. A. M. L. Van Delft, W. H. Gispen, J. L. Slangen, J. A. W. M. Weijnen and Tj. B. Van Wimersma Greidanus, who are all members of the Rudolf Magnus Institute.

D. DE WIED
Professor of Pharmacology,
Head of the Rudolf Magnus Institute
for Pharmacology

Acknowledgements

The Organizing Committee expresses its special thanks for the generous support by the following organizations:

Dutch Government, Department of Education and Science, The Hague
Farbe Werke Hoechst A.G., Frankfurt
Hoffmann–La Roche N.V., Mijdrecht
Merck Sharp and Dohme Nederland N.V., Haarlem
N.V. Organon, Oss
N.V. Philips Duphar, Amsterdam
The Dr. Saal van Zwanenberg Foundation, Oss
Schering Co., Bloomfield, N.J.
Smith, Kline and French Labs., Philadelphia, Pa.
Specia, Paris
Syntex Corp., Palo Alto, Calif.
The University of Utrecht
The Van Wijck Stam Casper Foundation, Utrecht

Contents

SESSION I

Effects of the Nervous System on Pituitary–Adrenal Activity

Chairman: G. W. HARRIS

University of Oxford, Department of Human Anatomy, South Parks Road, Oxford (U.K.)

The Limbic System and the Pituitary–Adrenal Axis

J. P. SCHADÉ

Netherlands Central Institute for Brain Research, Amsterdam

INTRODUCTION

The limbic system appears to be involved in activating or inhibiting basic drives as well as their concomitant hormone release. The anterior and medial hypothalamic areas are regarded as integrating centers for regulation of pituitary function (Sawyer *et al.*, 1968; Smelik, 1969). These hypothalamic regions are embedded in a dense meshwork of fibers, originating not only from neurons in other hypothalamic areas, but also from limbic and extralimbic systems (Nauta, 1958; De Groot, 1966).

Of particular importance for the study of control of the pituitary-adrenocortical system are the intrahypothalamic and intralimbic pathways which converge upon the anteromedial region. In this area, groups of neurons are located which produce and release a corticotrophin-releasing factor (CRF) which is essential for the release of ACTH by the pituitary.

The pool of CFR neurons is accessible to neural and humoral stimuli of excitatory and inhibitory nature. Therefore, it has been suggested that this pool is an integrative part of the "steroidstat", a homeostatic mechanism for keeping the glucosteroid content at a constant level (Schadé, 1969; Steiner *et al.*, 1969).

In the past decade, the introduction of axon degeneration techniques for the mapping of poorly myelinated systems, and the use of micro-electrodes for the investigation of the sensitivity of hypothalamic neurons, has facilitated the analysis of the role played by the hypothalamus in pituitary adreno-cortical relations. The finding of reciprocal neural pathways linking limbic areas with hypothalamic nuclear masses as well as certain brain stem areas, has necessitated a reappraisal of the neuronal control mechanisms of pituitary function.

No regulatory system can be adequately assessed until we appreciate the nature of physiological integration between the systems. Since we are dealing with the influence of the limbic system upon the pituitary-adrenal axis, an attempt should be made to integrate the functional properties of the two systems involved. The first principle, in such an understanding, is to know the morphological substratum with which one is dealing and its physiological properties. Since a rectilinear relationship may be assumed to exist between the CRF-producing neurons, the ACTH-producing cells in the anterior pituitary, and the corticosteroid-producing cells in the adrenals, the analysis of the limbic influence upon the pituitary-adrenal axis boils down to the functional interaction between the limbic system and the CRF-neurons in the hypothalamus.

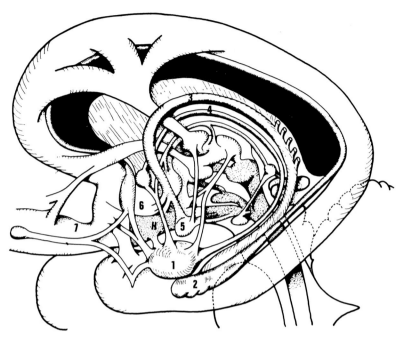

Fig. 1. Some limbic structures mentioned in the text. (Scheme after Needham and Dila, 1968)

1. amygdala   5. mammillary body
2. hippocampus   6. septum
3. fornix system   7. medial forebrain bundle
4. stria terminalis H. hypothalamus.

For this discussion we would like to have available a detailed anatomical scheme of the afferent and efferent connections between the limbic system and hypothalamus, and also an insight into the intrahypothalamic and intralimbic circuitry. Unfortunately, this information is not yet available. Since we are dealing with a multiloop control system in which rigid one-to-one or linear relations do not hold, it is essential to provide a structural frame of reference in order to draw up a simplified model. Therefore an attempt at system analysis of the limbic CRF-neuronal trajectory is being made. In this respect we have to deal with the following aspects of the problem:

(a) the characteristics of the substratum of the limbic regulatory system;

(b) its neurophysiological properties;

(c) the nature of the CRF-neuron pool and the reciprocal interaction between limbic system and CRF-pool.

PROPOSITION 1

The substratum of the limbic-hypothalamic (CRF-neuron pool – pituitary-adrenal) regulation consists of two classes of pathways with different integration levels, both classes of pathways having excitatory and inhibitory properties

Using histological and physiological methods, a number of limbic-hypothalamic pathways have been clarified. Especially important are the well-developed neuronal

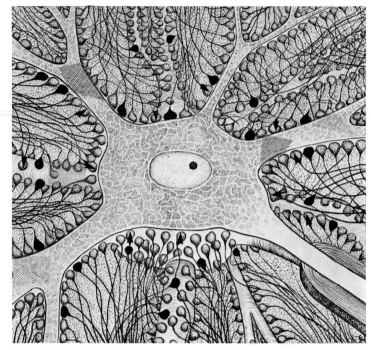

Fig. 2. Schematic model of the CRF-neuron (excitatory synapses: black; inhibitory synapses: arrow). The stippled and striped areas indicate parts of the receptive surface of the neuron which is sensitive to circulating factors.

trajectories between the amygdaloid complex and hippocampal formation on the one hand, and the neuronal pools of certain regions of the hypothalamus on the other hand (Bargmann and Schadé, 1963, 1964; Szentágothai *et al.*, 1968). The anterio-medial region: nodal area for the regulation of pituitary function and location of the CRF-neuron pool, receives afferent connections through the stria terminalis and the fimbria-fornix bundle. Furthermore, this hypothalamic area receives numerous short fiber bundles, a.o. from the periventricular system, mammillary bodies, medial fore-brain bundle, and the lateral and posterior hypothalamic regions.

On the basis of the functional properties, the pathways could be divided into two classes: the stria terminalis and fimbria-fornix bundle on the one hand, and all other connections on the other hand. In both classes fiber systems could be distinguished which either excite or inhibit the basic activity of the CRF-neuron pool (cf. Adey and Tokizane, 1967; Dallman and Yates, 1968).

The amygdaloid complex exerts an excitatory influence on the CRF-neuron pool, as illustrated by stimulation and ablation experiments (Mangili *et al.*, 1966; Gloor *et al.*, 1969). Stimulation of the amygdaloid nuclei activates ACTH-release; while bilateral destruction diminishes the activity of the pituitary adrenocortical axis.

The hippocampus and some other forebrain and rhinencephalic structures have been reported to inhibit the CRF-neuron pool. Stimulation within physiological

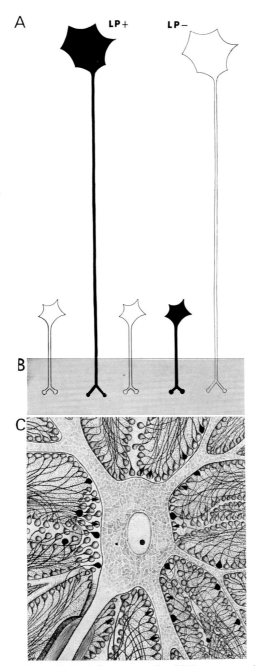

Fig. 3. Model of limbic and extralimbic influences on the CRF-neuron pool. A: limbic pyramidal system; LP+ fibers (e.g. from amygdala): limbic pyramidal system which excites CRF-neuron pool; LP− fibers (e.g. dorsal hippocampus): limbic pyramidal system which inhibits CRF-neuron pool; B: limbic extrapyramidal and other influences upon the CRF-neuron pool. The hierarchy of A is higher than that of B. The striped area of B indicates interneuron pools; C: CRF-neuron pool.

ranges of the dorsal hippocampus inhibits ACTH-release in the cat (Endröczi and Lissák, 1962). The reciprocal relationship between amygdaloid complex and hippocampus has also been demonstrated by bilateral lesions of the hippocampus. These latter experiments resulted in a high plasma corticoid level, indicating an excitation of the CRF-neuron pool.

It would now also be possible to explain the observations by Knigge and Hays (1963), who placed lesions in amygdala and hippocampus at different time intervals. After bilateral lesions in the amygdala were performed, the animals became unresponsive to certain stress-stimuli and no activation of ACTH-release was seen. Apparently, the inhibition by the hippocampal input of the CRF-neuron pool in conjunction with the background inhibition from other areas was so strong that no CRF was released. The additional destruction of the hippocampal area reestablished the discharge of ACTH because the decrease of inhibition resulted in a different activity level of the CRF-neuron pool which thereupon again could respond to the excitation caused by the stress-stimuli.

The amygdaloid complex and the hippocampal formation seem to play a major role in the regulation of the CRF-neuron pool, although many other limbic and extra-limbic pathways are known to be able to modulate the basic activity of this set of neurons (cf. Mangili et al., 1966).

PROPOSITION 2

The information flow along the limbic-hypothalamic pathways (connections between amygdala and hippocampus on the one hand and the CRF-neuron pool on the other) originate from integration centers

The amygdaloid complex is via the stria terminalis and the ventral amygdalo-fugal pathway connected with numerous neuron pools in the hypothalamus. Short latency responses are seen in the anterior part of the hypothalamus upon stimulation of various subdivisions of the amygdala. These potentials are indicative of a direct action upon the neurons of various areas (Gloor et al., 1969). The conduction velocity within the stria terminalis exceeds the value for the fibers of the direct amygdalofugal system. The amygdala consists, in part, of neurons which show changes in excitability upon neural stimuli of diverse sensory origin. It seems safe to assume that various subdivisions of the amygdaloid complex receive and transmit information of a complex nature; and therefore this area should be regarded as one of the major integration centers of the limbic system. The amygdala also diverges stimuli to many other limbic areas, e.g. the septum and the preoptic area. The experiments of Gloor and coworkers (1969) suggest that the firing patterns of many hypothalamic neurons could be modified by amygdaloid stimulation. These results show that the stimulus patterns of the amygdalohypothalamic pathway may, in part, determine the excitability level of neuron pools in the hypothalamus. As far as the CRF-neuron pool is concerned, the experiments, mentioned under proposition 1, indicate that the amygdala exerts an excitatory effect upon this particular hypothalamic function.

One can only speculate about the nature of the chemical transmission of this fiber system. It seems unlikely that monoaminergic neurotransmitters are involved (see Fuxe, 1964); but there is sufficient evidence that cholinergic mechanisms play a role in controlling the activity of CRF-neurons (Shute and Lewis, 1966). Steiner *et al.* (1969) found that acetylcholine, applied iontophoretically to steroid-sensitive neurons in the hypothalamus, markedly increased the firing rate. Thus, if the hippocampohypothalamic pathway, impinging upon the CRF-pool, is cholinergic, it should act via inhibitory neurons which synaptic action diminishes the firing rate of the CRF-neurons.

The amygdalohypothalamic connections are also involved in the control of food and water intake (Morgane, 1969). Experiments have shown, that for the regulation of these mechanisms, at least two neuron pools are responsible. Recently, Oomura and coworkers (1969) have shown that sets of neurons of these pools may either be activated or inhibited upon acetylcholine application. We may assume that the mechanisms ensuring homeostasis of the functions controlled by the pituitary-adrenocortical axis consist of two integrating centers; one of which is the CRF-neuron pool. The other reciprocal center, probably of a parasympathetic nature and located in the posterior hypothalamus, may also be under the control of the amygdaloid complex. To ensure a balanced neuronal input to both hypothalamic centers, the cholinergic pathway from the amygdala should then activate the neuron pool in the posterior hypothalamus. The findings of Oomura and coworkers do not contradict this hypothesis.

The same reasoning holds true for the hippocampal formation. Lack of space does not permit us to go into detail about this interesting problem. Adey and others (Adey 1967; Adey and Tokizane, 1967; McLardy, 1959) have shown that the neuronal aggregates of the hippocampus possess specific integrative properties. Neural stimuli of diverse origin converge upon single hippocampal neurons. The stream of hippocampal impulses arriving at the CRF neuron pool will be of an integrative nature. The ultimate effect on the CRF-neurons is mainly inhibitory, exerted in a direct way or via interneurons. This pathway may also be cholinergic.

PROPOSITION 3

The CRF-neuron pool, consisting of nerve cells with a large receptive surface, is accessible to neuronal and hormonal stimuli, and its nerve endings release CRF as a function of the integrated electrical activity

To evaluate the functional properties of the CRF-neuron pool, it is essential to discuss the structural and functional organization of the elements of this pool, the major neural and humoral influences on the elements, and the characteristics of the final common path.

There is sufficient evidence (cf. also the papers of other authors in this volume) that a group of neurons in the hypophysiotrophic area in the hypothalamus and its axons in the tuberoinfundibular tract should be regarded as the final common path for CRF-production and -release. The input of these cells consists of neural and humoral stimuli of diverse origin. Firstly therefore, we would like to make some comments as to the number of elements and the size of the receptive surface.

The neuronal population of the hypophysiotrophic area consists of small and medium size elements, which show a stellate- or spindle-shaped dendritic plexus. The dendrites are not very rich in spines, and the branches diverge in all directions or show a slight tendency to orient themselves along a given plane. Preliminary quantitative measurements of the size of the dendritic surface have revealed that the values range from 5000 to 22000 μ^2. Extrapolation of these values in respect to synaptic contacts, have resulted in estimates of 400 to 3000 synapses for a single hypothalamic neuron.

The total number of neurons in this particular area amounts to 125000–150000, of which a small percentage will belong to the CRF-neuron pool. These preliminary results, however, indicate that a large population of neurons, with a considerable receptive or integrative surface may be involved in the regulation of the pituitary-adrenocortical function.

This group of elements should not be regarded as a set of neurons with a fixed function, but rather as a statistical group with stochastic properties. Some neurons may have a low, others a high sensitivity to certain hormonal or neuronal stimuli. It seems also likely that small pools of inhibitory and excitatory interneurons belong to the CRF-neuron pool, since a major part of the limbic and extralimbic neuronal stimuli are mediated through intercalated neurons.

There is no question about the dual sensitivity for neurotransmitters; both excitatory and inhibitory chemical mediators have been shown to influence the receptive surface in the usual synaptic way (Steiner *et al.*, 1969). However, the elements of the CRF-neuron pool possess another specific property; corticosteroids and ACTH act upon the receptive surface by mimicking the synaptic input. At least a portion of the CRF-pool is sensitive both to neuronal and hormonal factors. These neurons are ideally suited as monitoring devices for the concentration of circulating steroids.

Under resting conditions, the firing patterns of the elements of the CRF-pool are rather low; between 1 and 10 imp./sec (Cross and Silver, 1966). A disturbance of the internal or external environment markedly enhances the basic activity, resulting in an increase of CRF-release. The exact relationship between input (neuronal and hormonal stimuli upon the receptive surface of the CRF-neurons) and the output (action potentials along the axons and subsequent CRF-release) is not known; but there is no reason to doubt that an increase in firing frequency results in an enhancement of CRF-release.

The structural and functional characteristics of the CRF-elements strongly indicate that the CRF-pool constitutes the substratum of the setpoint of neural control of the pituitary-adrenocortical axis. This setpoint is not a rigid system in view of the stochastical properties of the CRF-neuron pool. Adjustment of the setpoint may be provided by the integrated activity of some limbic structures (a.o. the amygdala and the hippocampus). The latter systems are able to raise or lower the excitability of the elements of the CRF-neuron pool. Another alternative may be that parts of the limbic system increase or decrease the gain of various feedback loops which partake in these homeostatic mechanisms. We have already mentioned the possibility that a neuron pool in the posterior hypothalamus acts as counterpart in a balanced system with the CRF-neuron pool. In a similar way, as has been shown for the neural regulation of glucose levels in the blood, a high activity in one center may be accompanied by a low activity in the other. Details of this mechanism have been worked out by computer simulation (Schadé and Smith, 1969).

A few words should be said about the hierarchy of the setpoint and the adjustment of the setpoint.

Although precise structural and physiological evidence is still lacking, there is some evidence that a rather specific organization of the receptive surface of the hypothalamic neurons exists. The cell body and the proximal parts of the dendritic branches seem to be involved in the collection of specific signals from the major limbic systems (e.g. amygdala and hippocampus).

In this context, the amygdalohypothalamic and the hippocampohypothalamic pathways may be regarded as the limbic "pyramidal" system, conveying signals with a high preference value. An increase or decrease in the firing rate, or shifts in the specific firing pattern, will immediately change the basic firing of the CRF-neuron pool. In this way, the setpoint will be shifted to a higher or lower level.

The more distant dendritic branches then collect information from the intra-hypothalamic sources, other limbic regions, and forebrain and midbrain areas. These stimuli, together with the hormonal factors of diverse origin, keep the elements of the CRF-neuron pool at appropriate levels of readiness to respond to the limbic pyramidal information. The information carried by these systems is analogous to the extra-pyramidal and spinal messages in providing the motoneurons with the appropriate back-ground activity. Although only a few building stones are available for a system analysis of hypothalamic functions, we readily gain insight into the input and output relations of complex homeostatic mechanisms. Biocybernetics may become a useful member of the science of neuroendocrinology (Wiener and Schadé, 1963).

REFERENCES

ADEY, W. R. (1967) Hippocampal states and functional relations with cortico-subcortical systems in attention and learning. *Progr. Brain Research*, **27**, 228–245.

ADEY, W. R. AND TOKIZANE, T. (Eds.) (1967) Structure and function of the limbic system. *Progr. Brain Research*, **27**.

BARGMANN, W. AND SCHADÉ, J. P. (Eds.) (1963) The rhinencephalon and related structures. *Progr. Brain Research*, **3**.

BARGMANN, W. AND SCHADÉ, J. P. (Eds.) (1964) Lectures on the diencephalon. *Progr. Brain Research*, **5**.

CROSS, B. A. AND SILVER, I. A. (1966) Electrophysiological studies on the hypothalamus. *Brit. Med. Bull.*, **22**, 254–260.

DALLMAN, M. F. AND YATES, F. E. (1968) Anatomical and functional mapping of central neural input and feedback pathways of the adrenocortical system. *Mem. Soc. Endocrinol.*, **17**, 39–72.

ENDRÖCZI, E. AND LISSÁK, K. (1962) Interrelations between paleocortical activity and pituitary-adrenocortical function. *Acta physiol. Acad. Sci. Hung.*, **21**, 257–263.

FUXE, K. (1964) Cellular localization of monoamines in the median eminence and the infundibular stem of some mammals. *Z. Zellforsch.*, **61**, 710–725.

GLOOR, P., MURPHY, J. T. AND DREIFUSS, J. J. (1969) Electrophysiological studies of amygdalo-hypothalamic connections. *Ann. N.Y. Acad. Sci.*, **157**, 629–641.

GROOT, J. DE (1966) Limbic and other neural pathways that regulate endocrine function. In: L. Martini and W. F. Ganong (Eds.), *Neuroendocrinology*, Vol. **1**, 81–106.

KNIGGE, K. M. AND HAYS, M. (1963) Evidence of inhibitive role of hippocampus in neural regulation of ACTH release. *Proc. Soc. Exptl. Biol. Med.*, **114**, 67–69.

MANGILI, G., MOTTA, M. AND MARTINI, L. (1966) Control of adenocorticotrophic hormone secretion. In: L. Martini and W. F. Ganong (Eds.), *Neuroendocrinology*, Vol. **1**, 298–370.

MCLARDY, T. (1959) Hippocampal formation of brain as detector-coder of temporal patterns of information. *Perspectives Biol. Med.*, **2**, 443–452.

MORGANE, P. J. (1969) The function of the limbic and rhinic forebrain-limbic midbrain systems and reticular formation in the regulation of food and water intake. *Ann. N.Y. Acad. Sci.*, **157**, 806–848.

NAUTA, W. J. H. (1958) Hippocampal projections and related neural pathways to the midbrain of the cat. *Brain*, **81**, 319–340.

NEEDHAM, C. W. AND DILA, C. J. (1968) Synchronizing and desynchronizing systems of the old brain. *Brain Res.*, **10**, 285–293.

OOMURA, Y., OOYAMA, H., YAMAMOTO, T. AND KOBAYASHI, N. (1969) Behavior of hypothalamic unit activity during electrophoretic application of drugs. *Ann. N. Y. Acad. Sci.*, **157**, 642–665.

SAWYER, C. H., KAWAKAMI, M., MEYERSON, B., WHITMOYER, D. I. AND LILLEY, J. J. (1968) Effects of ACTH, dexamethasone and asphyxia on electrical activity of the rat hypothalamus. *Brain Res.*, **10**, 213–226.

SCHADÉ, J. P. (1970) System analysis of some hypothalamic functions. I. Thermostat, Glucostat Steroidstat. In: L. Martini (Ed.), *Integration of endocrine and non-endocrine mechanisms in the hypothalamus.* Acad. Press, New York (In press).

SCHADÉ, J. P. AND SMITH, J. (1969) System analysis of some hypothalamic functions. II. Neural control of the pituitary-adrenocortical axis. *Curr. Mod. Biol.* (In press).

SHUTE, C. D. D. AND LEWIS, P. S. (1966) Cholinergic and monoaminergic pathways in the hypothalamus. *Brit. Med. Bull.*, **22**, 221–226.

SMELIK, P. G. (1969) The regulation of ACTH secretion. *Acta Physiol. Pharmacol. Neerl.*, **15**, 123–135.

SMITH, G. P. (1965) Neural control of the pituitary-adrenocortical system. In: W. S. Yamamoto and J. R. Brobeck (Eds.) *Physiological control and regulation.* Saunders, Philadelphia.

STEINER, F. A., RUF, K. AND AKERT, K. (1969) Steroid-sensitive neurons in rat brain: anatomical localization and responses to neurohumors and ACTH. *Brain Res.*, **12**, 74–85.

SZENTÁGOTHAI, J., FLERKO, B., MESS, B. AND HALÁSZ, B. (1968) *Hypothalamic control of the anterior pituitary, an experimental morphological study.* Akademiai Kiado, Budapest.

WIENER, N. AND SCHADÉ, J. P. (1963) *Progress in biocybernetics*, Vol. **1**, Elsevier, Amsterdam.

DISCUSSION

MARKS: Does all the regulation take place on the cell body or does there exist any regulation at the neurovascular junction as well?

SCHADÉ: In the model we need an integrating common final pathway. I believe that most of the integration takes place at this particular level. The possibility exists of a changing but steady background input into these neurons. The system is also able to adjust the setpoint.

HARRIS: One of the important questions at the present moment is, how much autonomous function over anterior pituitary secretion the hypothalamus has, when separated from all other regions of the CNS. I wonder, Dr. Schadé, if you would give us your views in this problem with respect to ACTH secretion.

SCHADÉ: If the hypothalamus is deprived of extra-hypothalamic influences, most of the integrating surface may be still intact. The system can thus be influenced by circulating factors, but it may not be able to adjust its setpoint very rapidly. A setpoint will be maintained by the background activity coming from various nuclei in the hypothalamus itself.

FELDMAN: The role of the neural input into the hypothalamus has been demonstrated by experiments in which stimuli have been applied to animals with deafferentation of the medial basal hypothalamus. It was found that in such animals there was a nearly complete inhibition of the response to auditory stimulation and a marked inhibition of the response to photic stimulation, when compared with intact animals. There was only a slight depression of the response to ether-venesection stress, but no inhibition to ether stress, anoxia or immobilization. These experiments may differentiate between two kinds of stresses. Those for which CNS input is essential to activate the pituitary, *e.g.* auditory stimulation, and stresses acting on the median eminence by humoral factors.

MARTINI: I would like to make a remark on Professor Harris' suggestion that information on the influence of the limbic system on the hypothalamic–pituitary–adrenal axis might be derived from experiments performed in animals with a "deafferented" hypothalamus. In this preparation also midbrain influences are eliminated, and these are rather important for the control of ACTH secretion.

I would also like to mention that following "deafferentation", the hypothalamic island contains CRF in amounts much higher than normal (Motta and Piva, unpublished data). This probably explains why "deafferented" animals have high levels of ACTH in their pituitary, and high levels of corticosterone in the general circulation. The data by Motta and Piva also indicate that CRF is synthesized by neurons which are located within the hypothalamic island.

The Hypothalamus and Pituitary ACTH Release

J. R. HODGES

Department of Pharmacology, Royal Free Hospital, School of Medicine, 8, Hunter Street, London (U.K.)

Our knowledge of the precise mechanisms which control the adrenocorticotrophic activity cf the pituitary gland is still far from complete but there can be no doubt that the hypothalamus plays a vital role. The release of ACTH in response to stress occurs with great rapidity. Fig. 2 shows the changes in the concentration of ACTH in the blood of rats subjected to the stress of laparotomy under ether anaesthesia. A significant rise in circulating corticotrophin occurs 1 min and a maximal level is reached $2\frac{1}{2}$ min after the beginning of anaesthesia. The adrenocorticotrophic activity in the blood then falls and is only just detectable 20 min after the stress. The rapidity with which the release of ACTH occurs is in accord with the existence of a neural or neurohumoral mechanism controlling the adrenocorticotrophic activity of the pituitary gland. A direct neural mechanism is unlikely to be involved since the adenohypophysis receives few nerve fibres (Harris, 1955).

It is now well known that the secretion of corticotrophin is dependent upon the functional integrity of the hypothalamus. The importance of the hypothalamus in this respect was made evident by the work of De Groot and Harris (1950) and Hume and Wittenstein (1950) who showed independently that electrical stimulation of the median basal hypothalamus causes ACTH secretion, and destruction of the same region prevents the release of the hormone in response to stress. The area involved is shown diagrammatically in Fig. 2.

Many objections have been made to the idea that the hypothalamus exerts a functional dominance over the adenohypophysis, mainly on the grounds that pituitary stalk section fails to produce any marked change in the activity of the adenohypophysis (Uotila, 1939; Cheng *et al.*, 1949). However, such objections were refuted by Harris (1949) who showed that regeneration of the vascular connections between the hypothalamus and the adenohypophysis occurs unless the operation of transection of the pituitary stalk is accompanied by the insertion of a plate to prevent revascularisation. The work of Harris and his colleagues made it clear that the vascular connections between the hypothalamus and the adenohypophysis (the hypophyseal portal vessels) are of prime importance in the control of pituitary adrenocorticotrophic activity. Attention was drawn to the existence of these blood vessels by Popa and Fielding (1930) who suggested incorrectly that the blood flows from the adenohypophysis to the hypothalamus. Not until several years later was it established that the principle flow occurs in the opposite direction (Green and Harris, 1947). The blood supply to the pituitary gland is shown diagrammatically in Fig. 3. Normal pituitary adreno-

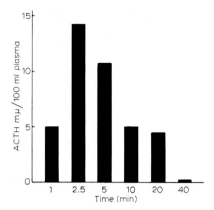

Fig. 1. Blood corticotrophin concentrations in the rat at various time intervals after laparotomy under ether anaesthesia.

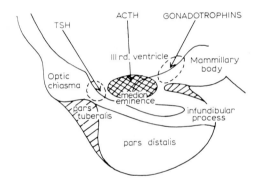

Fig. 2. Hypothalamic regions involved in adenohypophyseal function.

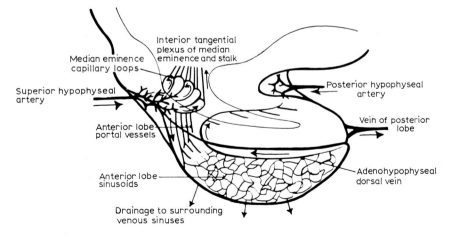

Fig. 3. Vasculature of the pituitary gland.

corticotrophic activity is dependent upon the hypothalamus and the hypophyseal portal blood vessels which carry transmitter substances from the median eminence to the gland.

Corticotrophin releasing factor (CRF) is secreted in the median basal hypothalamus and conveyed to the adenohypophysis by the hypophyseal portal vessels. The presence of such a factor in hypothalamic extracts and hypophyseal portal blood has often been demonstrated but many of the methods for its detection and estimation are open to criticism because of their lack of specificity. The use of rats treated with morphine, chlorpromazine, cortisol, dexamethasone (and various combinations of these substances) is based on the unjustifiable assumption that these drugs have no action on the hypothalamo-pituitary-adrenal system other than a specific inhibitory effect on the mobilisation of endogenous CRF. Bioassay methods using animals with hypothalamic lesions, or *in vitro* techniques involving ACTH synthesis by adeno-hypophyseal tissue, do not appear to be any more reliable.

A considerable amount of evidence has been advanced to suggest that CRF may be identical with vasopressin. Thus, rats in which the stress-induced release of ACTH has been abolished by hypothalamic lesions also exhibit diabetes insipidus and the release of ACTH can be elicited in these animals by vasopressin injections (McCann and Brobeck, 1954). On the other hand, it is unlikely that vasopressin is the neuro-humoral transmitter responsible for ACTH secretion because of the dissociation between antidiuretic and ACTH releasing activities in hypothalamic extracts. In fact, according to De Wied (1964), such extracts are devoid of pressor activity. However, vasopressin may play an important part in the sequence of events which lead to corticotrophin release. Hedge, Yates, Marcus and Yates (1966) showed that vaso-pressin causes ACTH secretion if it is injected into the median eminence but not if it is introduced directly into the adenohypophysis. Thus, it may provide a stimulus for the release of CRF.

The chemical nature of CRF is still not known. Several factors have been isolated from hypothalamic and pituitary tissue. Most of the active compounds are poly-peptides with structures not unlike either melanophore expanding hormone (αMSH) or lysine vasopressin. It has been suggested that one of these factors, α_2CRF, is a precursor of ACTH and another, βCRF, is the neurohumoral transmitter which stimulates corticotrophin release.

There can be no doubt that the secretion of corticotrophin in conditions of stress is dependent upon the release of a corticotrophin releasing factor from nerve endings in the hypothalamus. Since pituitary transplants fail to maintain normal adrenal function unless they are placed under the median eminence (Harris and Jacobsohn, 1950, 1952; Nikitovitch-Winer and Everett, 1957, 1958) it appears that the basal level of ACTH secretion is also under hypothalamic control. Anterior hypothalamic lesions abolish the diurnal variation in plasma corticosterone concentration (Slusher, 1964), indicat-ing that the hypothalamus is necessary for the circadian ACTH rhythm. On the other hand, it has often been suggested that the basal level of ACTH secretion may be independent of hypothalamic activity and may be controlled by corticosteroids in the blood. Certainly the mechanisms controlling ACTH release under non-stress and

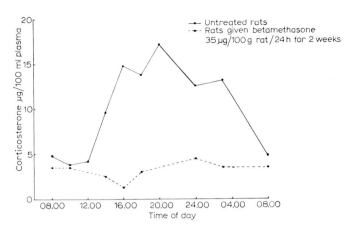

Fig. 4. Circadian rhythm in plasma corticosterone concentration in the male rat.

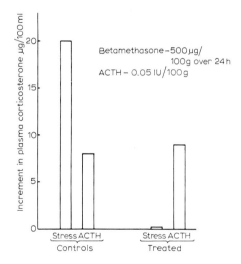

Fig. 5. Stress- and ACTH-induced increments in plasma corticosterone in betamethasone-treated rats.

stress conditions are functionally dissociable since small doses of corticosteroids suppress the marked circadian rise in plasma corticosterone without affecting the stress response (Zimmerman and Critchlow, 1967).

Fig. 4 shows the circadian rhythm in plasma corticosterone concentration in male rats. The concentration is lowest in the morning, rises steeply in the afternoon to reach a peak at about 20.00 h and then declines. The rhythm was completely obliterated by the inclusion of betamethasone in the animals' drinking water and this effect of betamethasone was entirely due to inhibition of ACTH release as is illustrated in Fig. 5. This shows plasma corticosterone concentrations in control and betamethasone-treated rats before and after exposure to stress or the injection of ACTH. Like the diurnal rise, the stress-induced increment in plasma corticosterone concentration was prevented by betamethasone treatment but the response to injected ACTH was not changed.

Since the mechanisms controlling circadian ACTH rhythm and stress-induced pituitary adrenocorticotrophic activity differ in their sensitivity to the inhibitory action of corticoids, we studied the recovery of these aspects of pituitary function after their inhibition by betamethasone treatment. Male rats were given betamethasone solution instead of drinking water for 24 h. The strength of the steroid solution was adjusted (on the basis of the results of a long series of preliminary experiments) to ensure that every animal received approximately 500 μg betamethasone/100 g during the 24-h period. The plasma corticosterone concentration was determined before and $\frac{1}{2}$ h after stress (exposure to ether vapour for 1 min) in control and treated animals at the end of the steroid treatment and 24 hours after stopping it. The experiments were done at 10 to 11 a.m. or 4 to 5 p.m. The results are shown in Fig. 6. In the untreated controls the stress-induced increment in plasma corticosterone concentration was the same in the morning and in the afternoon despite the difference in the pre-stress level of the steroid. Betamethasone treatment blocked completely the diurnal rise and the stress-induced increment in the plasma corticosterone concentration. Twenty-four hours after withdrawing the betamethasone, the diurnal rhythm was again present but the response to stress was still completely absent. These observations agree with the suggestion that the mechanisms controlling circadian ACTH rhythm and stress-induced ACTH release are dissociated, but indicate that the former is less sensitive to corticoids than the latter, in contrast to the findings of Zimmerman and Critchlow (1967).

Afferent nervous impulses to the hypothalamus are essential for unimpaired control of adrenocorticotrophic activity. The circadian ACTH rhythm is under the influence of afferent pathways different from those controlling the release of the hormone in response to stress (Halász, Slusher and Gorski, 1967; Halász, Vernikos–Danellis and

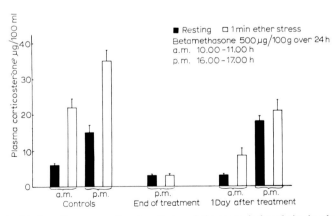

Fig. 6. The effect of betamethasone on the circadian and the stress-induced rise in plasma corticosterone concentration in the rat.

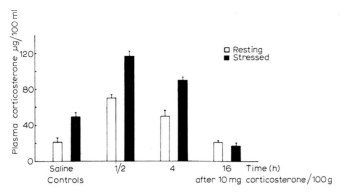

Fig. 7. The time delay between corticoid pre-treatment and inhibition of the stress-induced plasma corticosterone increment.

Gorski, 1967). Since the hypothalamus is part of the final common pathway for ACTH release the different sensitivities of the two mechanisms to the inhibitory action of corticosteroids suggest that the site of action of the corticosteroids is not in the hypothalamus as is generally believed. The presence of corticoid sensitive controllers in parts of the Central Nervous System, other than the hypothalamus, is also suggested by the marked dissociation between blood (and presumably hypothalamic) corticosteroid concentrations and the degree of inhibition of ACTH release. Fig. 7 shows the effect of stress on the plasma corticosterone concentration in rats pretreated with 10 mg of the steroid, injected subcutaneously. Stress caused a marked rise in plasma corticosterone in the saline-treated controls. It caused a similar rise in corticosterone-treated animals, despite the fact that the pre-existing plasma corticosterone concentration was very high indeed. The stress-induced increment was less 4 h later, by which time the plasma corticosterone concentration had fallen considerably. Sixteen hours after the steroid administration no rise in plasma corticosterone occurred in response to stress. Thus there was no inhibition of corticotrophin release when the plasma concentration of the steroid was raised, but complete inhibition when it had returned to the resting level. This lack of correlation between inhibition of ACTH release and blood corticosteroid concentration was also clearly demonstrated by Smelik (1963) using a different parameter of pituitary activity. The time delay before the appearance of any signs of pituitary inhibition suggests the existence of a corticoid sensitive controller of adrenocorticotrophic activity in some tissue not readily accessible to the systemic circulation.

It is clear that changes in the secretion rate of ACTH are dependent upon the functional integrity of the hypothalamus and afferent nervous pathways to it. In this brief account no attempt has been made to survey the literature. Instead, some experiments have been outlined, the results of which do not support the popular assumption that the hypothalamus is the site of a corticoid-sensitive controller of pituitary adrenocorticotrophic activity.

REFERENCES

CHENG, C. P., SAYERS, G., GOODMAN, L. S. AND SWINYARD, C. A. (1949) Discharge of ACTH from transplanted pituitary tissue. *Amer. J. Physiol.*, **159**, 426–434.

GREEN, J. D. AND HARRIS, G. W. (1947) The neurovascular link between the neurohypophysis and the adenohypophysis. *J. Endocrinol.*, **5**, 136–146.

GROOT, J. DE AND HARRIS, G. W. (1950) Hypothalamic control of the anterior pituitary gland and blood lymphocytes. *J. Physiol.*, **111**, 335–346.

HALÁSZ, B., SLUSHER, M. A. AND GORSKI, R. A. (1967) Adrenocorticotrophic hormone secretion in rats after partial or total interruption of neural afferents to the medial basal hypothalamus. *Neuroendocrinology*, **2**, 43–55.

HALÁSZ, B., VERNIKOS-DANELLIS, J. AND GORSKI, R. A. (1967) Pituitary ACTH content in rats after partial or total interruption of neural afferents to the medial basal hypothalamus. *Endocrinology*, **81**, 921–924.

HARRIS, G. W. (1949) Regeneration of hypophyseal portal vessels. *Nature*, **163**, 70.

HARRIS, G. W. (1955) *Neural control of the pituitary gland.* Arnold, London.

HARRIS, G. W. AND JACOBSOHN, D. (1950) Proliferative capacity of the hypophyseal portal vessels. *Nature*, **165**, 854.

HARRIS, G. W. AND JACOBSOHN, D. (1952) Functional grafts of the anterior pituitary gland. *Proc. Roy. Soc. B.*, **139**, 263–276.

HEDGE, G. A., YATES, M. D., MARCUS, R. AND YATES, F. E. (1966) Site of action of vasopressin in causing corticotrophin release. *Endocrinology*, **79**, 328–340.

HUME, D. M. AND WITTENSTEIN, G. J. (1950) The relationship of the hypothalamus to pituitary adrenocortical function. *Proc. First Clin. ACTH Conf.*, p. 134.

McCANN, S. M. AND BROBECK, J. R. (1954) Evidence for the role of supraopticohypophyseal system in regulation of adrenocorticotrophin secretion. *Proc. Soc. Exptl. Biol. Med.*, **87**, 318–324.

NIKITOVITCH-WINER, M. AND EVERETT, J. W. (1957) Resumption of gonadotrophic function in pituitary grafts following re-transplantation from kidney to median eminence. *Nature*, **180**, 1434–1435.

NIKITOVITCH-WINER, M. AND EVERETT, J. W. (1958) Functional restitution of pituitary grafts re-transplanted from kidney to median eminence. *Endocrinology*, **63**, 916–930.

POPA, G. T. AND FIELDING, U. (1930) A portal circulation from the pituitary to the hypothalamic region. *J. Anat. (Lond.)*, **65**, 88–91.

SLUSHER, M. A. (1964) Effects of chronic hypothalamic lesions on diurnal and stress corticosteroid levels. *Amer. J. Physiol.*, **206**, 1161–1164.

SMELIK, P. G. (1963) Relation between blood level of corticoids and their inhibiting effect on the hypophyseal stress response. *Proc. Soc. Exptl. Biol. Med.*, **113**, 616–619.

UOTILA, U. U. (1939) On the role of the pituitary stalk in the regulation of the anterior pituitary, with special reference to the thyrotropic hormone. *Endocrinology*, **25**, 605–614.

WIED, D. DE, SMELIK, P. G., MOLL, J. AND BOUMAN, P. R. (1964) On the mechanism of ACTH release. In: E. BAJUSZ and G. JASMIN (Eds.), *Major Problems in Neuroendocrinology.* Karger, Basel-New York, pp. 156–176.

ZIMMERMAN, E. AND CRITCHLOW, V. (1967) Effects of diurnal variation in plasma corticosterone levels on adrenocortical response to stress. *Proc. Soc. Exptl. Biol. Med.*, **125**, 658–663.

DISCUSSION

LEVINE: Would you be willing to modify your statement in that there may be many sites for the inhibitory action of corticosteroids on ACTH-release? Clearly there is evidence that if you implant a steroid in the median eminence directly, it has marked inhibitory effects on ACTH release, but there may be multiple sites.

HODGES: Yes I am. But I think that you would agree that one must also be very wary of the techniques in which steroids are implanted in various tissues because of their general diffusion.

LEVINE: No. I would not. Simply because we have evidence that the diffusion, at least of steroids placed in the median eminence, is very minimal if there is any at all. In fact, very minute quantities are even utilized over a long period of time. There is some evidence that estrogen does diffuse. If it diffuses, it would diffuse into the pituitary, but it is very unlikely that it would diffuse to any other CNS site.

HARRIS: Yet there is the point, I suppose, if the implant happens to be slightly in the third ventricle, your diffusion could be drastically altered.

FUXE: Have there been any autoradiographical studies on implants of labelled steroids, to check the diffusion in the brain?

MARTINI: Would Dr. Hodges accept as evidence that steroids may act on the hypothalamus the fact that, when you treat animals with adrenal steroids, CRF disappears from the hypothalamus?

HODGES: I would not dispute the fact that in certain doses any steroid may suppress ACTH release at the level of the pituitary gland, the hypothalamus, or some other site in the CNS. I am quite sure that all these things happen. With steroids like betamethasone and dexamethasone, of which the ACTH inhibitory activity is very potent compared with their biological properties in other respects one sees their pharmacological actions on the pituitary gland. Steroids administered to simulate physiological conditions appear to act neither on the anterior pituitary nor on the hypothalamus.

MARTINI: As far as Dr. Fuxe's comment is concerned, we have some data to answer his point. Recently, in a collaborative study with Dr. Kniewald we have studied the effect of the carrier material on the absorption of steroids from the brain.
The experiments were done with labelled testosterone. It was found that, if you place testosterone in the brain together with sucrose, testosterone will not be re-absorbed from the implantation site. On the contrary it will be easily re-absorbed if you place it together with cacao butter or with cholesterol.

HENKIN: The effect and localization of testosterone in the central nervous system is obviously different from that of other steroid hormones and it is difficult to extrapolate from one hormone to the other. Testosterone, progesterone, estrogen and cortisol have different lipid solubility and this, as well as other factors, affects their transport across the blood-brain barrier and into the brain as well. After injection into the peripheral circulation testosterone is taken up by the brain in a different manner from other steroid hormones. If progesterone distribution from peripheral circulation into the brain is evaluated its concentration in the brain is similar to that in fat. Cortisol distribution is also specific and its gets into the brain and it leaves the brain a manner peculiar to itself.

HARRIS: I think that the recent results of Dr. Dora Jacobsohn are of much interest in considering the action of different steroids on the brain.
She found that it was much more difficult to androgenize newborn female rats with testosterone itself as opposed to testosterone propionate.

HENKIN: Testosterone crosses the blood-brain barrier very rapidly and its concentration in the brain is two or even three times higher than in blood as soon as ten minutes after injection in the eviscerated animal.
Cortisol takes much more time to enter the brain. Progesterone and testosterone are similar in some ways in that both enter the brain quickly. Thus, there are time differences in the manner by which steroid hormones enter the central nervous system partially dependent upon the functional groups of these steroids, partially dependent upon their differences in lipid solubility and partially dependent upon other factors which we have not yet defined completely.

HARRIS: And how does testosterone compare with the propionate in this case?

HENKIN: We have not looked at that aspect of the problem.

LEVINE: As to testosterone, we have done some studies with labelled testosterone and testosterone propionate. The uptake by the newborn animal of the testosterone load is very rapid, within an hour or so; it is gone almost completely by eight hours, whereas the uptake of the testosterone propionate is much more slow and actually stays around much longer, for almost 48–72 hours. The myth of the single injection is the fact that you are giving a very prolonged acting substance in the propionate and not in the testosterone alone.

LARON: I would appreciate to hear more about the relationship between vasopressin and CRF. Is the evidence that injection of vasopressin into the pituitary does not release ACTH against the hypothesis of a CRF like activity of vasopressin, and in favour of an action of vasopressin on CRF?

HODGES: I was quoting work of Hedge, Yates, Marcus and Yates (Endocrinology, 1966, 79, 328–340). In this now classical paper they introduced vasopressin directly into the hypothalamus and elicited ACTH release. In contrast when they injected it directly into the adenohypophysis, it did not. The implication was that vasopressin played some part in the chain of events bringing about ACTH release. Dr. Smelik could perhaps give some more details since he has confirmed Yates' work.

SMELIK: I have just published a paper with Dr. Hedge on this subject (Neuroendocrinology, 1969, 4, 242–253). We are pretty sure at the moment that vasopressin is able to release CRF directly from the stores in the CRF neurons. Vasopressin causes a short-lasting pituitary-adrenal activation during dexamethasone blockade. This is dependent on the amount of CRF that is still present in the neuron, for if you deplete the CRF neurons first, then vasopressin in the same preparation has no effect any more.

Adrenocortical Feedback Control of Pituitary-Adrenal Activity

P. G. SMELIK

Department of Pharmacology, Free University, P.O. Box 7161, Amsterdam (The Netherlands)

When a functional system in a living organism has to operate properly, it can be expected that the level of activity is controlled continuously in accordance with the effects resulting from its action. This can be accomplished if the controlling center is informed, in a quantitative manner, by the output of the system. When the system is hormonal, that is: if the system's task is to liberate controlled amounts of a hormone into the general circulation, it is an obvious expectation that the level of circulating hormone will be the actual factor which feeds back on the controlling center in order to inform the system of its own achievements. That such an arrangement would also operate in the case of the hypothalamo-pituitary-adrenal axis, has been supposed for many years. In order to keep in check the activity of the system, the adrenocortical hormones should theoretically be capable of having two actions: if their level is too low, the system should be activated; and if the level is too high, the system should be blocked. In this way, a continuous adjustment of the system to the adrenals would exist. Such a negative feedback mechanism could in fact—again theoretically—be the only controlling device of the system; if it could be shown that a deficit in adrenocortical hormones would in itself represent a driving force for the system to operate. However, it would equally be possible that the factor which drives the system, is different from the circulating corticoid level, and exists independently of the presence of corticoids. In that case, the corticoids would only need to have an inhibitory action, and the system would operate maximally when no corticoids were present, because the drive is not inhibited any longer.

Of course, it could be a purely semantic question whether activation is the result of a central drive or a peripheral low level of corticoids. However, from a theoretical standpoint, it is more obvious to suppose that a driving force is not constituted by the absence of a peripheral factor, but by the pressure of activating inputs to the controlling center.

If this would be accepted, the most simple model for the hypothalamo-pituitary-adrenal axis would require the existence of a controlling center, which is capable of equating quantitatively incoming activating and inhibitory signals; and after summation, sends a releasing signal of an exactly determined intensity to the system elaborating the hormonal products.

Although the situation is, of course, much more complex, I think that essentially this happens. The model would predict that the normal resting levels of circulating corticoids continually keep in check the basal production of ACTH. There is not much evidence for this assumption. It is known that adrenalectomy results in an increase of ACTH levels in blood, but the only detailed studies so far are those of Brodish and Long (1956), in which they used the cross-circulation technique and assayed ACTH titers in blood for the adrenal ascorbic acid depletion in hypophysect-omized recipients. They showed that bilateral adrenalectomy results in an acute fall in circulating ACTH and then gradually ACTH levels rise to supranormal levels within a number of days. These surprising results do show that the absence of corticoids causes a disinhibition of pituitary corticotrophic function, but only very slowly. Apparently a sudden reduction in circulating corticoids is not an effective means at all to stimulate ACTH secretion; and the extremely long latency suggests that the mechanism cannot play an important physiological role.

Conversely, a rapid and dramatic rise in circulating corticosteroid levels inhibits ACTH secretion, but also here a considerable latency exists. Subcutaneous injection of corticosterone results in a peak level in the blood after some 30 min, but inhibition of the system occurs only after 2 h (Smelik, 1963a), and only if peripheral corticoid levels had reached supraphysiological values (Smelik, 1963b). Again, this suggests that the feedback mechanism has a rather low capacity and a slow action. It may account for the over-all stability of the system under resting conditions, circadian variations included. It cannot account for the rapid and short-lasting activation of the system which occurs when a stressful stimulus is presented.

We have been assuming that the pituitary-adrenal system is controlled by a center within the brain stem, which is capable of summating positive and negative incoming signals and sends the resultant signal to the pituitary. Among the positive signals, a cholinergic one may be of importance (Hedge and Smelik, 1968); among the negative stimuli a noradrenergic one may exist, although we could not obtain evidence for a role of monoaminergic transmission in this respect (Smelik, 1967). The controlling center should also be sensitive to the negative stimulus of the corticoids; and it seems logical that most people have assumed that the site of action of corticoid feedback is within the central nervous system. Since the structures regulating ACTH secretion appear to be located in the antero-basal part of the hypothalamus, it could be anticipated that this would also be the most sensitive area for corticoid inhibition. This has been substantiated by the results of implantation of crystalline corticoids into the brain stem. The most effective site of implantation appeared to be the area between the optic chiasm and the median eminence (Smelik and Sawyer, 1962; Smelik, 1965).

However, it has been argued by Bogdanove (1963) that perhaps hypothalamic implants are effective because the hormone is deposited near the portal vessel system; and that this might be the most efficient way to transport the substance to all cells of the anterior pituitary. This "implantation paradox" would imply that the pituitary itself would represent the actual site of the feedback action.

One way of testing this hypothesis would be to implant corticoids into the hypothalamus and then challenge the pituitary with a CRF preparation. If the block were on the pituitary level by transportation of the implanted material down the portal circulation, then the effect of CRF should be blocked.

Recently, we have worked with rats bearing implants of dexamethasone in the anterior part of the hypothalamus. In such animals, the usual adrenocortical response to stress is completely abolished one day after implantation. Similarly, the response to a number of naturally occurring ACTH-releasing substances is inhibited, e.g. adrenaline, acetylcholine, histamine, angiotensin, prostaglandin E1, and vasopressin. In contrast, the effect of a CRF preparation was not blocked, though somewhat reduced.

When the effect of the implant was followed with time, it appeared that: about 6 h after implantation, basal adrenal activity was induced, after 10 h the response to vasopressin was completely suppressed but that to CRF was normal, after 1 or 3 days a progressive reduction in the response to CRF could be observed.

This would suggest that, initially, the corticoid block is on the hypothalamic level; but that gradually the sensitivity of the pituitary-adrenal system decreases. Presumably this is due to the absence of the tonic hypothalamic influence on the system (Smelik, 1969).

Although we concluded from these and other studies that the feed-back action is primarily on the hypothalamus, we do not deny that the pituitary may be involved as well. This may depend on the dosage, since it has been shown that very high doses of corticoids, when given systemically, will block the effect of CRF preparations (De Wied, 1964). Such findings may cause some confusion in the literature, because they can be, and have been used, as evidence for or against either a hypothalamic or a pituitary site of action. Only if careful dose and time relationships are established experimentally, it will become clear that the conclusions are dependent on the experimental parameters; and that both structures can be affected, the hypothalamus being the most sensitive one.

REFERENCES

BOGDANOVE, E. M. (1963) Direct gonad-pituitary feedback: an analysis of effects of intra-cranial estrogenic depots on gonadotrophin secretion. *Endocrinology*, **73**, 696–712.

BRODISH, A. AND LONG, C. N. H. (1956) Changes in blood ACTH under various experimental conditions studied by means of a cross-circulation technique. *Endocrinology*, **59**, 666–676.

DE WIED, D. (1964) The site of the blocking action of dexamethasone on stress-induced pituitary ACTH release. *J. Endocrinol.*, **29**, 29–37.

HEDGE, G. A. AND SMELIK, P. G. (1968) Corticotrophin release: Inhibition by intra-hypothalamic implantation of atropine. *Science*, **159**, 891–892.

SMELIK, P. G. (1963a) Failure to inhibit corticotrophin secretion by experimentally induced increases in corticoid levels. *Acta Endocrinol.*, **44**, 36–46.

SMELIK, P. G. (1963b) Relation between the blood level of corticoids and their inhibiting effect of the hypophyseal stress response. *Proc. Soc. Exptl. Biol. Med.*, **113**, 616–619.

SMELIK, P. G. (1965) Effects of corticosterone implantation in the hypothalamus of rats on corticotrophin secretion. *Acta Physiol. Pharmacol. Neerl.*, **13**, 18.

SMELIK, P. G. (1967) ACTH secretion after depletion of hypothalamic monoamines by reserpine implants. *Neuroendocrinology*, **2**, 247–254.

SMELIK, P. G. (1969) The effect of a CRF preparation on ACTH release in rats bearing hypothalamic dexamethasone implants: a study on the "implantation paradox". *Neuroendocrinology*, in press.

SMELIK, P. G. AND SAWYER, C. H. (1962) Effects of implantation of cortisol into the brain stem or pituitary gland on the adrenal response to stress in the rabbit. *Acta Endocrinol.*, **41**, 561–570.

DISCUSSION

RINGOLD: We have recently studied the distribution of intravenously administered corticoids in the rat and are led to believe that some of the synthetic corticosteroids, which are extremely potent inhibitors of the adrenal axis, may exert their primary inhibitory activity at the pituitary level. One microgram of tritium-labelled steroid was injected into the tail vein of male adrenalectomized rats and groups of animals were sacrificed at time periods between 5 min and 2 h. Plasma, the pituitary, the hypothalamus, the cerebral cortex and the cerebral spinal fluid were each analyzed for organic extractable radioactivity and expressed as counts per mg tissue or fluid. Cortisol and corticosterone, which are only weakly suppressive, showed similar decay curves with plasma and pituitary radioactivity levels remaining close together. The hypothalamus and cortex showed lower levels of radioactivity with decay curves paralleling the plasma curve while the cerebrospinal fluid had a low level of steroid and a very shallow decay curve. Two synthetic steroids were also studied, $6\alpha,9\alpha$-difluoro-16α-methylhydrocortisone, and 6α-fluoro-16α-methylhydrocortisone, which exhibit marked adrenal suppression in the rat in common with the 16-methyl steroids dexamethasone and betamethasone. These were found to have slow plasma decay curves, but, relative to plasma, the concentration of radioactive steroid in the hypothalamus, cortex and cerebrospinal fluid were not markedly different from the cortisol and corticosterone cases. However, the pituitary showed a very marked concentration gradient with 5–10 times the specific activity of the plasma and a delayed clearance. Thus corticosteroids which exhibit marked inhibition of the hypothalamic–pituitary–adrenal axis possess distribution characteristics which lead to concentration in the pituitary and suggest this organ as an important site of the feedback mechanism.

HODGES: I would like to know how you reconcile your belief that the hypothalamus is the site of action of a corticoid-sensitive controller, with the complete lack of association between the blood level of corticosteroids and the inhibition of ACTH release. I suppose that the hypothalamic corticoid level follows the blood level fairly quickly.

SMELIK: Concerning the delay, I could not give an adequate answer. Perhaps something should happen first with the corticosteroids in the brain cells before action takes place. Whether this is a matter of slow uptake somewhere in the cells or a conversion to some other compounds, or a chemical exchange, I have no idea. However it is not a matter of solubility. The time course of the effect of pure dexamethasone implants is exactly the same as of implants of dexamethasone phosphate, which is of course completely water soluble.

BOHUS: I think that the type of stimulus, unilateral adrenalectomy, immobilization, or any other stimulus is also an important factor as far as the feedback regulation of the pituitary adrenal axis is concerned. The time course of plasma steroid levels follows a pattern that depends on the type of stimulus.

The Role of "Short" Feedback Mechanisms in the Regulation of Adrenocorticotropin Secretion

M. MOTTA, F. PIVA* AND L. MARTINI

Department of Pharmacology, University of Milan, 32 Via Vanvitelli, 20129 Milan (Italy)

INTRODUCTION

It is now well established that the anterior pituitary gland is regulated by two different types of feedback mechanisms. One, which might be called the "classic" feedback system, was discovered several years ago: in this system the controlling (inhibiting or activating) signal is represented by the hormones produced by the peripheral target glands (thyroid, adrenal cortex, gonads). The second mechanism, was discovered more recently and is usually referred to as the "short" or the "auto" or the "internal" feedback mechanism: in this particular system the controlling signal is provided by the pituitary hormones themselves (Mess and Martini, 1968; Motta, Fraschini and Martini, 1969).

The existence of a control mechanism of the "short" type has been demonstrated for all the hormones manufactured in the anterior pituitary gland, as well as for the Melanocyte Stimulating Hormone (MSH) which, in several species of animals, is secreted by the intermediate lobe (Table 1). It is an interesting fact that a "short" system is involved also in the control of the secretion of those pituitary hormones (growth hormone, prolactin and MSH) which do not have a peripheral target gland, and which consequently are not regulated by traditional feedback mechanisms.

The receptors sensitive to the signals of the "classic" feedback mechanisms are localized either in the brain (mainly in the median eminence of the hypothalamus), or in the anterior pituitary (Mangili *et al.*, 1966; Motta *et al.*, 1969); those sensitive to "short" feedback messages normally reside in the brain. Intrapituitary receptors for these types of signals have been postulated only as far as Growth Hormone (GH) is concerned (Motta *et al.*, 1969).

This paper will provide a concise review of the data which suggest that a "short" feedback mechanism may play a physiological role in the control of the secretion of the Adrenocorticotropin (ACTH). A more detailed discussion may be found in the chapter by Motta *et al.* (1969).

---

* Ford Foundation Fellow.

TABLE I

TABLE I

PITUITARY HORMONES CONTROLLED BY "SHORT" FEEDBACK MECHANISMS

ACTH	Halász and Szentágothai, 1960
	Motta *et al.*, 1965
LH	Dávid *et al.*, 1966
	Corbin and Cohen, 1966
FSH	Corbin and Story, 1967
	Fraschini *et al.*, 1968
TSH	Motta *et al.*, 1969
GH	Müller and Pecile, 1966
	Katz *et al.*, 1967
Prolactin	Clemens and Meites, 1968
MSH	Kastin and Schally, 1967

EVIDENCE SUGGESTING THE EXISTENCE OF A "SHORT" FEEDBACK MECHANISM FOR THE CONTROL OF ADRENOCORTICOTROPIN SECRETION

Stressful stimuli induce a greater secretion of ACTH in adrenalectomized rats if the initial plasma level of the hormone is low rather than high, suggesting that high levels of circulating ACTH reduce the reactivity of the hypothalamic-pituitary axis (Hodges and Vernikos, 1958; 1959). Chronic treatment of adrenalectomized animals with exogenous ACTH increases pituitary ACTH stores (Kitay *et al.*, 1959). Exogenous ACTH, administered to adrenalectomized rats, blocks the fall of pituitary ACTH usually induced by stress (Kitay *et al.*, 1959). The presence in the body of a pituitary tumor secreting ACTH prevents the increase in plasma and pituitary ACTH levels that usually occurs after adrenalectomy (Vernikos–Danellis and Trigg, 1967). Stress-induced increases in plasma ACTH in adrenalectomized animals bearing tumors of this type are not as great as those found in adrenalectomized rats with no tumors (Vernikos–Danellis and Trigg, 1967).

Additional support for the hypothesis that ACTH may directly intervene in the control of its own secretion has been recently provided by Dallman and Yates (1968). They have evaluated the effects of chronic ACTH pretreatment, performed in normal rats, on the acute secretion of ACTH induced by several types of stresses. Stimuli were applied 24 h after the last injection of ACTH, at a time when plasma corticosterone levels had returned to normal. Stresses such as noise and ether were partially inhibited by ACTH pretreatment, while others (scald, laparotomy, etc.) were not. The conclusion from these studies was that ACTH can block stress-induced increases in ACTH secretion; however, the inhibition seems to depend on the type of the stimulus. Dallman and Yates (1968) postulated a direct effect of ACTH on the brain. However, when exogenous corticoids are administered, stress responses remain blocked for several hours after plasma corticoid levels have returned to normal (Gavazzi *et al.*, 1962; Smelik, 1963). Presumably this occurs because corticoids remain bound to their brain receptors (Henkin *et al.*, 1967). Therefore, the inhibition of stress responses reported by Dallman and Yates (1968) might be the consequence of the accumulation in the brain of endogenous corticoids. In order to overcome this argument, Dallman and Yates (1968) have studied the inhibitory effects of pretreatment with ACTH in normal animals in which the receptors for the steroid feedback mechanism had theoretically been completely saturated by the administration of high doses of dexamethasone. They found, in confirmation of Mangili et al. (1965), that histamine and laparotomy activated ACTH release even in the presence of high doses of dexamethasone; but that the stimulating activity of these stresses was inhibited if dexamethasone-treated animals were also given ACTH. Dallman and Yates (1968) concluded that the hypothalamic-pituitary-adrenal axis normally receives two types of inputs; one which is corticosteroid-sensitive and can be saturated by dexamethasone; and one which is corticosteroid-insensitive but can be blocked by treatment with ACTH.

LOCALIZATION OF RECEPTORS SENSITIVE TO ADRENOCORTICOTROPIN

The evidence available suggests that the basal hypothalamus represents the most important receptor area for the "short" feedback effect of ACTH. In pioneer work, Halász and Szentágothai (1960) implanted anterior pituitary tissue in the infundibular recess of the third ventricle of the rat, and found a depressing effect of such implants on adrenal function. Motta et al. (1965) implanted solid ACTH into several areas of the brain and into the pituitary of normal male rats. The animals were then subjected to a mild environmental stress. ACTH proved effective in depressing blood corticosterone levels and in inhibiting the response to the mild stress, but only when placed in the median eminence region. Implants of ACTH in the frontal cerebral cortex or the pituitary were completely ineffective, as were implants of Luteinizing Hormone (LH) in the median eminence (Table 2). Exactly the same degree of inhibition was observed when either a crude or a synthetic ACTH preparation (beta 1–24 corticotropin) was implanted in the median eminence. These results provide one of the few

TABLE II

EFFECT OF IMPLANTS OF ACTH IN THE MEDIAN EMINENCE (ME), THE ANTERIOR PITUITARY (PIT) AND THE CEREBRAL CORTEX (CC) OF MALE RATS[1]

Groups[2]	Adrenal weight (mg)	Plasma corticosterone (µg/100 ml)
Controls	43.1 ± 4.2	19.1 ± 1.25
ME-sham (18)	41.2 ± 2.2	18.4 ± 1.60
ME-ACTH (USP Reference Standard) (24)	44.0 ± 2.8	9.1 ± 0.78[3]
ME-ACTH (synthetic) (8)	43.1 ± 2.2	10.7 ± 0.84[3]
Pit-ACTH (USP Reference Standard) (12)	43.7 ± 2.8	18.1 ± 2.02
CC-ACTH (USP Reference Standard) (12)	43.4 ± 1.6	19.4 ± 2.00
ME-LH (NIH-B 1 bovine) (8)	42.2 ± 2.7	19.2 ± 1.04

[1] Values are means ± S.E.
[2] Number of rats in parentheses.
[3] $P \leqslant 0.001$ vs. ME-sham.

demonstrations, so far available, that a "short" feedback effect can be obtained with a hormone absolutely devoid of contamination. Since beta 1–24 corticotropin has complete ACTH activity (Desaulles and Rittel, 1968), the data also suggest that the feedback effect is a property of ACTH as such. There is not necessarily any discrepancy between these results and those more recently reported by Davidson, Jones and Levine (1968), who have found that ACTH implants performed in the median eminence of normal male rats do not reduce "basal" levels of corticosterone and do not inhibit the response of the pituitary-adrenal axis to a strong stimulus (ether anesthesia). It is abvious that the conditions of the experiments of Davidson *et al.* (1968) differ considerably from those of Motta and her co-workers (1965); the latter investigators never evaluated the effects of ACTH implants in animals under resting conditions or exposed to major stresses.

The participation of the hypothalamus in the "short" feedback effect of ACTH has been assessed also in other ways. Adrenalectomy has been shown to increase the concentration of the Corticotropin Releasing Factor (CRF) in the hypothalamus (Vernikos–Danellis, 1965; Motta *et al.*, 1968). A further increase in CRF content is obtained if hypophysectomy is added to adrenalectomy (Motta *et al.*, 1968; Seiden and Brodish, 1969). Since CRF also appears in the circulation after hypophysectomy (Schapiro *et al.*, 1958; Eik–Nes and Brizzee, 1958; Brodish and Long, 1962), these results suggest that the elimination of the inhibiting feedback signal, normally provided by ACTH, activates the synthesis as well as the release of its hypothalamic mediator (Motta *et al.*, 1968). Treatment of adrenalectomized-hypophysectomized animals with exogenous ACTH reduces CRF stores to the level found following adrenalectomy alone; but even high doses of ACTH will not reduce the hypothalamic content of CRF to pre-adrenalectomy levels (Motta *et al.*, 1968). This suggests that CRF is under a dual feedback control via corticoids and ACTH. A similar conclusion has been reached by Chowers *et al.* (1967).

Support for a neural component in the feedback effect of ACTH has been obtained also from histological, neuropharmacological, behavioral, and electrophysiological studies (Table 3).

These will not be reviewed in detail here, since there are other sections of this book specifically devoted to these aspects. A summary of these findings has been recently provided by Motta *et al.* (1969) and by De Wied (1969).

CLINICAL IMPLICATIONS OF THE EXISTENCE OF A "SHORT" FEEDBACK MECHANISM FOR THE CONTROL OF ADRENOCORTICOTROPIN SECRETION

The existence of a "negative" feedback effect of ACTH on its own secretion has potential clinical implications. For instance, if the "short" feedback effect of ACTH is present in humans, one might expect that the administration of ACTH to patients on long-term corticoid therapy would result in a further depression of the reactivity of the hypothalamic-pituitary axis. A few clinical data have appeared which indicate this to be the case. ACTH has been shown to restore adrenal size and responsiveness in steroid-treated patients (Sandberg *et al.*, 1957); yet, despite ACTH treatment, the

TABLE III

EVIDENCE FOR THE EXISTENCE OF ACTH-SENSITIVE ELEMENTS IN THE BRAIN

Histological evidence
  Effects of ACTH on hypothalamic nuclei and on hypothalamic neurosecretion in adrenalectomized animals (Castor *et al.*, 1951; Peczely, 1966).

Behavioral evidence
  Effects of ACTH on avoidance learning (De Wied, 1969).
  Effects of ACTH on extinction of conditioned behavior (De Wied, 1969).
  Effects of ACTH on locomotor phenomena (Ferrari *et al.*, 1963).
  Effects of ACTH on sexual behavior (Bertolini *et al.*, 1968, 1969).

Neuropharmacological evidence
  Effects of ACTH on electroshock threshold in normal and adrenalectomized rats (Woodbury and Vernadakis, 1967; Wasserman *et al.*, 1965).
  Effects of ACTH on epilepsy in children (Klein and Livingstone, 1950; Millichap and Jones, 1964).

Electrophysiological evidence
  Effects of ACTH on EEG in patients with Addison's disease or congenital adrenal hyperplasia (Milcu *et al.*, 1964).
  Effects of ACTH on EEG in normal, hypophysectomized and adrenalectomized rats (Torda and Wolff, 1952).
  Effects of ACTH on electric potentials of the median eminence in rabbits (Kawakami *et al.*, 1966).
  Effects of ACTH on electric potentials of the midbrain reticular formation, the amygdala, the hippocampus (Kawakami *et al.*, 1966).
  Effects of ACTH on electric potentials of the septum, the somatomotor cortex, the thalamus in normal and adrenalectomized rats (Korányi *et al.*, 1966; Monnier, 1953).
  Effects of ACTH on electric potentials of the arcuate nucleus, baso-lateral hypothalamus and zona incerta (Sawyer *et al.*, 1968).
  Effects of ACTH on electric potentials of hypothalamic neurones (Steiner *et al.*, 1969).

adrenals of these patients revert to the hypo-functional state as soon as ACTH is discontinued (Liddle, Estep, Kendall, Williams and Townes, 1959). In addition, subjects pretreated with ACTH for three days, and tested with either metyrapone or vasopressin (two potent stimuli of ACTH secretion in untreated subjects) (Martini, 1966) immediately after discontinuation of ACTH administration, show a decreased endogenous release of ACTH (Plager and Cushman, 1962; Sussman *et al.*, 1965).

ACKNOWLEDGMENTS

The experimental work described in this paper was supported by funds of the Department of Pharmacology of the University of Milan and by the following grants: 67-530 of the Ford Foundation, New York, N.Y.; AM 10119-01, AM 10119-02, AM 10119-03 and AM 11783-01 of the National Institutes of Health, Bethesda, Maryland; 61052-69-C-0028 of the European Office of Aerospace Research, Brussels, Belgium.
  Bibliographic assistance was received from the UCLA Brain Information Network.

REFERENCES

BERTOLINI, A., GESSA, G. L., VERGONI, W. AND FERRARI, W. (1968) Induction of sexual excitement with intraventricular ACTH; permissive role of testosterone in the male rabbit. *Life Sci.*, **7**, 1203–1206.

BERTOLINI, A., VERGONI, W., GESSA, G. L. AND FERRARI, W. (1969) Induction of sexual excitement by the action of adrenocorticotrophic hormone in brain. *Nature*, **221**, 667–669.

BRODISH, A. AND LONG, C. N. H. (1962) ACTH-releasing hypothalamic neurohumor in peripheral blood. *Endocrinology*, **71**, 298–306.

CASTOR, C. W., BAKER, B. L., INGLE, D. J. AND LI, C. H. (1951) Effect of treatment with ACTH or cortisone on anatomy of the brain. *Proc. Soc. Exptl. Biol. Med.*, **76**, 353–357.

CHOWERS, I., CONFORTI, N. AND FELDMAN, S. (1967) Effects of corticosteroids on hypothalamic corticotropin releasing factor and pituitary ACTH content. *Neuroendocrinology*, **2**, 193–199.

CLEMENS, J. A. AND MEITES, J. (1968) Inhibition by hypothalamic prolactin implants of prolactin secretion, mammary growth and luteal function. *Endocrinology*, **82**, 878–881.

CORBIN, A. AND COHEN, A. I. (1966) Effect of median eminence implants of LH on pituitary LH of female rats. *Endocrinology*, **78**, 41–46.

CORBIN, A. AND STORY, J. C. (1967) "Internal" feedback mechanism: response of pituitary FSH and of stalk-median eminence follicle stimulating hormone-releasing factor to median eminence implants of FSH. *Endocrinology*, **80**, 1006–1012.

DALLMAN, M. F. AND YATES, F. E. (1968) Anatomical and functional mapping of central neural input and feedback pathways of the adrenocortical system. *Mem. Soc. Endocrinol.*, **17**, 39–72.

DÁVID, M. A., FRASCHINI, F. AND MARTINI, L. (1966) Control of LH secretion: role of a "short" feedback mechanism. *Endocrinology*, **78**, 55–60.

DAVIDSON, J. M., JONES, L. E. AND LEVINE, S. (1968) Feedback regulation of adrenocorticotropin secretion in "basal" and "stress" conditions: acute and chronic effects of intrahypothalamic corticoid implantation. *Endocrinology*, **82**, 655–663.

DESAULLES, P. A. AND RITTEL, W. (1968) Adrenocorticotrophic activity of synthetic peptide sequences related to ACTH. *Mem. Soc. Endocrin.*, **17**, 125–137.

DE WIED, D. (1969) Effects of peptide hormones on behavior. In: *Frontiers in Neuroendocrinology*, W. F. Ganong and L. Martini (Eds.) Oxford University Press, New York, pp. 97–140.

EIK-NES, K. B. AND BRIZZEE, K. R. (1958) Some aspects of corticotrophin secretion in the trained dog. I. The presence of corticotrophin releasing factor in the blood stream of dogs shortly after hypophysectomy. *Acta Endocrinol.*, **29**, 219–223.

FERRARI, W., GESSA, G. L. AND VARGIU, L. (1963) Behavioral effects induced by intracisternally injected ACTH and MSH. *Ann. N.Y. Acad. Sci.*, **104**, 330–345.

FRASCHINI, F., MOTTA, M. AND MARTINI, L. (1968) A "short" feedback mechanism controlling FSH secretion. *Experientia*, **24**, 270–271.

GAVAZZI, G., MANGILI, G., MARTINI, L. AND PECILE, A. (1962) Action de la dexaméthasone sur les taux plasmatiques de corticostérone chez le rat. *Actualité Endocrinol.*, **3**, 169–172.

HALÁSZ, B. AND SZENTÁGOTHAI, J. (1960) Control of adrenocorticotrophin function by direct influence of pituitary substance on the hypothalamus. *Acta Morphol. Acad. Sci. Hung.*, **9**, 251–261.

HENKIN, R. I., WALKER, M. D., HARLAN, A. B. AND CASPER, A. G. T. (1967) Dynamics of transport of cortisol from peripheral blood into cerebrospinal fluid (CSF), central and peripheral nervous system and other tissues of the cat. *Program of the Forty-Ninth Meeting of the Endocrine Society*, p. 92.

HODGES, J. R. AND VERNIKOS, J. (1958) Influence of circulating adrenocorticotrophin on the pituitary adrenocorticotrophic response to stress in the adrenalectomized rats. *Nature*, **182**, 725.

HODGES, J. R. AND VERNIKOS, J. (1959) Circulating corticotrophin in normal and adrenalectomized animals after stress. *Acta Endocrinol.*, 30, 188–196.

KASTIN, A. J. AND SCHALLY, A. V. (1967) Autoregulation of release of melanocyte stimulating hormone from the rat pituitary. *Nature*, **213**, 1238–1240.

KATZ, S., MOLITCH, M. AND MCCANN, S. M. (1967) Feedback of hypothalamic growth hormone (GH) implants upon the anterior pituitary (AP). *Program of the Forty-Ninth Meeting of the Endocrine Society*, p. 86.

KAWAKAMI, M., KOSHINO, T. AND HATTORI, Y. (1966) Changes in EEG of the hypothalamus and limbic system after administration of ACTH, SU-4885 and Ach in rabbits with special reference to neurohumoral feedback regulation of pituitary-adrenal system. *Jap. J. Physiol.*, **16**, 551–569.

KITAY, J. I., HOLUB, D. A. AND JAILER, J. W. (1959) Inhibition of pituitary ACTH release: an extra-adrenal action of exogenous ACTH. *Endocrinology*, **64**, 475–482.

KLEIN, R. AND LIVINGSTONE, S. (1950) The effect of adrenocorticotropic hormone in epilepsy. *J. Pediat.*, **37**, 733–742.

KORÁNYI, L., ENDRÖCZI, E. AND TÁRNOK, F. (1966) Sexual behavior in the course of avoidance conditioning in male rabbits. *Neuroendocrinology*, **1**, 144–157.

LIDDLE, G. W., ESTEP, H. L., KENDALL, J. W., JR., WILLIAMS, W. C., JR. AND TOWNES, A. W. (1959) Clinical application of a new test of pituitary reserve. *J. Clin. Endocrinol.*, **19**, 875–894.

MANGILI, G., MOTTA, M., MUCIACCIA, W. AND MARTINI, L. (1965) Midbrain, stress and ACTH secretion. *Europ. Rev. Endocrin.*, **1**, 247–253.

MANGILI, G., MOTTA, M. AND MARTINI, L. (1966) Control of adrenocorticotropic hormone secretion. In: *Neuroendocrinology*, L. MARTINI and W. F. GANONG (Eds.), Academic Press, New York, vol. I, pp. 297–370.

MARTINI, L. (1966) Neurohypophysis and anterior pituitary activity. In: *The Pituitary Gland*, G. W. HARRIS and B. T. DONOVAN (Eds.), Butterworths, London, vol. III, pp. 535–577.

MESS, B. AND MARTINI, L. (1968) The central nervous system and the secretion of anterior pituitary trophic hormones. In: *Recent Advances in Endocrinology*, V. H. T. JAMES (Ed.), J. and A. Churchill, London, pp. 1–49.

MILCU, S. M., DEMETRESCU, M. AND NICOLESCU-CATARGI, A. (1964) The cortico-subcortical action of hypophyseal trophic hormones. *Rev. Roum. Endocrin.*, **1**, 297–306.

MILLICHAP, J. G. AND JONES, J. D. (1964) Acid-base, electrolyte and amino-acid metabolism in children with petit mal. Etiologic significance and modification by anti-convulsant drugs at the ketogenic diet. *Epilepsia*, **5**, 239–247.

MONNIER, M. (1953) *Rev. Méd. Suisse Romande*, **32**, 511–518. Quoted by S. N. MILCU, M. DEMETRESCU and A. NICOLESCU-CATARGI (1964) in *Rev. Roum. Endocrin.*, **1**, 297–306.

MOTTA, M., MANGILI, G. AND MARTINI, L. (1965) A "short" feedback loop in the control of ACTH secretion. *Endocrinology*, **77**, 392–395.

MOTTA, M., FRASCHINI, F., PIVA, F. AND MARTINI, L. (1968) Hypothalamic and extra-hypothalamic mechanisms controlling adrenocorticotrophin secretion. *Mem. Soc. Endocrinol.*, **17**, 3–18.

MOTTA, M., FRASCHINI, F. AND MARTINI, L. (1969) "Short" feedback mechanisms in the control of anterior pituitary function. In: *Frontiers in Neuroendocrinology*, W. F. GANONG and L. MARTINI (Eds.), Oxford University Press, New York, pp. 211-253.

MÜLLER, E. E. AND PECILE, A. (1966) Influence of exogenous GH on endogenous growth hormone release. *Proc. Soc. Exptl. Biol. Med.*, **122**, 1289–1291.

PECZELY, P. (1966) Effect of ACTH on the hypothalamic neurosecretion of the pigeon *(Columba livia domestica L.)*. *Acta Biol. Acad. Sci. Hung.*, **17**, 291–310.

PLAGER, J. E. AND CUSHMAN, P. (1962) Suppression of the pituitary-ACTH response in man by administration of ACTH or cortisol. *J. Clin. Endocrinol.*, **22**, 147–154.

SANDBERG, A. A., EIK-NES, K., MIGEON, C. J. AND KOEPF, G. F. (1957) Plasma 17-OHCS in hyper-function suppression and deficiency of adrenal cortical function. *J. Lab. Clin. Med.*, **50**, 286–296.

SAWYER, C. H., KAWAKAMI, M., MEYERSON, B., WHYTMOYER, D.I. AND LILLEY, J. J. (1968) Effects of ACTH, dexamethasone and asphyxia on electrical activity of the rat hypothalamus. *Brain Res.*, **10**, 213–226.

SCHAPIRO, S., MARMORSTON, J. AND SOBEL, H. (1958) Steroid feedback mechanism. *Am. J. Physiol.*, **192**, 58–62.

SEIDEN, G. AND BRODISH, A. (1969) Differential effects of hypophysectomy and adrenalectomy on hypothalamic CRF content. *Program of the Fifty-First Meeting of the Endocrine Society*, p. 92.

SMELIK, P. G. (1963) Relation between blood level of corticoids and the inhibiting effect on the hypophyseal stress response. *Proc. Soc. Exptl. Biol. Med.*, **113**, 616–619.

STEINER, F. A., RUF, K. AND AKERT, K. (1969) Steroid-sensitive neurones in rat brain: anatomical localization and responses to neurohumours and ACTH. *Brain Res.*, **12**, 74–85.

SUSSMAN, L., LIBRIK, L. AND CLAYTON, G. W. (1965) Effect of prior ACTH administration on ACTH release in man. *Metabolism*, **14**, 583–589.

TORDA, C. AND WOLFF, H. G. (1952) Effects of various concentrations of adrenocorticotrophic hormone on electrical activity of brain and on sensitivity to convulsion-inducing agents. *Am. J. Physiol.*, **168**, 406–413.

VERNIKOS-DANELLIS, J. (1965) Effect of stress, adrenalectomy, hypophysectomy and hydrocortisone on the corticotrophin-releasing activity of rat median eminence. *Endocrinology*, **76**, 122–126.

VERNIKOS-DANELLIS, J. AND TRIGG, L. N. (1967) Feedback mechanisms regulating pituitary ACTH secretion in rats bearing transplantable pituitary tumors. *Endocrinology*, **80**, 345–350.

WASSERMAN, M. J., BELTON, N. R. AND MILLICHAP, J. G. (1965) Effect of corticotropin (ACTH) on experimental seizures. *Neurology*, **15**, 1136–1141.
WOODBURY, D. M. AND VERNADAKIS, A. (1967) Influence of hormones on brain activity. In: *Neuro-endocrinology*, L. MARTINI and W. F. GANONG (Eds.), Academic Press, New York, vol. II. pp. 335–375.

DISCUSSION

MIRSKY: Is the inhibition due solely to the inhibition of release or is it also due to an inhibition of synthesis?

MARTINI: I think it is an inhibition of release; treatment of adrenalectomized animals with ACTH results in an increase in pituitary ACTH stores.

DE WIED: Did you study the effect of implantation in the ME of ACTH analogues like MSH, to investigate the specificity of the short feedback action of ACTH?

MARTINI: No, we did not study this.

MARKS: What is the time course of the ACTH short feedback inhibition?

MARTINI: No studies have been devoted so far to study this parameter.

MARKS: If I remember your experiments well, you studied the effects of ACTH implants at 5 days; why didn't you use shorter intervals?

MARTINI: We simply followed the protocol of an earlier experiment with dexamethasone implants.

HODGES: If ACTH has a direct inhibitory effect on the release of ACTH, these observations have great clinical significance. Some clinicians "tail off" patients after long-term corticoid treatment by injecting them with ACTH, assuming that when the adrenal response to exogenous ACTH is normal, the hypothalamo–pituitary–adrenal response to stress is also normal. In fact the patients are probably worse off than they were before.

MARTINI: There are at least a couple of papers which indicate that in patients treated with corticoids for a long time, the addition of ACTH results in a reduction rather than in an increase of the ability of the pituitary–adrenal system to respond to stressful stimulations, to the metopyrone test and to vasopressin administration.

McEWEN: Are the effects of ACTH implants and steroid implants reversible?

MARTINI: Yes, they are. It is interesting that when we measured the amount of ACTH present in the needle, 5 days after the implants had been left in the brain, practically no ACTH had escaped. ACTH acts presumably by some kind of "contact effect".

LEVINE: There is evidence that chronic treatment with ACTH alters both the levels of circulating steroids and the time course of steroid elevation. A single injection of ACTH results in a peak elevation of steroids at 15 min. After 3 days of ACTH injections, the peak steroid response is reduced and does not occur until 45 min after ACTH treatment.

MIRSKY: Dr. Martini, has there been any *in vitro* work to determine whether the ACTH *per se* acts on the pituitary?

MARTINI: I only know of one set of results by Dr. Fand; unfortunately they have never been published *in extenso*. He incubated pituitary tissue *in vitro*, adding different amounts of ACTH. He found that the number of basophilic cells in the incubated pituitaries were reduced in proportion to the amounts of ACTH which were added.

On the Subcellular Localization of Corticotropin-Releasing Factor (CRF) in the Rat Median Eminence

A. H. MULDER*

Rudolf Magnus Institute for Pharmacology, University of Utrecht, Medical Faculty, Vondellaan 6, Utrecht (The Netherlands)

According to a hypothesis, originally advanced by Harris and co-workers in the early 1950's (Harris, 1955) the control of anterior pituitary function by the central nervous system is mediated by neurohumors ("Releasing Factors"), which are elaborated in the hypothalamus and transported to the pituitary via the portal vessel system. In the past fifteen years, experimental evidence which supports this postulate has accumulated, and has been reviewed by Ganong (1963), Fortier (1966), McCann, Dhariwal and Porter (1968) and others. In fact, a number of different releasing factors have been extracted from the median eminence (ME) region of the hypothalamus, and have been partially purified (Guillemin, 1964). The available evidence suggests, that the corticotropin-releasing factor (CRF) is a peptide, possibly related to the neurohypophysial hormone vasopressin. Vasopressin is also present in the hypothalamus and, although it is found in relatively small amounts (Lederis, 1962), it has been attributed a specific role in the regulation of ACTH secretion (De Wied, 1961; Smelik, Gaarenstroom, Konijnendijk and De Wied, 1962). It was deemed of interest therefore to investigate the localization of both CRF and pressor activity in the ME at the subcellular level.

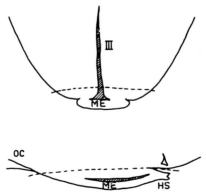

Fig. 1. Transversal and sagittal section through the median eminence region of the rat hypothalamus. The piece of tissue, which was used in the experiments is indicated by dotted lines. ME = median eminence; OC = optical chiasm; HS = remnant of the hypophyseal stalk; III = third ventricle.

---

* Present address: Department of Pharmacology, Free University, Van der Boechorststraat 7, Amsterdam, The Netherlands.

References p. 40

TABLE I

Protein was determined by the method of Lowry *et al.* (1951), cytochrome c oxidase by the method of
Cooperstein and Lazarow (1951).

Fraction	Protein (%)	Cyt.c ox. (RSA)	CRF activity as cort. prod. in vitro ($\mu g/100$ mg/h) *
600 $\times$ 12 g.min sed.	15.1	1.0	12.9 $\pm$ 0.8 (5)**
4 500 $\times$ 15 g.min sed.	32.0	1.9	17.0 $\pm$ 0.6 (7)
9 000 $\times$ 15 g.min sed.	17.2	1.3	13.3 $\pm$ 2.5 (7)
55 000 $\times$ 30 g.min sed.	13.9	0.2	13.3 $\pm$ 1.5 (7)
55 000 $\times$ 30 g.min sup.	21.8	—	10.4 $\pm$ 1.4 (7)

* 3 ME equivalents injected i.v.
** Mean $\pm$ standard error of the mean.

ME tissue from female rats of an inbred Wistar strain, weighing 140–180 g, was
used for the preparation of homogenates. In each experiment 40 to 50 pieces of ME
tissue (Fig. 1), with a total weight of 200–250 mg, were collected immediately after
decapitation of the animals. Homogenates (10%, w/v) in 0.4 M sucrose were made
using the Potter–Elvehjem technique (clearance 0.20–0.25 mm). The homogenates
were fractionated by differential and density gradient centrifugation. In general, the
600 $\times$ 12 g.min supernatant S1 (obtained by centrifugation of the homogenate at
600 g for 12 min) was used as the starting material. Homogenization and centrifugation procedures were carried out at 0–4° C.

Extracts from the subcellular fractions were prepared by acidification to pH 1 with
2 N hydrochloric acid. To determine their CRF activity, the neutralized extracts were
injected intravenously into female rats of 140–160 g, anesthetized with pentobarbital
and pretreated with chlorpromazine to block unspecific stimulation of ACTH release
(De Wied, 1967). Decapitation of the animals occurred 15 min after injection of the
extracts. The adrenals were quickly removed, cut into quarters, and incubated in a
Krebs–Ringer bicarbonate–glucose medium at 37° C for one hour in a Dubnoff
metabolic shaking incubator. After extraction with dichloromethane, the amount of
corticosteroids produced by the adrenals *in vitro* was determined spectrophotometric-
ally (Van der Vies, Bakker and De Wied, 1960). Pressor activity was estimated by
measuring the rise in blood pressure after i.v. injection of the extracts into male rats of
180–200 g, anesthetized with urethane and pretreated with dibenzyline (Dekanski,
1952), using arginine–vasopressin (AVP) as a standard.

Injection of 1 ME equivalent of an extract of S1 caused a corticosteroid production
in vitro of 15–20 $\mu g/100$ mg/h. The corresponding control values obtained from animals
injected with 0.4 M sucrose varied between 5 and 7 $\mu g/100$ mg/h. It was found that S1
extracts, when tested on hypophysectomized rats, contained no significant ACTH
activity. The pressor activity of the S1 averaged 11.0 $\pm$ 1.3 mU of AVP per ME
equivalent; this activity could be destroyed almost completely by treatment with

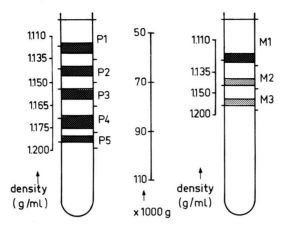

Fig. 2. Position of the subfractions in the centrifuge tubes after gradient centrifugation of the 10 000 ×
20 g.min fractions. The middle scale indicates the centrifugal force at different points along the tubes.
After resuspension in 0.8 M sucrose the 10 000 × 20 g.min sediment was layered on a discontinuous
gradient (left side) consisting of 5.0 ml 1.5 M, 1.5 ml 1.3 M, 2.0 ml 1.2 M, 1.5 ml 1.1 M and 1.5 ml
1.0 M sucrose. The sucrose concentration in the 10 000 × 20 g.min supernatant was brought to
0.8 M with 2.0 M sucrose and this fraction was layered on a gradient of 7.5 ml 1.5 M, 1.5 ml 1.1 M
and 1.5 ml 1.0 M sucrose respectively. Both gradients were spun for 3 hours at 28 000 r.p.m. in an
International B-35 Ultracentrifuge, swing-out rotor SB-269.

thioglycollate. In the assay system used, the CRF activity of AVP was detectable only
if the dose injected exceeded 30 mU.

Preliminary differential centrifugation experiments, one of which is shown in Table
I, indicated that the CRF-containing particles constitute a very heterogeneous population varying in size between large mitochondria and small microsomes. Therefore an
attempt was made to concentrate and eventually isolate the CRF-containing particles
by centrifugation on discontinuous sucrose density gradients. A crude mitochondrial
fraction, sedimented by centrifugation of S1 at 10 000 × 20 g.min, contained about
60% of the total CRF activity. After resuspending this fraction in 0.8 M sucrose it
could be further separated into five subfractions (P1–P5) on a gradient of 1.0–1.5 M
sucrose. From the postmitochondrial supernatant three subfractions (M1–M3) were
obtained by centrifugation on an essentially similar gradient (Fig. 2). The subfractions
were collected by puncturing the bottom of the centrifuge tubes.

For electronmicroscopy, part of the subcellular fractions was centrifuged at 150 000
× 30 g.min. The pellets were fixed with 2% glutaraldehyde in 0.1 M phosphate solution, pH 7.4. After postfixation with 0.1% osmium tetroxide, the pellets were con-
trasted with 1% uranyl acetate and dehydrated with an alcohol series. Randomly
chosen parts from the centre and periphery of the loosened pellets were separately
embedded in Epon-812. Ultra thin sections were cut with a LKB ultramicrotome.
These sections were postcontrasted with lead citrate according to the method of
Reynolds (1963) and studied with a Siemens Elmiskop I electron microscope. Pinched-
off nerve endings ("synaptosomes") were found present in subfractions P2–P5.
Myelin was exclusively found in the subfraction P1 and the bulk of the mitochondria in
subfractions P4 and P5. Various granules and small membrane fragments were mostly

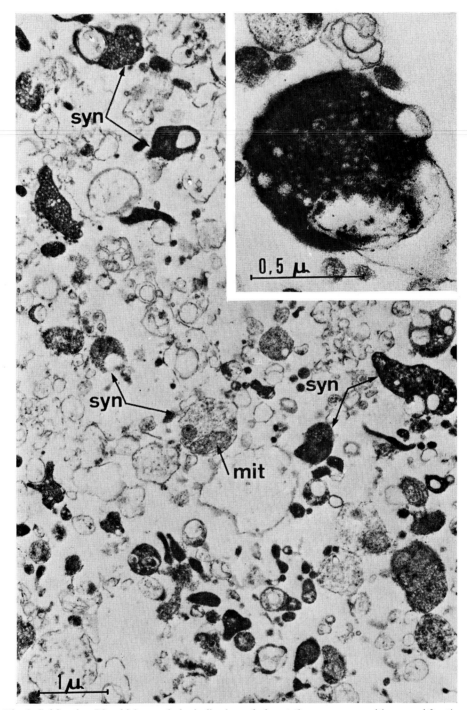

Fig. 3. Subfraction P2, which morphologically showed almost the same composition as subfraction P3. These subfractions contained several nerve endings ("synaptosomes" = syn) besides membrane fragments and some granules. In one of the nerve endings a mitochondrion (mit) can be seen.
Inset: A nerve ending from subfraction P3 at a higher magnification, showing very clearly the "synaptic cleft" with remnants of the postsynaptic membrane.

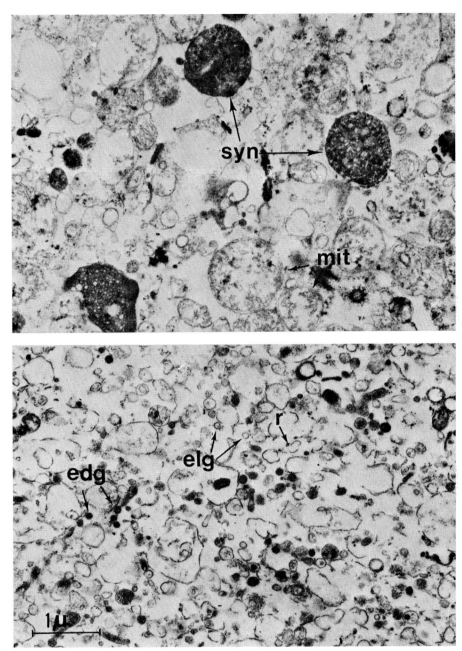

Fig. 4. Upper part: Subfraction P5, containing mainly mitochondria (mit) and large nerve endings (syn). Lower part: subfraction M2, containing small membrane fragments, ribosomes (r) and different granules (edg: electron-dense granules; elg: electron-lucent granules).

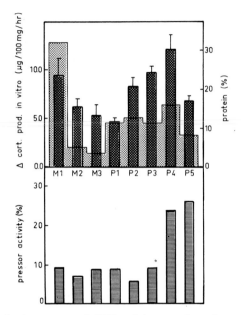

Fig. 5. Subcellular distribution pattern of CRF activity, protein and pressor activity after gradient centrifugation of the 10 000 × 20 g.min fractions. The CRF activity is expressed as the increase in the corticosteroid production *in vitro* above the control value (5.9 ± 0.5 μg/100 mg/h). This control value was obtained from animals which were injected with 0.4 M sucrose. From each subfraction 4.4 ME equivalents were injected i.v. into pentobarbital/chlorpromazine pretreated rats. Each value is the mean of 4–6 animals ± the standard error of the mean.

concentrated in subfractions M1–M3. Typical pictures of three of the subfractions are shown in Figs. 3 and 4.

After gradient centrifugation, 50–60% of the total CRF-activity was found in the subfractions P2–P5. These subfractions also contained the nerve endings. The distribution pattern obtained from one of the experiments is shown in Fig. 5.

These results suggest that in a homogenate, CRF is localized partly in nerve endings and partly in granules. Nevertheless, the relative specific activities (RSA)* in the nerve endings containing subfractions P2–P5 were found to be rather low (≤ 1.5) and furthermore, the RSA values obtained were found not to differ considerably from each other. This indicates that in none of these subfractions, a significant specific concentration of CRF activity had occurred (the RSA values can be roughly estimated from Fig. 5, in which both the corticosteroid production *in vitro* and the percentages of protein are presented). Obviously, CRF-containing nerve endings, with respect to their sedimentation characteristics, constitute a very heterogeneous population, which cannot be easily concentrated by conventional centrifugation techniques. In general, this situation is not uncommon in subcellular localization studies of brain tissue (Whittaker, 1965, 1968). This is connected with the morphological and functional complexity of this tissue.

---

* The RSA is defined as the ratio between the activity in a subfraction expressed as the percentage of total activity and the percentage of protein present.

TABLE II

EFFECT OF HYPOTONIC SHOCK ON CRF ACTIVITY

S1 was divided into two equal portions, which were centrifuged at 10 000 × 20 g.min. One sediment was subjected to osmotic shock by resuspension in 1 mM phosphate solution, pH 7.6, at 0° C. The other sediment was resuspended in 0.4 M sucrose and served as a control. Both samples were centrifuged at 10 000 × 20 and 150 000 × 60 g.min respectively. Before centrifugation, the sucrose concentration in the hypotonically treated fraction was brought to 0.4 M with 1.2 M sucrose.

Fraction	Protein (mg/g)	CRF activity as cort. prod. in vitro (μg/100 mg/h)
Control		
10 000 × 20 g.min sed.	37.2	16.5 ± 1.2 (4)*,†
150 000 × 60 g.min sed.	10.0	5.4 ± 0.7 (5)**
150 000 × 60 g.min sup.	0.8	5.3 ± 0.6 (4)**
After hypotonic shock		
10 000 × 20 g.min sed.	20.8	6.0 ± 0.6 (6)*
150 000 × 60 g.min sed.	13.4	11.7 ± 0.4 (3)**
150 000 × 60 g.min sup.	13.6	14.4 ± 2.1 (4)**
0.4 M sucrose		5.5 ± 0.3 (4)

  * 2.6 ME equivalents injected i.v.
** 4.0 ME equivalents injected i.v.
  † Mean ± standard error of the mean.

A fact, which emerges clearly from the gradient experiments, is that in the subfractions P2–P5 the distribution pattern of the pressor activity differs from that of the CRF activity. High RSA values, with respect to the pressor activity, were found in P4 and P5. Rather high RSA values, with regard to both pressor and CRF activities, were also obtained from the granule-rich subfractions M2 and M3.

The results of the gradient experiments lead to the assumption that CRF is localized in nerve endings and stored in granules within these endings. If this assumption is correct, it should be possible to isolate a granule fraction rich in CRF activity by osmotic disintegration of the nerve endings, provided that the binding of CRF to the granules is a strong one. Therefore the crude mitochondrial fraction, sedimented at 10 000 × 20 g.min, was subjected to hypotonic shock by resuspension of this fraction in a 1 mM phosphate solution. After such treatment, the 10 000 × 20 g.min sediment no longer contained CRF activity (Table II). Of the activity lost from the crude mitochondrial fraction 40–50% was found in the small-particle fraction, which sedimented at 150 000 × 60 g.min from the 10 000 × 20 g.min supernatant. The rest of the CRF activity was recovered in the 150 000 × 60 g.min supernatant. No CRF activity could be demonstrated in the control 150 000 × 60 g.min fractions, obtained after resuspending the crude mitochondrial fraction in 0.4 M sucrose. Apparently most of the CRF activity in the crude mitochondrial fraction is localized in rather large particles, presumably nerve endings, which seem to be fairly stable.

These results strongly suggest that CRF is, at least partly, granule-bound within nerve endings. Thus, with respect to storage and release, there seems to exist a marked resemblance between CRF and vasopressin. Furthermore, CRF, like vasopressin, probably is a peptide. However, the localization of both substances in different nerve endings indicates that production, transport and release of CRF and vasopressin take place in separate neurons within the hypothalamus.

ACKNOWLEDGEMENT

I wish to thank Dr. J. J. Geuze of the Department of Histology and Medical Electron microscopy for his indispensable help.

REFERENCES

COOPERSTEIN, S. I. AND LAZAROW, A. (1951) A microspectrophotometric method for the determination of cytochrome-oxidase. *J. Biol. Chem.*, **189**, 665–670.

DEKANSKI, J. (1952) The quantitative assay of vasopressin. *Brit. J. Pharmacol.*, **7**, 567–572.

FORTIER, C. (1966) Nervous control of ACTH-secretion. In: *The Pituitary Gland, vol. II*, G. W. HARRIS AND B. T. DONOVAN (Eds.), Butterworths, London, pp. 195–235.

GANONG, W. F. (1963) The central nervous system and the synthesis and release of adrenocorticotropic hormone. In: *Advances in Neuroendocrinology*, A. V. NALBANDOV (Ed.), University of Illinois Press, Urbana, pp. 92–149.

GUILLEMIN, R. (1964) Control of pituitary hormone secretion. Hypothalamic factors releasing pituitary hormones. *Rec. Progr. Hormone Res.*, **20**, 89–130.

HARRIS, G. W. (1955) *Neural Control of the Pituitary Gland*, Arnold Ltd., London.

LEDERIS, K. (1962) The distribution of vasopressin and oxytocin in hypothalamic nuclei. In: *Neurosecretion, Mem. Soc. Endocrinol.*, **12**, H. HELLER AND R. B. CLARK (Eds.), Academic Press, London pp. 227–236.

LOWRY, O. H., ROSEBROUGH, N. J., FARR, A. L. AND RANDALL, R. J. (1951) Protein measurement with the Folin Phenol reagent. *J. Biol. Chem.*, **193**, 265–275.

McCANN, S. M., DHARIWAL, A. P. S. AND PORTER, J. C. (1968) Regulation of the adenohypophysis. *Ann. Rev. Physiol.*, **30**, 589–640.

REYNOLDS, E. S. (1963) The use of lead citrate at high pH as an electronopaque stain in electron microscopy. *J. Cell Biol.*, **17**, 208–212.

SMELIK, P. G., GAARENSTROOM, J. H., KONIJNENDIJK, W. AND DE WIED, D. (1962) Evaluation of the role of the posterior lobe of the hypophysis in the reflex secretion of corticotrophin. *Acta Physiol. Pharmacol. Neerl.*, **11**, 20–33.

VIES, J. VAN DER, BAKKER, R. F. M. AND DE WIED, D. (1960) Correlated studies on plasma free corticosterone and on adrenal steroid formation rate *in vitro*. *Acta Endocrinol.*, **34**, 513–523.

WHITTAKER, V. P. (1965) The application of subcellular fractionation techniques to the study of brain function. *Progr. Biophys. Mol. Biol.*, **15**, 41–98.

WHITTAKER, V. P. (1968) The morphology of fractions of rat forebrain synaptosomes separated on continuous sucrose density gradients. *Biochem. J.*, **106**, 412–417.

WIED, D. DE (1961) The significance of the antidiuretic hormone in the release mechanism of corticotrophin. *Endocrinology*, **68**, 956–970.

WIED, D. DE (1967) Corticotrophin releasing factor (CRF); evaluation of assays. In: *Drugs of Animal Origin*, A. LEONARDI AND J. WALSH (Eds.), Ferro Edizioni, Milano, pp. 157–166.

DISCUSSION

HARRIS: Is there any evidence as to what type of granules the CRF is contained in? Is it possible to hazard a guess as to whether it's the smaller electron-translucent granules or the larger electron-dense granules as seen with the electron microscope?

MULDER: I do not think that there is much agreement yet among investigators about the correlation between the morphological appearance of the various granules in the hypothalamus and their function. This is particularly true for the granules with a diameter between 50 and 150 mμ. It is more or less accepted that the small electron-translucent granules, the "synaptic vesicles", contain acetylcholine and that vasopressin and oxytocin are contained within the neurosecretory granules, which have a diameter of 150–200 mμ. In answer to your question: I suppose that the CRF activity is contained in granules with a diameter of 100–120 mμ, but I want to stress that this is only a guess.

MIRSKY: Is it possible that the dissociation observed between vasopressin and the CRF could be due to the dissociation of the neurophysin–vasopressin complex in the process of isolation? The dissociation is very rapid under the most gentle conditions and you do get dissociation especially at pH 7.4.

MULDER: I think that this possibility can be rejected merely on the grounds of the low sensitivity of the CRF test for vasopressin. As you have seen, the fractions P2, P3 and P4, which have the highest CRF activity, contain a low pressor activity and the amounts of vasopressin injected are no more than 4 to 5 mU. In the CRF test which we have used, these small doses of vasopressin will have no effect, since vasopressin causes ACTH release in this test only if the dose injected exceeds 30 mU.

LARON: Did you test the isolated granules with CRF activity for other releasing factor activities?

MULDER: No, so far I did not.

MARTINI: I was impressed to see in one of your first slides that you find CRF activity in all sorts of fractions (containing nuclei, mitochondria, microsomes, etc.). We have obtained similar results in experiments carried on with Dr. Clementi and Dr. Motta aimed at clarifying which intracellular structures store the FSH-releasing factor. Apparently there is a wide-spread distribution; this in part answers also the question asked by Dr. Laron.

MULDER: First of all, as to the particulate composition, the subcellular fractions prepared by the usual centrifugation techniques generally are far from homogeneous. In brain homogenates subcellular distribution patterns are even more complicated by the fact that there seems to exist no straight correlation between the size and sedimentation characteristics of the nerve endings on the one hand and their functional type on the other. In fact, there will be found a considerable sedimentation overlap of nerve endings with nuclei, mitochondria, microsomal membrane fragments and granules. Of course this results in a high degree of cross-contamination among the different subcellular fractions. Therefore, in answer to your question, Dr. Martini, I am of the opinion that the rather diffuse subcellular distribution pattern of the CRF activity is due to cross-contamination, which is a consequence of the presumed localization of CRF in nerve endings and granules. In addition, I doubt whether without fundamental improvements of the current centrifugation technique one can ever obtain a good separation between the functionally different types of nerve endings and granules.

Central Monoamine Neurons and Pituitary–Adrenal Activity

KJELL FUXE, HANS CORRODI, TOMAS HÖKFELT AND GÖSTA JONSSON

Department of Histology, Karolinska Institute, Stockholm 60, Research Laboratories of AB Hässle, Göteborg and Department of Pharmacology, University of Göteborg (Sweden)

For many years, it has been known that drugs interfering with central monoamine neuro-transmission, such as reserpine, chlorpromazine, and amphetamine, produce marked changes in ACTH secretion* (see reviews by Ganong and Lorenzen, 1967; De Wied, 1967; Gold and Ganong, 1967). These findings led to the view that monoaminergic mechanisms participate in the control of ACTH secretion. This view was supported by many studies reporting certain decreases in brain NA levels after various types of acute stress (for references see, *e.g.*, Glowinski and Baldessarini, 1966). However, many reports on the effects of psychoactive drugs are in disagreement; and a decrease in NA levels in acute stress has not been found in several other studies.

In order to further elucidate the role of central monoamine neurons in the regulation of pituitary–adrenal activity, we have started experiments to study amine turnover in central monoamine neurons in endocrine states with various degrees of ACTH secretion. The amine turnover was estimated with the help of three different amine synthesis inhibitors: an inhibitor of the tyrosine hydroxylase, α-methyl-p-tyrosine (H 44/68), of the tryptophan hydroxylase, α-propyldopacetamide (H 22/54), and of the dopamine-β-oxidase (FLA 63) using a combined biochemical and histochemical amine analysis (for review, see Andén, Corrodi and Fuxe, 1969a). Since the rate of amine depletion is highly dependant on the nervous impulse flow, this approach will give an indication of the neural activity in the central monoamine neurons, which will be helpful when assessing their possible functional role in the regulation of ACTH secretion.

POSSIBLE ROLE OF CENTRAL NA NEURONS IN ACTH REGULATION

In *immobilization* stress (the rats are wrapped in wire nets) there is an increased rate of amine depletion after H 44/68 treatment in practically all the NA nerve terminal systems of the brain and of the spinal cord (Figs. 1, 2; Tables 1–3; Corrodi *et al.*, (1968). These findings indicate an increased activity in the central NA neurons. No

---

* *Abbreviations used*: ACTH = Adrenocorticotropic hormone, ADH = Antidiuretic hormone, CRF = Corticotropin-releasing factor, LHRF = Luteinizing hormone-releasing factor, CA = Catecholamine, DA = Dopamine, 5-HIAA = 5-Hydroxyindoleacetic acid, 5-HT = 5-Hydroxytryptamine, 5-HTP = 5-Hydroxytryptophan, MAO = Monoamine oxidase, NA = Noradrenaline.

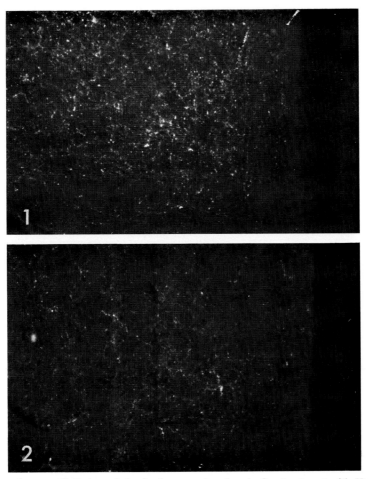

Fig. 1. Nuc. dorso-medialis hypothalami of a normal male rat after treatment with H 44/68 (250 mg/kg, i.p., 4 hours before killing). A large number of mainly moderately fluorescent NA nerve terminals are seen. × 120.

Fig. 2. Same area and treatment as described in text to Fig. 1 except that the rat was exposed to immobilization stress for 4 hours. Now mainly weakly fluorescent NA terminals are seen and less fluorescent terminals are present due to an increased rate of NA depletion. × 120.

drop in the NA levels was observed, probably due to the fact that increased synthesis had compensated for the increase in NA release.

Also in hypophysectomized rats, in which the amine turnover in the central NA neurons is reduced and possibly relatively unresponsive due to lack of hormonal stimuli from endocrine organs, except the pituitary gland, there is a stress-induced activation of the central NA neurons (unpublished data). Signs of increased NA turnover have also been observed in other types of stress, such as *muscular exhaustion* (Gordon, Spector, Sjoerdsma and Udenfriend, 1966) and *electric shock* (Thierry, Javoy, Glowinski and Kety, 1969; Bliss, Ailion and Zwanziger, 1968). However, we have failed to observe an increase in central NA turnover after exposure of the animals to cold (Corrodi, Fuxe and Hökfelt, 1967b) as reported by other workers

TABLE 1

DA AND NA IN RAT BRAIN IN PER CENT OF NORMAL VALUES

(DA = 0.65 ± 0.016 μg/g; NA = 0.45 ± 0.009 μg/g; n = 10). Means ± s.e.m. 250 mg/kg of H 44/68 was given i.p. and the animals were put into the wire cage for 4 or 8 hours. n = Number of experiments.

Treatment		n	DA in %	NA in %
untreated		10	100.0 ± 2.5	100.0 ± 2.0
stress		6	91.2 ± 4.4	92.7 ± 3.4
H 44/68	4 h	9	29.5 ± 2.7	46.3 ± 1.6[1]
stress + H 44/68	4 h	10	28.0 ± 1.4	33.7 ± 1.5[2]
Statistical significance between [1] and [2]: $p < 0.001$				
untreated		10	100.0 ± 2.5	100.0 ± 2.0
stress		6	99.8 ± 2.3	93.7 ± 3.0
H 44/68	8 h	6	21.3 ± 2.8	33.6 ± 0.4[1]
stress + H 44/68	8 h	6	23.5 ± 5.3	24.5 ± 2.2[2]
Statistical significance between [1] and [2]: $p < 0.005$				

From Corrodi, Fuxe and Hökfelt, 1968.

TABLE 2

NA IN RAT BRAIN IN PER CENT OF NORMAL VALUES

(NA = 0.45 ± 0.009 μg/g; n = 10). Means ± s.e.m. The dopamine-β-oxidase inhibitor, FLA 63 was given i.p. and the rats were put into the wire net for 6 hours. n = number of experiments. Student's t test (From Corrodi *et al.*, to be published).

Treatment	n	NA in %
untreated	10	100 ± 2.0
stress	6	92.7 ± 3.4
FLA 63 10 mg/kg	12	55.2 ± 1.8[1]
FLA 63 10 mg/kg + stress	12	34.7 ± 2.0[2]
FLA 63 25 mg/kg	4	30.8 ± 1.0[3]
FLA 63 25 mg/kg + stress	4	16.0 ± 1.3[4]
Statistical significance between [1-2] and [3-4]: $p < 0.001$		

(Gordon *et al.*, 1966). In a hot environment (+40°C), however, there is a marked activation of the central NA neurons (Corrodi *et al.*, 1967b) which may suggest that the NA neurons are also involved in thermo-regulation. At a temperature of 32°C there may be a selective activation of the hypothalamic NA nerve terminals (Iversen and Simmonds, 1969). Also in *sham rage behaviour*, produced either by electrical stimulation of the amygdaloid cortex (Fuxe and Gunne, 1964), or by acute brain stem transection, (Reis and Fuxe, 1968a) there is a marked increase in amine turnover in the various NA nerve terminal systems of the brain, *e.g.*, in the hypothalamus, limbic system and the reticular formation. All these stressful conditions are probably associated with increased ACTH secretion of various degrees (see Ganong, 1963; Mangili, Motta and Martini, 1966).

TABLE 3

EFFECT OF IMMOBILIZATION STRESS, ADRENALECTOMY AND GLYCOCORTICOIDS ON THE
RATE OF FLUORESCENCE DISAPPEARANCE FROM THE HYPOTHALAMIC NA NERVE TERMINALS
OF MALE RATS AFTER TREATMENT WITH H 44/68 (250 mg/kg, i.p.)

A semi-quantitative estimation of the fluorescence intensity has been made: 3+ = strong intensity;
2+ = moderate intensity; 1+ = weak intensity; ½+ = very weak intensity. Number of rats within
parentheses.

Treatment	Fluorescence intensity		Effect on the rate of NA depletion
	Without H 44/68	With H 44/68	
normal	3+ (35)	1+ (8) 2+ (28)	—
immobilization stress 4 hours	3+ (10)	½+(4)1+ (30)2+ (3)	acceleration
immobilization stress + chlordiazepoxide 30 mg/kg	3+ (6)	1+ (2)2+ (7)	blockade of acceleration
immobilization stress + dexamethasone (100 μg/100 g) 3 min before the stress	3+ (8)	1+ (8)2+ (1)	acceleration
adrenalectomy, 10 days	3+ (10)	1+ (12)2+ (3)	acceleration
adrenalectomy, 10 days + cortisol (solucortef; 2.5 mg/100 g) for 2 days	3+ (6)	1+ (3)2+ (9)	blockade of acceleration

In studies on the NA turnover in immobilization stress, it has been found that
minor tranquillizers, such as chlordiazepoxide, were able to block the stress-induced
activation of the central NA neurons (see Table 1, Corrodi, Fuxe and Hökfelt, to be
published). These drugs are also known to modify ACTH secretion (see Gold and
Ganong, 1967). It may be that the "anti-stress" effects of these drugs are mediated at
least partly via a blockade of the activation of the central NA neurons. Acute treatment with the synthetic glycocorticoid, dexamethasone (100 μg/100 g rat), on the
other hand, did not cause a blockade of the increase in the NA turnover found in
immobilization stress (Fuxe, Hökfelt and Lidwall, unpublished data). This glycocorticoid is known to exert a strong negative feed-back action on ACTH secretion,
probably mainly by way of an action on the brain (Smelik and Sawyer, 1962, Smelik,
1969) but probably also on the anterior pituitary (De Wied, 1964), at least with the
dose used in the present study. These results do not in any way imply, however, that
the NA neurons are not involved in ACTH regulation, since the negative feed-back
action of the steroid on the brain may be insufficient to block the stress-induced activation of the peptidergic neurons containing the corticotrophin-releasing factor (see
Ganong, 1963, Mangili et al., 1966).

It is not known if the increase in NA turnover in various types of stress is related to
the increased ACTH secretion. A good experiment would be to see if drugs (e.g.
chlordiazepoxide) (see Corrodi et al., 1968, and unpublished data) which block the
selective activation of the central NA neurons (DA and 5-HT neurons are not activated)
in immobilization stress also influence the increase in ACTH secretion found in this
type of stress. Chlordiazepoxide per se does not affect the NA turnover in the brain nor

TABLE 4

EFFFCT OF FLA 63 ON THE ULCERATION OF THE RAT STOMACH MUCOSA INDUCED BY
IMMOBILIZATION STRESS

(Corrodi *et al.*, to be published)

Treatment	Time interval (hours)	n (total number of animals)	n_{ulc} (number of animals with ulcers)	$\dfrac{\% \, n_{ulc} \cdot 100}{n}$
controls (saline)	2	11	1.5	13
	4	11	6	55
	6	30	21	70
FLA 63 5 mg/kg, i.p.	2	4	0.5	12
	4	4	0	0
	6	4	0	0
FLA 63 10 mg/kg, i.p.	2	4	2	50
	4	4	2	50
	6	12	2.5	20

the turnover of DA or 5-HT (Corrodi, Fuxe and Hökfelt, 1967a). We know, however, that the NA released in sham rage is a necessary requirement for this type of behaviour (Reis and Fuxe, 1968a, b) and for the appearance of gastric ulcers in immobilization stress (Table 4; Corrodi, Fuxe, Hökfelt and Lidwall, unpublished data). Thus, it has been found that protriptyline, which is a potent blocker of the membrane pump in the NA neurons, markedly increases the number of sham rage attacks; and haloperidol, which acts by blocking central DA and NA receptors completely abolishes the sham rage behaviour. In the case of the ulcer formation in immobilization stress, this effect of stress was, to a large extent, blocked by a potent dopamine-β-oxidase inhibitor (FLA63).—When discussing the functional significance of increased release of NA in stress for ACTH secretion, it is necessary to consider the fact that reserpine, which decreases monoamine transmission by blocking the uptake–storage mechanism in the amine granules of all the central monoamine neurons (see Dahlström, Fuxe and Hillarp, 1965; Carlsson, 1966), and chlorpromazine which causes blockade of central NA and DA receptors (Carlsson and Lindqvist, 1963; Corrodi, Fuxe and Hökfelt, 1967a, Andén; Corrodi, Fuxe and Hökfelt, 1967), both produce hypersecretion of ACTH and decrease of the CRF stores in the median eminence (see Bhattacharya and Marks, 1969). If these effects are related to blockade of central CA neurotransmission, it would mean that the NA released from the various NA nerve terminal systems of the brain would all aim to inhibit the secretion of ACTH. This view is also supported by the fact that amphetamine and methamphetamine, which act by releasing extra-granular amine stores from DA and NA neurons (Carlsson, Fuxe, Hamberger and Lindqvist, 1966) have been reported by some workers to inhibit ACTH secretion (see Lorenzen, Wise and Ganong, 1965); and recently dopa with or without monoamine oxidase inhibition has also been found to cause an inhibition of ACTH secretion

(Ganong, 1969). All these pharmacological experiments would favour the view that increased release of NA from the NA neurons in stress acts to inhibit ACTH secretion. Thus, probably both excitatory and inhibitory pathways, with regard to ACTH secretion, are activated in stressful situations. The function of the central NA neurons would be to prevent excessive secretion of ACTH.

However, the results obtained with psychoactive drugs have to be interpreted with caution, particularly in view of the fact that many authors report different results. Thus, it has been found that a stress-induced increase in ACTH secretion is not changed by combined treatment with reserpine and α-methyltyrosine (Carr and Moore, 1968) which certainly blocks central CA neurotransmission. Furthermore, data have recently been obtained that reserpine-induced stimulation of the pituitary–adrenal axis is not related to depletion of monoamines, since reserpine elicited the same response also in animals pretreated with reserpine plus α-methyl-tyrosine (Hirsch and Moore, 1968). Furthermore, Smelik's findings (1967) on the lack of effect of reserpine implants in the hypothalamus on ACTH secretion, certainly demonstrate that intact function of the hypothalamic NA nerve terminals at least is not crucial in regulation of ACTH secretion. However, the NA neurons may still play an important role. The CRF release from the hypothalamus is probably regulated by excitatory and inhibitory afferents and by the glycocorticoid and ACTH level in the blood (Mangili et al., 1966, Motta, Fraschini and Martini, 1969). The balance between these various nervous and hormonal inputs to the CRF-producing neurons probably undergo marked changes; and it is quite possible that the NA afferent input to various parts of the brain plays an important role in ACTH regulation in at least certain special situations.

Under all conditions the NA pathways play an important physiological role for the behavioral performance in the alarm reaction (see Reis and Fuxe, 1968a, b). In view of the dense NA innervation of the preganglionic sympathetic and parasympathetic nuclei (Fuxe, 1965), it can directly influence the activity in the whole part of the peripheral autonomic nervous system and the adrenaline secretion from the adrenal medulla. This view is also supported by the fact that when catapresan, which probably stimulates central NA receptor sites (Andén, Corrodi, Fuxe, Hökfelt, Hökfelt, Rydin and Svensson, 1969b), is given to reserpine–apomorphine (a DA receptor-stimulating agent) (Andén, Fuxe, Hökfelt and Rubensson, 1967) pretreated rats, there is a marked behavioral activation of the rats. The rats run rapidly round and out of the cages (Andén et al., 1969b).

To further investigate the possible role of NA neurons in ACTH secretion, the effect of adrenalectomy on the turnover of the central NA neurons was studied. As in stress, the ACTH secretion is increased in adrenalectomized rats, in this case probably due to removal of the negative feed-back of the glycocorticoids. Ten days after adrenalectomy there was an increased rate of amine depletion in most of the NA nerve terminal systems of the brain after treatment with a tyrosine hydroxylase inhibitor or a dopamine-β-oxidase inhibitor as revealed both histochemically (Table 3) and biochemically. These findings suggest that there is an increased turnover and activity of the NA neurons not only in stress but also after adrenalectomy. An increase in NA turnover after adrenalectomy (6 days) has also been observed by Javoy, Glowinski and Kordon (1968). These workers report that this effect is not present 2–3 days after adrenalectomy. In order to see if there is any relation between the increased ACTH secretion and the increase in NA neuron activity after adrenalectomy, the rats were injected with cortisol (2.5 mg/100 g) 24 and 4 hours before injection of the amine synthesis inhibitor. It was found that cortisol, at least partly, blocked the increased NA turnover found after adrenalectomy (see Table 3; Fuxe *et al.*, unpublished data). Thus, when the increase in ACTH secretion is decreased, also the increase in NA turnover is at least partly blocked. The site of steroidal "negative" feed-back is probably mainly localized in the hypothalamus and the limbic system; it may, to a certain extent, also be localized to the mesencephalon (see review by Ganong, 1963, Mangili *et al.*, 1966).

The following speculation can be given to explain the turnover changes in the NA neurons following adrenalectomy with or without cortisol treatment. The CRF-containing neurons gradually increase their activity after adrenalectomy due to decreased "negative" feed-back by the glycocorticoids. If we assume that these neurons have collaterals, the CRF neurons could initiate impulse activity in a nervous chain ending in the reticular formation, *i.a.* on the NA cell bodies of the rhombencephalon. In this way information on pituitary–adrenal activity could reach the NA neurons, and the turnover in the NA neurons would be increased, as was observed in the present experiments, possibly to avoid excessive ACTH secretion. When hydrocortisone, on the other hand, is given, the glycocorticoid "negative" feed-back decreases the activity of the CRF neurons and the activity of the neuronal chain postulated above returns to normal and so does the activity in the NA neurons. Of course, it cannot be excluded that cortisol normally acts directly on the NA neurons, *e.g.* by influencing tyrosine hydroxylase or dopamine-β-oxidase activity. It is possible that ACTH itself may have an indirect influence on the activity of the NA neurons, since it is probable that it exerts a "negative" feed-back on the CRF neurons (Motta *et al.*, 1969), and it has potent actions on animal behavior by an action on the brain (De Wied, 1969). However, treatment of, *e.g.*, hypophysectomized rats, which have a markedly decreased NA turnover (Fuxe, Hökfelt and Jonsson, unpublished data) with ACTH β1-24 from 2.5 mU to 10 mU per rat and per day for 2 days, did not change the NA turnover as observed histochemically (unpublished data). Normal rats or adrenalectomized rats have not been studied in this respect, however.

Preliminary studies on brain slices from normal rats treated with cortisol (5 mg/100 g) for 3 days indicate that cortisol does not interfere with the accumulation of (^{3}H)NA (10^{-7}M) in the hypothalamus (unpublished data). This indicates that since cortisol does not change the brain NA levels, the membrane pump in the NA neurons is not blocked by cortisol.

It should be pointed out that nuc. supraopticus is densely innervated by NA nerve terminals (Fuxe, 1965). In all types of stress described above and also under osmotic (hypo- or hypertonic) stress (Andén, Fuxe and Hökfelt, unpublished data) these terminals are activated as well as the other nerve terminals of the brain. The NA neurons, therefore, probably participate in the neural control of ADH secretion, which is of interest when discussing ACTH regulation, since ADH may in certain situa-

TABLE 5

5-HT IN RAT BRAIN IN PER CENT OF NORMAL VALUES 16 h AFTER p-CHLOROPHENYLALANINE
METHYLESTER HYDROCHLORIDE (H 69/17, 300 mg/kg, i.p.)

Means $\pm$ s.e.m. The animals were kept in the wire cage for 16 hours. n = number of experiments.

Treatment	n	5-HT in %
untreated controls	10	100.0 $\pm$ 3.5
stress	3	105.9 $\pm$ 12.8
H 69/17	3	46.4 $\pm$ 10.0
stress + H 69/17	4	43.6 $\pm$ 2.8

From Corrodi, Fuxe and Hökfelt, 1968.

TABLE 6

5-HT IN RAT BRAIN IN PER CENT OF NORMAL VALUE

(0.45 $\pm$ 0.015 μg/g of wet weight n = 10). Means $\pm$ s.e.m. 500 mg/kg of H 22/54 was given i.p. and
the animals put into the wire cages for 3 hours. n = number of experiments.

Treatment	n	5-HT in %
untreated animals	10	100.0 $\pm$ 3.5[1]
stress	12	80.0 $\pm$ 6.8[2]
H 22/54	11	43.5 $\pm$ 2.5
stress + H 22/54	13	39.3 $\pm$ 2.4

Statistical significance between [1] and [2]: $p < 0.025$. From Corrodi, Fuxe and Hökfelt, 1968.

tions cause release of ACTH, possibly from the median eminence (see Smelik, 1969).

POSSIBLE ROLE OF CENTRAL DA NEURONS IN ACTH REGULATION

Various types of stress and adrenalectomy have not been found to obviously change
the turnover in the tubero-infundibular DA neurons of female and male rats, which
are also unaffected by cortisol in very high doses (normal and castrated rats; 100 mg/
rat for 3 days, see Fuxe and Hökfelt, 1967; Fuxe, Hökfelt and Nilsson, 1969a). These
neurons, therefore, probably do not participate in the regulation of ACTH secretion.
This view is supported by the fact that reserpine implants in the median eminence do
not cause any change in the ACTH secretion (Smelik, 1967). Instead, the tubero-
infundibular DA neurons have been shown to be involved in gonadotrophin regulation, probably mainly by inhibiting the release of LHRF from the median eminence
(Fuxe, Hökfelt and Nilsson, 1967a, b, 1969a, b; Fuxe and Hökfelt, 1967, 1969 a, b).
    The turnover in the nigro-neostriatal DA neurons has not been found to be in-
fluenced by immobilization stress (Table 1; Corrodi et al., 1968) or by adrenalectomy
(unpublished data). Therefore, it is not probable that they participate in ACTH

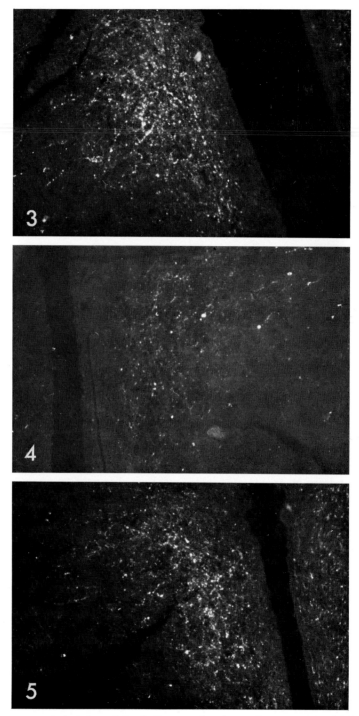

Fig. 3. Nuc. paraventricularis hypothalami of a normal male rat after treatment with H 44/68 (see text to Fig. 1). Mainly moderately fluorescent NA nerve terminals are seen. × 120.

Fig. 4. Nuc. paraventricularis hypothalami of a male rat 10 days after adrenalectomy and 4 hours after treatment with H 44/68 (see text to Fig. 1). Now mainly weakly fluorescent NA nerve terminals are seen and less fluorescent NA terminals are present due to an increased rate of NA depletion. × 120.

Fig. 5. Same treatment and area as in Fig. 4, except that cortisol was given (2.5 mg/100 g) 24 and 4 hours before killing. The number and intensity of the fluorescent NA nerve terminals is similar to that found in the normal male rat after treatment with H 44/68. Thus, the increased rate of NA depletion found after adrenalectomy is at least partially blocked. × 120.

regulation. This view is not in disagreement with the fact that in electric shock experiments the DA turnover has been found to be increased (Bliss *et al.*, 1968; Thierry *et al.*, 1969). This is probably related to the fact that in this type of stress the animal exhibits considerable locomotion.

POSSIBLE ROLE OF CENTRAL 5-HT NEURONS IN ACTH REGULATION

In immobilization stress (Corrodi *et al.*, 1968, Table 6) it has been found that there is a 20% depletion of 5-HT after 3 hours of stress. However, after 16 hours of stress there is no longer any depletion of brain 5-HT. The depletion of 5-HT observed after 3 hours was probably not due to an increased nervous impulse flow in the 5-HT neurons, since the rate of 5-HT depletion found after the tryptophan hydroxylase inhibitors α-propyldopacetamide (H 22/54) and *p*-chlorophenylalanine methylester (Koe and Weissman, 1967) was not significantly changed as found both histo- and biochemically (Tables 5, 6). Recently it has been found that cortisol (5 mg/kg, i.p.) produces a short-lasting depletion of brain 5-HT which was in the same order of magnitude as observed in the present experiments (Green and Curzon, 1969). This 5-HT depletion could be prevented by treatment with a tryptophan pyrrolase inhibitor (allopurinol). These authors, therefore, suggested that the 5-HT depletion caused by cortisol was due to an activation of the tryptophan pyrrolase resulting in increased formation of formylkurenine and decreased amounts of tryptophan reaching the brain with a concomitant decline of 5-HT synthesis. This view was supported by the fact that the 5-HIAA levels were decreased as well (Curzon and Green, 1968). It may, therefore, be that in immobilisation stress the rapid and short-lasting decline of 5-HT levels is due to the increased amounts of cortisol released from the adrenal cortex. Obviously after 16 hours of stress, this mechanism is no longer at work or is counteracted by another unknown mechanism. This hypothesis, which of course needs much more experimental support, is of great interest since by such a mechanism, pituitary–adrenal activity could participate in the control of 5-HT neuro-transmission and herewith in the control of mood (Carlsson, Corrodi, Fuxe and Hökfelt, 1969; Fuxe and Ungerstedt, 1968).

Other types of stress such as *electric shock* have been found to cause increased 5-HT levels rather than decreased 5-HT levels (Thierry, Fekete and Glowinski, 1968); and signs of increased 5-HT turnover have been obtained (Thierry *et al.*, 1968, Bliss *et al.*, 1968). These results clearly indicate that the type of stress used is of great importance for determining the activity in the various monoamine neuron systems under stressful conditions. The difficulties involved are furthermore illustrated by the fact that it has been reported, contrary to our results, that restraint stress causes increased brain 5-HT levels (De Schaepdryver, Preziosi and Scapagnini, 1969).

Taken together, the results from the studies on 5-HT turnover in stressed rats indicate that the 5-HT neurons do not play an essential role in corticotrophin regulation in this situation. This view is further supported by the findings that marked changes in 5-HT levels caused by MAO inhibitors, tryptophan-hydroxylase inhibitors, tryptophan deficiency and *p*-chloramphetamine do not change the degree of adrenocortical activation in stress (Dixit and Buckley, 1969, De Schaepdryver *et al.*, 1969). When studying the effect of stress on 5-HT neurons it has to be remembered that any change in body temperature may influence the activity in the central 5-HT neurons. Thus, in a hot environment, the activity of the 5-HT neurons will increase, whereas it will decrease in cold (Corrodi *et al.*, 1967 b). These studies certainly indicate that the 5-HT neurons are involved in thermo-regulation in agreement with the studies of Feldberg and Myers (1963). Thus, if body temperature is changed in stress, this could influence the amine turnover in the 5-HT neurons. This might be an explanation for the differences in results reported by several authors.

Most workers agree that the brain 5-HT levels are not changed to any significant degree by adrenalectomy (see McKennee *et al.*, 1966). This is also in agreement with our fluorescence histochemical findings. No changes in fluorescence intensity are observed 10 days after adrenalectomy in the central 5-HT neurons (cell bodies and terminals).

Daily injections of cortisol (0.74 mg/kg) for 5 days into normal or adrenalectomized rats did not cause any change in the 5-HT levels (McKennee *et al.*, 1966). Using high daily doses of cortisol, however, Kato and Valzelli (1958) found increases in brain 5-HT levels. Obviously, effects on the tryptophan pyrrolase are at least, mainly, of some importance only in acute experiments. In long-term experiments, cortisol must affect the central 5-HT neurons by another mechanism and in another way (see below).

In turnover studies on 5-HT neurons following adrenalectomy, positive results have been obtained. The results seem to indicate that there is a reduced turnover of amine in the 5-HT neurons of adrenalectomized rats (10 days) as seen both histo- and biochemically (unpublished data). The decrease in 5-HT turnover is also evident from the fact that accumulation of 5-HT following monoamine oxidase inhibition is reduced both in 5-HT cell bodies and nerve terminals following adrenalectomy. The 5-HT turnover is restored to normal after daily treatment with cortisol for two days. The action of the glycocorticoids on the 5-HT turnover may either be indirect by way of, *e.g.*, increasing the excitatory nervous input onto the 5-HT cell bodies, or direct by way of *e.g.*, increasing tryptophan hydroxylase activity. Thus, it may be that also the 5-HT neurons participate in ACTH regulation, possibly by an inhibitory action on ACTH secretion, since *inter alia* drugs such as α-ethyltryptamine, which is known to inhibit ACTH secretion (Ganong, 1969), stimulates 5-HT receptor sites in the brain and the spinal cord (Meek and Fuxe, unpublished data). Furthermore, the results indicate that the negative feedback action of glycocorticoids on the brain may partly be mediated via activation of central 5-HT neurons.

Studies on the accumulation of (^{3}H)5-HT in brain slices indicate no marked change in the degree of accumulation as observed after daily treatment *in vivo* with cortisol (5 mg/100 g) for 2 days.

It should also be pointed out that the 5-HT neuron system participates in the innervation of the preganglionic sympathetic and parasympathetic nerve cell bodies; as an example, the 5-HT innervation of the sympathetic lateral column may be taken (Carlsson, Falck, Fuxe and Hillarp, 1964). Evidence has been obtained that 5-HTP inhibits the increase in adrenaline secretion from the adrenal medulla caused by insulin-induced hypoglycemia (Andén, Carlsson and Hillarp, 1964). The preganglionic nerve cell bodies to the adrenal medulla may therefore receive an inhibiting 5-HT input.

CONCLUSIONS

There is evidence from amine turnover studies and pharmacological studies that central NA neurons may participate in the regulation of ACTH secretion from the anterior pituitary. The interpretation is given that the NA neurons may exert an inhibitory influence which, at least in certain situations, could be of importance for regulation of ACTH secretion. This interpretation is supported by the fact that steroid-sensitive neurons in the hypothalamus are, to a large extent, inhibited by NA (Steiner *et al.*, 1969).

It is not likely that the tubero-infundibular DA neurons and the nigro-neostriatal DA neurons participate in ACTH regulation.

The central 5-HT neurons probably do not directly participate in ACTH regulation with regard to stress responses. However, the 5-HT neurons may still play a role in the regulation of ACTH secretion, since 5-HT turnover is reduced by adrenalectomy and restored again to normal by subacute treatment with glycocorticoids. The increased 5-HT turnover caused by prolonged treatment with glycocorticoids may be of importance both for the negative feedback action on ACTH secretion caused by these steroids and for their actions on the affective state.

ACKNOWLEDGEMENTS

This work has been supported by a small NIH Grant (1 R03 NH 16825-01) and by Grants (14X-715-05B, 14X-1015-05, B70-14X-2295-03, B70-14X-2887-01) from the Swedish Medical Research Council.

REFERENCES

ANDÉN, N.-E., CARLSSON, A. AND HILLARP, N.-Å. (1964) Inhibition by 5-hydroxytryptophan of insulin-induced adrenaline depletion. *Acta pharmacol. toxicol.*, **21**, 183–186.

ANDÉN, N.-E., CORRODI, H. AND FUXE, K. (1969a) Turnover studies using synthesis inhibition. In: *Metabolism of Amines in the Brain*, G. HOOPER (Ed.), Macmillan, London, pp. 38–47.

ANDÉN, N.-E., CORRODI, H., FUXE, K. AND HÖKFELT, T. (1967) Increased impulse flow in bulbospinal NA neurons by catecholamine receptor blocking agents. *Europ. J. Pharmacol.*, **2**, 59–64.

ANDÉN, N.-E., FUXE, K., HÖKFELT, T. AND RUBENSSON, A. (1967) Evidence for dopamine receptor stimulation by apomorphine. *J. Pharm. Pharmacol.*, **19**, 335–337.

ANDÉN, N.-E., CORRODI, H., FUXE, HÖKFELT, K. HÖKFELT, B., RYDIN, C. AND SVENSSON, T. (1969b) Evidence for a central noradrenaline receptor stimulation by catapresan. *Life Sci.*, in press.

BHATTACHARYA, A. N. AND MARKS, B. H. (1969) Reserpine- and chlorpromazine-induced changes in hypothalamo-hypophyseal-adrenal system in rats in the presence and absence of hypothermia. *J. Pharmacol. Exptl. Ther.*, **165**, 108–116.

BLISS, E. L., AILION, J. AND ZWANZIGER, J. (1968) Metabolism of norepinephrine, serotonin and dopamine in rat brain with stress. *J. Pharmacol. Exptl. Ther.*, **164**, 122–134.

CARLSSON, A. (1966) Drugs which block the storage of 5-hydroxytryptamine and related amines. In: *Handbook of Experimental Pharmacology*, Vol. 19, Springer Verlag, Berlin, Heidelberg, Göttingen, pp. 529–592.

CARLSSON, A., CORRODI, H., FUXE, K. AND HÖKFELT, T. (1969) Effect of antidepressant drugs on the depletion of intraneuronal brain 5-hydroxytryptamine stores caused by 4-methyl-α-ethyl-meta-tyramine. *Europ. J. Pharmacol.*, **5**, 357–366.

CARLSSON, A., FALCK, B., FUXE, K. AND HILLARP, N.-Å. (1964) Cellular localization of monoamines in the spinal cord. *Acta physiol. scand.*, **60**, 112–119.

CARLSSON, A., FUXE, K., HAMBERGER, B. AND LINDQVIST, M. (1966) Biochemical and histochemical studies on the effects of imipramine-like drugs and (+)-amphetamine on central and peripheral catecholamine neurons. *Acta physiol. scand.*, **67**, 481–497.

CARLSSON, A. AND LINDQVIST, M. (1963) Effect of chlorpromazine or haloperidol on formation of 3-methoxytyramine and normetanephrine in mouse brain. *Acta pharmacol. toxicol.*, **20**, 140–144..

CARR, L. A. AND MOORE, K. E. (1968) Effects of reserpine and α-methyltyrosine on brain catecholamines and the pituitary-adrenal response to stress. *Neuroendocrinol.*, **3**, 285–302.

CORRODI, H., FUXE, K. AND HÖKFELT, T. (1967a) The effect of neuroleptics on the activity of central catecholamine neurons. *Life Sci.*, **6**, 767–774.

CORRODI, H., FUXE, K. AND HÖKFELT, T. (1967b) A possible role played by central monoamine neurons in thermo-regulation. *Acta physiol. scand.*, **71**, 224–232.

CORRODI, H., FUXE, K. AND HÖKFELT, T. (1968) The effect of immobilization stress on the activity of central monoamine neurons. *Life Sci.* **7**, 107–112.

CURZON, G. AND GREEN, A. R. (1968) Effect of hydrocortisone on rat brain 5-hydroxytryptamine. *Life Sci.*, **7**, 657–663.

DAHLSTRÖM, A., FUXE, K. AND HILLARP, N.-Å. (1965) Site of action of reserpine. *Acta pharmacol.*, **22**, 277–292.

DE SCHAEPDRYVER, A., PREZIOSI, P. AND SCAPAGNINI, U. (1969) Brain monoamines and adreno-cortical activation. *Brit. J. Pharmacol.*, **35**, 460–467.

DE WIED, D. (1964) The site of blocking action of dexamethasone on stress-induced pituitary ACTH release. *J. Endocrinol.*, **29**, 29–37.

DE WIED, D. (1967) Chlorpromazine and endocrine function. *Pharmacol. Rev.*, **19**, 251–288.

DE WIED, D. (1969) Effects of peptide hormones on behaviour. In: *Frontiers in Neuroendocrinology*, W. F. GANONG AND L. MARTINI (Eds.), Oxford University Press, New York, London, Toronto, pp. 97–140.

DIXIT, B. N. AND BUCKLEY, J. P. (1969). Brain 5-hydroxytryptamine and anterior pituitary activation by stress. *Neuroendocrinol.*, **4**, 32–41.

FELDBERG, W. AND MYERS, R. D. (1963) A new concept of temperature regulation by amines in the hypothalamus. *Nature (Lond.)*, **200**, 1325.

FUXE, K. (1965) Evidence for the existence of monoamine neurons in the central nervous system. IV. The distribution of monoamine nerve terminals in the central nervous system. *Acta physiol. scand.*, 64, Suppl. **247**, 39–85.

FUXE, K. AND GUNNE, L. M. (1964) Depletion of the amine stores in brain catecholamine terminals on amygdaloid stimulation. *Acta physiol. scand.*, **62**, 493–494.

FUXE, K. AND HÖKFELT, T. (1967) The influence of central catecholamine neurons on the hormone secretion from the anterior and posterior pituitary. In: *Neurosecretion*, F. STUTINSKY (Ed.), Springer Verlag, New York, pp. 165–177.

FUXE, K. AND HÖKFELT, T. (1969a) Monoaminergic afferent input to the hypothalamus and the dopamine afferent input to the median eminence. *3. Int. Congr. Endocrinol. Mexico 1968*, in press.

FUXE, K. AND HÖKFELT, T. (1969b) Catecholamine in the hypothalamus and the pituitary gland. In: *Frontiers in Neuroendocrinology*, W. F. GANONG AND L. MARTINI (Eds.), Oxford University Press, New York, London, Toronto, pp. 47–96.

FUXE, K., HÖKFELT, T. AND NILSSON, O. (1967a) Activity changes in the tubero-infundibular DA neurons of the rat during various states of the reproductive cycle. *Life Sci.*, **6**, 2057–2061.

FUXE, K., HÖKFELT, T. AND NILSSON, O. (1967b) Changes in amine levels of the tubero-infundibular dopamine neuron system during implantation in rats. *Excerpta med. int. Congr. Ser.*, **133**, 541–542.

FUXE, K., HÖKFELT, T. AND NILSSON, O. (1969a) Castration, sex hormones and tubero-infundibular dopamine neurons. *Neuroendocrinology*, in press.

FUXE, K., HÖKFELT, T. AND NILSSON, O. (1969b) Factors involved in the control of the activity of the tubero-infundibular DA neurons, especially during pregnancy and lactation. *Neuroendocrinology*, in press.

FUXE, K. AND UNGERSTEDT, U. (1968) Histochemical studies on the effect of (+)-amphetamine, drugs of the imipramine group and tryptamine on central catecholamine and 5-hydroxytryptamine neurons after intraventricular injection of catecholamines and 5-hydroxytryptamine. *Europ. J. Pharmacol.*, **4**, 135–144.

GANONG, W. F. (1963) The central nervous system and the synthesis and release of adrenocorticotropic hormone. In: *Advances in Neuroendocrinology*, A. V. NALBANDOV (Ed.), University of Illinois Press, Urbana, pp. 92–149.

GANONG, W. F. (1969) Control of ACTH and MSH secretion. Report presented at congress on "*Integration of endocrine and non endocrine mechanism in the hypothalamus*" in Stresa, May 1969.

GANONG, W. F. AND LORENZEN, L. C. (1967) Brain neurohumors and endocrine function. In: *Neuroendocrinology*, (Vol. 2,) L. MARTINI AND W. F. GANONG (Eds.), Academic Press, New York, London, pp. 583–640.

GLOWINSKI, J. AND BALDESSARINI, R. J. (1966) Metabolism of norepinephrine in the central nervous system. *Pharm. Rev.*, **18**, 1201–1238.

GOLD, E. M. AND GANONG, W. F. (1967) Effects of drugs on neuroendocrine processes. In: *Neuroendocrinology*, (Vol. 2), L. MARTINI AND W. F. GANONG (Eds.), Academic Press, New York, pp. 377–438.

GORDON, R., SPECTOR, S., SJOERDSMA, A. AND UDENFRIEND, S. (1966) Increased synthesis of norepinephrine and epinephrine in the intact rat during exercise and exposure to cold. *J. Pharmacol. Exptl. Ther.*, **153**, 440–447.

GREEN, A. R. AND CURZON, G. (1969) Decrease of 5-hydroxytryptamine in the brain provoked by hydrocortizone and its prevention by allopurinol. *Nature*, **220**, 1095–1097.

HIRSCH, G. H. AND MOORE, K. E. (1968) Brain catecholamines and the reserpine-induced stimulation of the pituitary-adrenal system. *Neuroendocrinol.*, **3**, 398–405.

IVERSEN, L. L. AND SIMMONDS, M. A. (1969) Studies of catecholamine turnover in rat brain using ^{3}H-noradrenaline. In: *Metabolism of Amines in the Brain*, G. HOOPER (Ed.), Macmillan, London, pp. 48–54.

JAVOY, F., GLOWINSKI, J. AND KORDON, C. (1968) Effects of adrenalectomy on the turnover of norepinephrine in the rat brain. *Europ. J. Pharmacol.*, **4**, 103–104.

KATO, R. AND VALZELLI, L. (1958) Cortisone e 5-idrossitriptamina cerebrale. *Bull. Soc. ital. Biol. Sperm.*, **34**, 1402.

KOE, B. K. AND WEISSMAN, A. (1968) The pharmacology of *para*-chlorophenylalanine, a selective depletor of serotonin stores. *Adv. Pharmacol.*, **6**, B, 29–47.

LORENZEN, L. C., WISE, B. L. AND GANONG, W. F. (1965) ACTH-inhibiting activity of drugs related to α-ethyltryptamine: relation to pressor activity. *Federation Proc.*, **24**, 128.

MANGILI, G., MOTTA, M. AND MARTINI, L. (1966) Control of adrenocorticotropic hormone secretion. In: *Neuroendocrinology*, (Vol. 1), L. MARTINI AND W. F. GANONG (Eds.), Academic Press, New York, pp. 297–370.

MCKENNEE, C. T., TIMIRAS, P. S. AND QUAY, W. B. (1966) Concentrations of 5-hydroxytryptamine in rat brain and pineal after adrenalectomy and cortisol administration. *Neuroendocrinol.*, **1**, 251–256.

MOTTA, M., FRASCHINI, F. AND MARTINI, L. (1969) "Short" feedback mechanisms in the control of anterior pituitary function. In: *Frontiers in Neuroendocrinology*, W. F. GANONG AND L. MARTINI (Eds.), Oxford University Press, New York, London, Toronto, pp. 211–253.

REIS, D. J. AND FUXE, K. (1968a) Depletion of noradrenaline in brainstem neurons during sham rage behaviour produced by acute brainstem transection in cat. *Brain Res.*, **7**, 448–451.

REIS, D. J. AND FUXE, K. (1968b) Evidence that brain noradrenalin release is essential for sham rage behavior produced by acute brainstem transection in cat. *Transact. Amer. Neurol. Ass.*, **93**, 268–270.

SMELIK, P. G. (1967) ACTH secretion after depletion of hypothalamic by reserpine implants. *Neuroendocrinology*, **2**, 247–254.

SMELIK, P. G. (1969) Integrative hypothalamic responses to stress. Report presented at the congress on "*Integration of endocrine and non endocrine mechanisms in the hypothalamus*" in Stresa, May 1969.

SMELIK, P. G. AND SAWYER, H. (1962) Effects of implantation of cortisol into the brain stem or pituitary gland on the adrenal response to stress in the rabbit. *Acta Endocrinol.*, **41**, 561–570.

STEINER, F. A., RUF, K. AND AKERT, K. (1969) Steroid-sensitive neurones in rat brain: anatomical localization and responses to neurohumours and ACTH. *Brain Res.*, **12**, 74–85.

THIERRY, A.-M., FEKETE, M. AND GLOWINSKI, J. (1968) Effects of stress on the metabolism of noradrenaline, dopamine and serotonin (5-HT) in the central nervous system of the rat. (II). Modifications of serotonin metabolism. *Europ. J. Pharmacol.*, **4**, 384–289.

THIERRY, A. M., JAVOY, F., GLOWINSKI, J. AND KETY, S. S. (1969) Effects of stress on the metabolism of norepinephrine, dopamine and serotonin in the central nervous system of the rat. I. Modifications of norepinephrine turnover. *J. Pharmacol. Exptl. Ther.*, in press.

DISCUSSION

SMELIK: Do you imply that all NA fiber systems in the brain behave in the same way during stress, or during treatment with different substances? Is it not possible that in some area of the brain the system is activated whilst there is an inhibition in another area?

FUXE: To me it does not seem to be like that, actually I think that one has to be aware of the fact that these NA neurons have enormous collateral connections, which means that one single NA neuron might invade the spinal cord, cerebellum, hypothalamus and the limbic system.

There are two ascending pathways, one innervating mainly cortical areas, the other mainly the hypothalamus (pre-optic area). There might be a possibility of a specificity here.

McEWEN: We (Azmitia and McEwen, 1969) have recently observed that tryptophan hydroxylase levels are under control of corticosterone in the midbrain of the rat. The enzyme levels drop after adrenalectomy and are restored by corticosterone. We also believe that your results with prolonged stress, where you observed no change in 5-HT levels, can be explained by a compensatory increase of enzyme level induced by stress levels of corticosterone since we recently have found increases in tryptophan hydroxylase levels with chronic stress in normal, but not in adrenalectomized, rats. This increased enzyme level can then provide 5-HT to supply the increased demand for 5-HT under stress.

FUXE: Our data are in complete agreement with these results. The 5-HT turnover is decreased by adrenalectomy and increased again by cortisol treatment. I do not think that we can say at the moment whether it is a direct or indirect action of the glycocorticoids on the 5-HT and NA neurons.

McCLURE: Would you mind speculating about the effects if one would administer dexamethasone?

FUXE: Considering adrenalectomy experiments I would speculate that you would have similar results as obtained with cortisol. But it is difficult to postulate effects in stress experiments. Very much depends on the type of stress you are using. If the nervous afferent excitatory input becomes too large for the CRF neuron, the negative feedback of the dexamethasone will not be able to exert its action, as this action is counteracted by the nervous impulses.

McCLURE: I asked you this question because we are highly interested in this area. You mentioned the effect of disorders; we are successfully treating some of our depressed patients with a combination of dexamethasone and anti-depressant medication.

FUXE: It is fascinating to hear this, because it fits nicely with the view that 5-HT neurons are very important with regard to mood.

HARRIS: I wonder if I might ask you the same question that I have put before to Dr. Mulder. Have you any views on the chemical nature of the vesicles in the nerve terminals in the median eminence?

FUXE: Well, I think that according to Hökfelt's studies it is relatively safe to say that in the median eminence the main bulk of dopamine is stored in the so-called synaptic vesicles. It is, however, premature to say if dopamine in the median eminence has the same properties as in the neostriatum.

MILKOVIĆ: We have analyzed the serotonin concentration in the brains of rats bearing ACTH-secreting tumors. No change in brain serotonin concentration was observed. The adrenal glands of these rats were very much enlarged by the chronic hypersecretion of ACTH from tumor. Adrenalectomy (10 days) in these ACTH-secreting tumor rats was not followed by any change in brain serotonin concentration. We found, however, that the serotonin concentration decreased, sometimes with more than 20%, following stress. This even occurred in fetal rats.

Psychopharmacological Effects and Pituitary–Adrenal Activity[1]

B. H. MARKS, M. M. HALL[2] AND A. N. BHATTACHARYA[3]

Department of Pharmacology, Ohio State University College of Medicine, Columbus, Ohio (U.S.A.)

The past two decades have witnessed a great increase in our ability to affect animal behavior by the administration of chemical agents. In this same time period, we have learned much about the identity, distribution, synthesis, metabolism, release and uptake of monoamines in brain neurons. We have become accustomed to call these monoamines "neurotransmitters", although the relationship between the liberation of these amines at specific synapses by nerve impulses and the occurrence of specific post-synaptic events in the brain is still not clear in most instances. Accepting, as we must, some degree of ambiguousness about "neurotransmitter" phenomena, we still find that when we approach the discussion of drugs that affect behavior, such a discussion is commonly framed in terms of these putative neurotransmitters. Here difficulty is added to difficulty, because in many instances there remain outstanding areas of uncertainty about the action of even the most common psychotropic drugs on the synthesis, release, re-uptake and metabolism of monoamines or upon the interaction of monoamines with post-synaptic receptors. Consequently, the cause and effect relationship between the actions of specific psychotropic drugs on monoamines and their effect upon behavior is still often problematical.

Despite all these problems, it is still desirable to discuss the effect of some important psychopharmacological agents on the regulation of ACTH secretion. This is due to the fact that most drugs that affect emotional behavior and mood produce marked and often persistent effects on the secretion of ACTH as well as alterations in other pituitary functions. It should be obvious, though, that any conclusions reached in this discussion undoubtedly will represent an oversimplification due to insufficient knowledge of the detailed operation of the system.

Several generalizations appear to be tenable in reviewing the present state of knowledge of this area. First, the effect of psychopharmacologic agents can in general be attributed to actions upon the nervous system, rather than to effects upon the pituitary gland (Gold and Ganong, 1967). This is not to say that drug-induced changes in pituitary metabolism may not affect the ability to release ACTH. Inhibitors such as ethionine have been shown to block ACTH secretion (Marks and Vernikos-Danellis, 1963) and the phosphodiesterase inhibitors caffeine and theophylline may augment

[1] Supported in part by grants AM-05110 and AM-13606 from the National Institutes of Health.
[2] NIH Trainee in training program GM-01417.
[3] Present address: Department of Physiology, School of Medicine, University of Pittsburgh, Pittsburgh, Pennsylvania 15213.

References pp. 68–69

ACTH secretion by acting upon the pituitary (Vernikos-Danellis and Harris, 1968), suggesting that the availability of biological energy and the generation of cyclic AMP may be important in ACTH secretion. A number of drugs and monoamines to be discussed have been tested for their direct action upon the pituitary and have been found to be inactive, although occasional indications of direct actions of psychotropic drugs upon the pituitary have been found (Bohus and De Wied, 1966).

The second generalization is that many of the drugs found to stimulate ACTH secretion after a single administration have also been found to inhibit stress-induced ACTH secretion under various conditions (Gold and Ganong, 1967). This is true particularly of chlorpromazine and reserpine. This inhibition has been explained as being due either to errors of experimental design or to pituitary exhaustion (Maickel, Westermann and Brodie, 1961; Smith, Maickel and Brodie, 1963). We feel that this phenomenon is more likely to be due to disordered regulation of the neuroendocrine apparatus, as we shall see later, or to neural inhibitory activity upstream from the hypothalamus (Bhattacharya and Marks, 1969a; De Wied, 1967). Reduction of pituitary ACTH content does not appear to be a valid explanation for insensitivity to stress, since a repeated stress has been found to elicit marked ACTH secretion at times when the pituitary content was greatly reduced. The ability of the pituitary to release ACTH appears to depend more on its ability to synthesize ACTH rapidly than on the pre-existing content of the hormone (Vernikos-Danellis, 1963). Some psychotropic drugs which stimulate ACTH secretion have been reported not to be followed by inhibition (Anichkov, 1968).

The third generalization is that an ideal method for examining the effect of drugs on the ACTH neuro-endocrine system does not exist. Since the most immediate effect of psychopharmacologic agents would be exerted upon the release of CRF into the hypophyseal portal vascular system, an ideal index of drug responses would be the measurement of rate of CRF release (McCann and Porter, 1969). Since this is not yet practical, we must compromise by measuring the CRF content of the hypothalamus and either blood ACTH content or the adrenal corticosterone response to the circulating ACTH. A combination of these measurements should give us an index of the instantaneous state of the CRF–ACTH neuro-endocrine system.

Information will be presented about the effect of reserpine, chlorpromazine, pargyline and amphetamine upon the neuro-endocrine system regulating ACTH secretion emphasizing measurements of CRF and of corticosterone. The method used for the measurement of CRF in rats is shown schematically in Fig. 1 (Bhattacharya and Marks, 1969a). Basically, median eminence fragments were extracted with acid. The lypohilized and reconstituted extracts were then incubated with pituitary halves from normal female donor rats. The ACTH released into the medium was biologically assayed by measuring its effect on the adrenal corticosterone content of dexamethasone-blocked assay rats. Within a limited range, the ACTH released is proportional to the amount of CRF in the incubation medium. Even large amounts of monoamines do not produce ACTH secretion if added to the pituitary incubation medium. Table 1 is one such experiment. This suggests that alteration of monoamine content of the hypothalamus by drugs should not influence the ability to measure CRF.

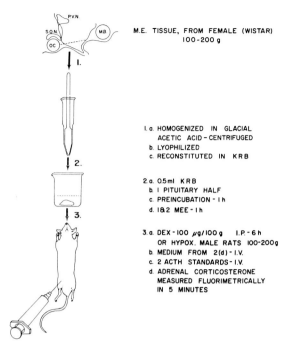

Fig. 1. Schematic outline of method of CRF assay in rats. The tissue from experimental animals removed and assayed for CRF is indicated by the dotted line in the drawing of the midline section of the rat hypothalamus. MB — mammillary body; OC — optic chiasm: P.V.N. — paraventricular nucleus; S.O.N. — supraoptic nucleus.

TABLE 1

EFFECT OF EPINEPHRINE AND NOREPINEPHRINE ON RELEASE OF ACTH BY ANTERIOR PITUITARY TISSUE *in vitro* IN THE PRESENCE OF MEDIAN EMINENCE (ME) EXTRACT

Addition	ME/Pituitary half	ACTH release mU/mg/h/ME
Control 10 μl saline/pituitary half	1	1.7 (1.6–2.0)*
Epinephrine 25 μg/pituitary half in 10 μl saline	1	1.6 (1.2–2.2)
Norepinephrine 25 μg/pituitary half in 10 μl saline	1	1.5 (1.0–2.0)

* Fiducial limits of error, $P = 0.95$.

Like many others (Gold and Ganong, 1967), we have documented the marked stimulation of ACTH secretion seen after a single injection of chlorpromazine or reserpine in rats (Bhattacharya and Marks, 1969a). Fig. 2 shows the time course of the changes in plasma corticosterone concentration and Fig. 3 the changes in adrenal

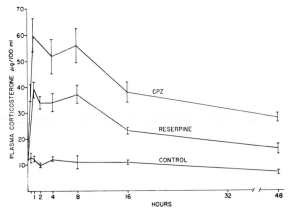

Fig. 2. Response of plasma corticosterone concentration to a single intraperitoneal injection of chlorpromazine (CPZ) — 25 mg/kg, reserpine — 5 mg/kg, or saline — 2 ml/kg. Each point is the mean, and the vertical line the standard error, of a group of 6–8 female rats weighing approximately 150 g.

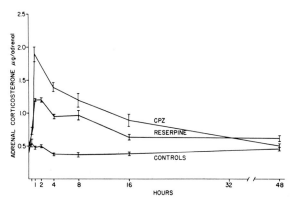

Fig. 3. Response of adrenal corticosterone content to a single intraperitoneal injection of chlorpromazine (CPZ) — 25 mg/kg, reserpine — 5 mg/kg, or saline — 2 ml/kg. Each point is the mean, and the vertical line the standard error, or a group of 6–8 female rats weighing approximately 150 g.

corticosterone. We tend to place greater emphasis on the adrenal corticosterone responses as indications of the change in blood ACTH content, since factors such as alteration in blood volume or circulation, protein binding of corticosteroids, and rate of hepatic corticosteroid metabolism may influence the plasma concentration of corticosterone independent of changes in ACTH. These factors may be influenced by reserpine and chlorpromazine treatment.

The contribution which changes in the hypothalamus make to these events described above is seen in the measurement of the CRF content following chlorpromazine or reserpine administration. Fig. 4 shows that the CRF content of the ventral hypothalamus fell dramatically. The return to the control state is related in time to the restoration of the normal adrenal corticosterone content. One can say that the pituitary and adrenal secretory responses are secondary to a degree of hypersecretion of CRF sufficient to produce rather marked and prolonged depletion of this hypo-

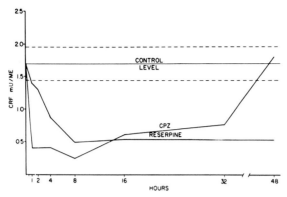

Fig. 4. Response of the CRF content of the ventral hypothalamus to a single intraperitoneal injection of chlorpromazine (CPZ) — 25 mg/kg, reserpine — 5 mg/kg, or saline — 2 ml/kg. Each point represents a biological assay of the pooled hypothalamic tissue from 6–8 female rats. The control level is the mean of 5 assays from saline-injected rats at various times after injection and the dashed line above and below the control is one standard deviation from the mean. The units of CRF are expressed as mU of ACTH released per mg pituitary tissue per median eminence per hour of incubation.

TABLE 2

EFFECT OF AMBIENT TEMPERATURE ON THE CRF CONTENT IN THE MEDIAN EMINENCE (ME) TISSUE OF RESERPINE- AND CHLORPROMAZINE-TREATED RATS

Treatment	CRF[1] content in rats at:	
	24°C	31°C
	mU/ME	
Saline controls (0.2 ml/100 g i.p.) 8 h	1.7[2] (1.4–1.9)[3]	1.5 (1.1–2.1)
Reserpine (5 mg/kg i.p.) 8 h	0.50 (0.2–1.4)	0.58 (0.25–1.3)
Chlorpromazine (25 mg/kg i.p.) 8 h	0.26 (0.12–0.55)	0.33 (0.08–1.2)

[1] CRF activity expressed as mU of ACTH released per mg of pituitary tissue per hour per median eminence extract.
2 Analysis of variance confirmed that the CRF content of median eminence tissue of control and drug-treated groups were significantly different ($P < 0.05$).
[3] Fiducial limits of error $P = 0.95$.

physiotropic hormone. We interpret the blockade of further stresses by suggesting that the CRF secretion is already spontaneously maximal, due to removal of inhibitory controls by the action of reserpine or chlorpromazine. This is similar to the conclusion reached by Giuliani et al. (1966) after studying the interaction between reserpine and dexamethasone (Giuliani, Motta and Martini, 1966). This marked effect on CRF content of the hypothalamus bears no relationship to the hypothermia seen with these drugs. Maintaining rats at 31°C ambient temperature prevents any fall in rectal temperature after chlorpromazine or reserpine treatment. Under these conditions, the same depletion of CRF is seen (Table 2) (Bhattacharya and Marks, 1969a). The stimulation of adrenal corticosterone secretion is also unaffected by this change in body temperature.

References pp. 68–69

TABLE 3

EFFECT OF PARGYLINE PRETREATMENT ON THE RESERPINE-INDUCED CHANGES IN PLASMA, ADRENAL CORTICOSTERONE, PITUITARY ACTH, AND CRF CONTENT IN RATS

Treatment	Plasma corticosterone (μg/100 ml ± SE)	Adrenal corticosterone (μg/adrenal±SE)	Pituitary ACTH mU/mg	CRF[4] (mU/ME)
A. Controls	12 ± 0.44[1] (8)[2]	0.52 ± 0.01[1] (8)[2]	17 (12–20)[3]	1.8 (1.5–2.1)[3]
B. Reserpine (5 mg/kg, i.p. 8 h)	37 ± 3.7 (8)	0.97 ± 0.07 (8)	10 (5.9–17)	0.50 (0.2–1.4)
C. Pargyline (50 mg/kg, i.p. 16 h) plus Reserpine (5 mg/kg, i.p. 8 h)	15 ± 0.67 (8)	0.55 ± 0.01 (8)	12 (10–13)	1.5 (1.3–1.8)

[1] Plasma and adrenal corticosterone values for groups A and C not significantly different.
[2] Number of animals used per observation.
[3] Fiducial limits of error, $P = 0.95$.
[4] CRF activity expressed as mU of ACTH released per mg of pituitary tissue per hour per median eminence extract.

TABLE 4

EFFECT OF PARGYLINE PRETREATMENT ON RESERPINE AND ACUTE STRESS-INDUCED PLASMA CORTICOSTERONE CHANGES IN RATS

Treatment[1]	Plasma corticosterone (μg/100 ml ± S.E.)	
	Unstressed	Stressed[3]
Normal controls	12 ± 1.5 (10)[2]	40 ± 3.6** (10)
Pargyline	9.0 ± 0.95 (4)	17 ± 4.1** (4)
Reserpine	37 ± 3.7 (8)	38 ± 1.4 (8)
Pargyline + reserpine	7.5 ± 0.55 (4)	20 ± 0.19** (4)

[1] All drugs given intraperitoneally; pargyline, 50 mg/kg, 24 h; reserpine, 5 mg/kg, 8 h.
[2] Number of animals used per observation. Difference unstressed compared to stressed significant at ** < 0.001.
[3] Ether-laparotomy stress-rats sacrificed after 15 minutes.

Since the effect of reserpine is well known to be associated with depletion of brain catecholamines and 5-hydroxytryptamine, it seems reasonable to ask if drug treatment which augments brain monoamine content and activity can reverse these neuroendocrine effects. This experiment was done by pretreating rats with pargyline, a monoamine oxidase inhibitor, before the administration of reserpine. Pargyline increases the brain content of catecholamine and 5-hydroxytryptamine. Along with

TABLE 5

EFFECT OF AMPHETAMINE PRETREATMENT ON ACUTE STRESS-
INDUCED PLASMA CORTICOSTERONE CHANGES IN RATS

Treatment[1]	Plasma corticosterone ($\mu g/100\ ml \pm S.E.$)	
	Unstressed	Stressed
Normal controls	12 ± 1.5 (10)[2]	40 ± 3.6* (10)
Amphetamine	4.5 ± 0.9 (4)	28 ± 1.8* (4)

[1] Drug given intraperitoneally; 5 mg/kg, 4 h.
[2] Number of animals used per observation. Difference unstressed compared to stressed significant at * < 0.01.

the reversal of the behavioral effects of reserpine, this treatment reversed the changes in the neuro-endocrine system regulating ACTH secretion (Table 3) (Bhattacharya and Marks, 1969b). Not only did pargyline alter the steady state level of pituitary–adrenal activity after reserpine administration, but it markedly reduced the burst of ACTH secretion in response to the acute stress of ether and laparotomy. This is seen in Table 4 (Bhattacharya and Marks, 1969b). It is obvious that the inhibition of the acute stress response cannot be due to a deficiency of CRF or ACTH. Consequently, it must be proposed that it is possible for drugs to generate neural inhibitory effects on CRF release by altering the activity or availability of either catecholamines or 5-hydroxytryptamine in the brain. This postulate was tested by examining the effects of amphetamine administration on the ability of rats to respond to an acute stress. Amphetamine is known to increase physiologically active and available norepinephrine in the brain (Glowinski and Axelrod, 1965). We find that a single administration of amphetamine not only reduced the resting level of plasma corticosterone, but reduced the elevation of corticosterone following an acute stress (Table 5) (Bhattacharya and Marks, 1969b). These results with monoamine oxidase inhibitors and with amphetamine have been observed in other species by a number of investigators. The ACTH inhibition is not related to peripheral blood pressure responses to drugs of this type, as had been proposed (Gold and Ganong, 1967), since the duration of pretreatment is such as to be well beyond the period of these initial peripheral responses. This inhibition of ACTH secretion is instead associated with behavioral alerting and increased gross motor behavior in rats that we relate to increased availability of brain monoamines, particularly catecholamines.

We felt, after the above experiments, that we needed a more direct way to demonstrate the effect of presumed neuro-transmitters upon the pituitary adrenal system. This we have recently attempted by administering catecholamines and carbachol into the ventricular system of the rat brain (Noble, Wurtman and Axelrod, 1967). Carbachol was selected because of its stability in the presence of the various brain cholinesterases. These experiments were done in pentobarbital-anesthetized

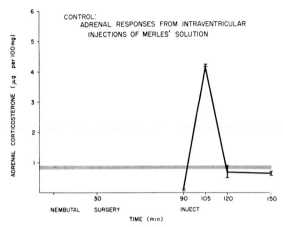

Fig. 5. Adrenal corticosterone concentration responses following injection into the cerebral ventricular system of 25 μl of Merles' solution, an artificial cerebrospinal fluid. Time is measured from the time of pentobarbital administration (35 mg/kg i.p.). Surgery is making a skin incision and drilling a hole through the calvarium. Inject is the time of intraventricular injection. Female rats, weight 150 g. The cross-hatched bar is the adrenal corticosterone concentration mean ± S.E. of a group of normal rats.

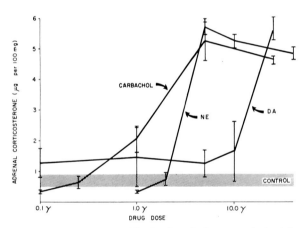

Fig. 6. The adrenal corticosterone responses 30 min after the intraventricular injection of carbachol, norepinephrine (NE) or dopamine (DA) in the doses indicated. Points are means and the vertical lines S.E. All doses were injected in 25 μl of Merles' solution. The cross-hatched zone is the mean ± S.E. 30 min after injecting 25 μl of Merles' solution.

rats, using the protocol of Fig. 5, which shows the effect of 25 μl of an artificial cerebrospinal fluid (Glowinski and Axelrod, 1965). Fifteen minutes after the control injection there is a sharp rise in adrenal corticosterone content, indicating that the procedure of injecting causes ACTH release. Thirty and sixty minutes after intraventricular injection, however, the adrenal corticosterone has returned to the level of normal rats. This is the time period in which one may conveniently examine the effects of monoamines injected into the ventricular system. Fig. 6 shows the available information on the dose–response relationships of carbachol, norepinephrine and dopamine when injected intraventricularly. All three of these amines stimulate ACTH

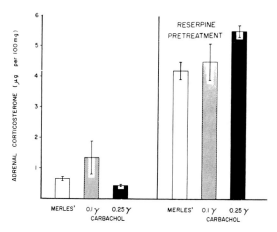

Fig. 7. The adrenal corticosterone responses 60 min after the intraventricular injection of carbachol into normal or reserpine-pretreated (2.5 mg/kg − 16 h) female rats. All injections were made in 25 μl of Merles' solution. White bars are controls, cross-hatched bars 0.1 μg carbachol and black bars 0.25 μg carbachol. Vertical lines are S.E.

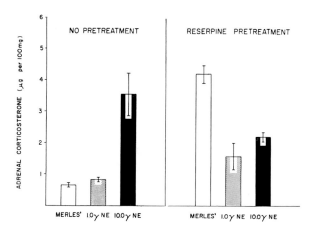

Fig. 8. The adrenal corticosterone responses 60 min after the intraventricular injection of norepinephrine (NE) into normal or reserpine-pretreated (2.5 mg/kg − 16 h) female rats. All injections were made in 25 μl of Merles' solution. White bars are controls, cross-hatched bars 1.0 μg NE and black bars 10 μg NE. Vertical lines are S.E.

secretion, but the dose−response relationships of the catecholamines are uncharacteristically steep, suggesting some kind of threshold phenomenon. The minimally effective doses of catecholamines for stimulation of ACTH secretion are very high—greater than the content of these amines in the whole rat brain. This may mean that the ACTH release from these high doses of catecholamines may be due to transport out of the brain where they may produce actions similar to those from peripherally injected catecholamines (Vernikos-Danellis, 1969).

In order to look at more specific central neuropharmacologic response of these amines, the effect of low doses of these substances was examined in rats pretreated with reserpine in order to establish a steady state of moderate ACTH hypersecretion.

References pp. 68–69

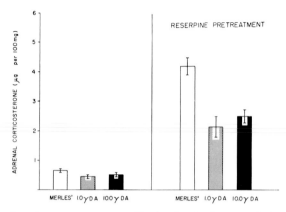

Fig. 9. The adrenal corticosterone responses 60 min after the intraventricular injection of dopamine (DA) into normal or reserpine-pretreated (2.5 mg/kg — 16 h) female rats. All injections were made in 25 μl of Merles' solution. White bars are controls, cross-hatched bars 1.0 μg DA and black bars 10 μg DA. Vertical lines are S.E.

If one accepts the postulate that the action of reserpine on brain monoamines produces a state of unrestrained CRF secretion, then supplying the missing inhibitory neural factor should rapidly terminate this hypersecretion with its resultant elevated adrenal corticosterone. Fig. 7 shows that one hour after being administered intraventricularly to such animals carbachol produced only augmentation of ACTH release, the augmentation being significant with 0.25 μg carbachol. Fig. 8 shows that as little as 1.0 μg of norepinephrine in this same situation produced a marked suppression of ACTH release and Fig. 9 that dopamine also reduced ACTH secretion, although to a lesser extent than equivalent doses of norepinephrine. These minimally effective doses of amines, it should be emphasized, have little effect on ACTH secretion in normal (*i.e.*, non-reserpine-pretreated) rats and produce no effect on heart rate or blood pressure of rats when administered intraventricularly.

These studies suggest that there may be both cholinergic stimulatory mechanisms and adrenergic inhibitory mechanisms in the hypothalamus involved in the regulation of ACTH secretion. The blocking effects of atropine implants in the hypothalamus (Hedge and Smelik, 1968) supports the view that a cholinergic mechanism must be involved in the stimulation of CRF release. On the other hand, reserpine implants in the median eminence region failed to alter ACTH release (Smelik. 1967) in response to various stimuli, including reserpine or chlorpromazine administration. This must indicate that the adrenergic inhibitory mechanism which we see must be outside of the immediate region of the median eminence or may be in a larger and more diffuse neural field than can be affected by a small drug implant. This adrenergic inhibitory mechanism must be readily accessible by diffusion from the third ventricle, however, perhaps in the periventricular gray matter.

Not all studies support the concept of a cholinergic stimulatory and an adrenergic inhibitory process for ACTH regulation. In guinea pigs, regional injections into the hypothalamus either of carbachol or of norepinephrine stimulates ACTH secretion, but both of these drugs are ineffective in midbrain-transected animals, suggesting

TABLE 6

EFFECT OF αMT OR PCPA ON THE RESERPINE-INDUCED DEPLETION
OF HYPOTHALAMIC CRF CONTENT

Treatment	Time (h)	CRF content mU/ME[1]
L-Tyrosine	16	1.7 (1.3 –2.3)[2]
L-αMT	16	2.0 (1.5 –2.6)
DL-Phenylalanine	48	1.8 (1.6 –2.0)
DL-PCPA	48	1.6 (1.3 –2.0)
Reserpine	8	0.50 (0.2 –1.4)
αMT + reserpine	16 + 8	0.68 (0.43–1.0)
PCPA + reserpine	48 + 8	0.54 (0.44–0.65)

[1] CRF content is expressed as mU of ACTH released per mg pituitary tissue per hour per extract from one median eminence.
[2] Results of CRF assays include, in parentheses, the 95% confidence limits. L-tyrosine and L-αMT were administered i.v. −200 mg/kg; DL-phenylalanine and DL-PCPA were given i.p. 316 mg/kg; reserpine i.p. 5 mg/kg. L-Tyrosine and DL-phenylalanine injections were used as controls for the αMT and PCPA groups respectively.

that the effects involve reflex mechanisms (Naumenko, 1968). Serotonin, however, causes ACTH secretion upon injection into the hypothalamus of intact and midbrain-sectioned guinea pigs, so that Naumenko has proposed that the terminal neurons regulating CRF release are serotonergic. These studies deserve to be repeated, allowing more time for the animals to recover from the surgical shock and neural trauma associated with the midbrain transection. The intraventricular administration of serotonin in the rat brain neither stimulates nor inhibits ACTH secretion consistently in normal rats or in reserpine-pretreated rats (Hall and Marks, unpublished observations). This fails to support the role proposed for serotonin in the control of ACTH secretion (Westermann, Maickel and Brodie, 1962) after reserpine.

Many investigators (Hirsch and Moore, 1968; Carr and Moore, 1968; Preziosi, Scapagnini and Nistico, 1968; De Schaepdryver, Preziosi and Scapagnini, 1969) have found that depleting brain monoamines by preventing amine synthesis with such drugs as alpha methyl tyrosine and p-chlorophenylalanine does not affect the ability to secrete ACTH in response to various stresses or in response to reserpine administration. We have found that these inhibitors of monoamine synthesis do not alter CRF content of the hypothalamus and do not prevent the depletion of CRF produced by reserpine administration (Table 6). This kind of observation has frequently been the basis for the conclusion that brain monoamines have little to do with the regulation of ACTH secretion, but we must regard this as negative evidence of uncertain significance for the time being. The degree of depletion of brain amines is often small enough (De Schaepdryver et al., 1968) that one may suppose that the residual amine is sufficient to maintain reasonably normal neural activity. We would agree with Hirsch and Moore (1968) that reserpine-induced ACTH secretion may be a result of unopposed central cholinergic neuron activation, but the persistence

References pp. 68–69

and magnitude of the response must be in part due to the simultaneous depletion of inhibitory monoaminergic influences.

Obviously, psychopharmacologic agents such as reserpine, chlorpromazine, monoamine oxidase inhibitors and amphetamine have profound effects on ACTH secretion. Whether our current knowledge of the mechanism of action of these drugs permits us to interpret their neuro-endocrine effects in detail in terms of monoamine changes is doubtful. It is, however, reasonably consistent with our observations to propose that, in the rat, psychopharmacologic agents may initiate marked and persistent changes in the rate of CRF release by acting upon neural mechanisms in the brain which control this process. Those drugs which produce cholinergic effects or which block central adrenergic activity increase the rate of CRF secretion. Those drugs which augment adrenergic activity or which block central cholinergic processes reduce the rate of CRF secretion. Changes in pituitary and adrenal activity are secondary to these neuro-endocrine control mechanisms.

REFERENCES

ANICHKOV, S. V. (1968) Highlights of Soviet pharmacology. In: *Ann. Rev. Pharmacol.*, Vol. 8, Annual Reviews, Inc., Palo Alto, Calif., pp. 25–38.

BHATTACHARYA, A. N. AND MARKS, B. H. (1969a) Reserpine- and chlorpromazine-induced changes in hypothalamo-hypophyseal-adrenal system in rats in the presence and absence of hypothermia. *J. Pharmacol. Exptl. Ther.*, **165**, 108–116.

BHATTACHARYA, A. N. AND MARKS, B. H. (1969b) Effects of pargyline and amphetamine upon acute stress responses in rats. *Proc. Soc. Exptl. Biol. Med.*, **130**, 1194–1198.

BOHUS, B. AND DE WIED, D. (1966) Facilitatory and inhibitory influences of the central nervous system on the pituitary-adrenal axis: a study with chlorpromazine. *Abstract First International Symposium on Biorhythms in Clinical and Experimental Endocrinology*, pp. 21–22.

CARR, L. A. AND MOORE, K. E. (1968) Effects of reserpine and alpha-methyltyrosine on brain catecholamines and the pituitary adrenal responses to stress. *Neuroendocrinology*. **3**, 285–302.

DE SCHAEPDRYVER, A., PREZIOSI, P. AND SCAPAGNINI, U. (1969) Brain monoamines and adrenocortical activation. *Brit. J. Pharmacol.*, **35**, 460–467.

DE WIED, D. (1967) Chlorpromazine and endocrine function. *Pharmacol. Rev.*, **19**, 251–288.

GIULIANI, G., MOTTA, M. AND MARTINI, L., (1966) Reserpine and ACTH secretion. *Acta Endocrinol.*, **51**, 203–209.

GLOWINSKI, J. AND AXELROD, J. (1965) Effect of drugs on the uptake, release and metabolism of ^{3}H-norepinephrine in rat brain. *J. Pharmacol. Exptl. Ther.*, **149**, 43–49.

GOLD, E. M. AND GANONG, W. F. (1967) Drug effects on neuroendocrine processes. In *Neuroendocrinology*, Vol. II, L. MARTINI AND W. F. GANONG (Eds.), Academic Press, New York and London, p. 386.

HEDGE, G. A. AND SMELIK, P. G. (1968) Corticotropin release: inhibition by intrahypothalamic implantation of atropine. *Science*, **159**, 891–892.

HIRSCH, G. H. AND MOORE, K. E. (1968) Brain catecholamines and the reserpine-induced stimulation of the pituitary-adrenal system. *Neuroendocrinology*, **3** 398–405.

MAICKEL, R. P., WESTERMANN, E. O. AND BRODIE, B. B. (1961) Effects of reserpine and cold-exposure on pituitary-adrenocortical function in rats. *J. Pharmacol. Exptl. Ther.*, **134**, 167–175.

MARKS, B. H. AND VERNIKOS-DANELLIS, J. (1963) Effect of acute stress on the pituitary gland: action of ethionine on stress-induced ACTH release. *Endocrinology*, **72**, 582–587.

MCCANN, S. M. AND PORTER, J. C. (1969) Hypothalamic pituitary stimulating and inhibiting hormones. *Physiol. Rev.*, **49**, 240–284.

NAUMENKO, E. V. (1968) Hypothalamic chemoreactive structures and the regulation of pituitary-adrenal function. Effects of local injections of norepinephrine, carbachol and serotonin into the brain of guinea pigs with intact brains and after mesencephalic transection. *Brain Res.*, **11**, 1–10.

Noble, E. P., Wurtman, R. J. and Axelrod, J. (1967) A simple and rapid method for injecting H³-norepinephrine into the lateral ventricle of the rat brain. *Life Sci.*, **6**, 281–291.

Preziosi, P., Scapagnini, U. and Nistico, G., (1968) Brain serotonin depletors and adrenocortical activation. *Biochem. Pharmacol.*, **17**, 1309–1313.

Smelik, P. G. (1967) ACTH secretion after depletion of hypothalamic monoamines by reserpine implants. *Neuroendocrinology*, **2**, 247–254.

Smith, R. L., Maickel, R. P. and Brodie, B. B. (1963) ACTH-hypersecretion induced by pheno-thiazine tranquilizers. *J. Pharmacol. Exptl. Ther.*, **839**, 185–190.

Vernikos-Danellis, J. (1963) Effect of acute stress on pituitary gland: changes in blood and pituitary ACTH concentrations. *Endocrinology*, **72**, 574–581.

Vernikos-Danellis, J. and Harris, C. G., III. (1968) The effect of *in vitro* and *in vivo* caffeine, theophylline and hydrocortisone on the phosphodiesterase activity of the pituitary, median eminence, heart and cerebral cortex of the rat. *Proc. Soc. Exptl. Biol. Med.*, **128**, 1016–1021.

Vernikos-Danellis, J. (1969) The pharmacological approach to the study of mechanisms regulating ACTH secretion. In: *The Pharmacology of Hormonal Polypeptides and Proteins*. L. Martini (Ed.), in press.

Westermann, E. O., Maickel, R. P. and Brodie, B. B. (1962) On the mechanism of pituitary-adrenal stimulation by reserpine. *J. Pharmacol. Exptl. Ther.*, **138**, 208–217.

DISCUSSION

Smelik: Would not a blockade of CRF synthesis be a more obvious explanation for the CRF deple-tion by chlorpromazine or reserpine?

Marks: I think that what you say is quite true, but we will not be able to prove it until we have a way to measure CRF secretion directly.

De Wied: You showed that amphetamine tends to reduce ACTH release and stress-induced ACTH release. However, does not amphetamine also stimulate the discharge of ACTH, depending on the time of observation?

Marks: This may have something to do with peripheral receptor mechanisms. Our animals are unanesthetized and this is different from a number of other people's experimental situations. I think that stimulation is only a very temporary thing with amphetamine.

Hodges: Although you consider that the hormone content of an endocrine gland is no reflection of its functional capacity, you use changes in adrenal corticosterone content as the index of pituitary ACTH release. Do you think this is a reliable index?

Marks: Yes, I think it is. I must say that in almost all experiments we tend to measure both plasma and adrenal corticosterone simultaneously. I have not always shown them both. It is very unusual for the two measurements not to be very much in agreement.

Smelik: Referring to Dr. Hodges' remark: The situation in the adrenal cortex is different from the situation in the pituitary or the hypothalamus, since there is no proof of release from corticoid stores in the adrenals. In your case the adrenal content may be more reliable than plasma corticosterone; although I would personally prefer the *in vitro* production of corticosteroids by excised adrenal glands over these two measures.

Levine: The problem of content and release is very important in the question of measurement. Re-cently, Dr. Vernikos-Danellis and I have shown that ACTH content in the pituitary can be depleted by 50% without any effect on circulating ACTH or on plasma corticosterone.

Mirsky: I do want to add to that last statement the plea that a distinction be made between synthesis and release. Too frequently, the word secretion is meant to imply both, but recent experiences with *in vitro* islets, or even with pieces of pancreas have caused us to be very careful about whether we refer to releasers as distinct from agents which stimulate synthesis,

MARKS: The relationship of monoamines to these processes is something that we still have to work out. I said that the addition of monoamines to culture mediums of pituitary does not seem to affect the amount released. It is very well possible that the additional monoamines may affect the ability of the pituitary to synthesize.

Feedback Control of Pituitary–Adrenal Activity in Fetus

S. MILKOVIĆ, KARMELA MILKOVIĆ, ILINKA SENČAR AND
JASNA PAUNOVIĆ

Laboratory for Experimental Medicine, General Hospital "Dr Mladen Stojanović", Vinogradska cesta 29, Zagreb and Institute of General Biology, Medical Faculty, University of Zagreb (Yugoslavia)

There is no longer doubt about the dependence of growth and differentiation of fetal adrenal glands on the adrenocorticotropic activity of the fetal pituitary (Jost, 1966; K. Milković and Milković, 1966) or about the dependence of the fetal adrenal responsiveness to stress on fetal ACTH (K. Milković and Milković, 1966; S. Milković and Milković, 1969). In view of the technical difficulties there are not sufficient data on the onset of adrenocorticotropic activity of the fetal pituitary. In rat, activity begins between the 17th and 18th day of intrauterine development (S. Milković and Milković, 1969), while in other species this question remains to be solved.

This paper shows the dependence of growth and functional differentiation of the fetal adrenal glands on the weight and secretory activity of the mother's adrenal glands as well as the results of an attempt to determine the quantitative participation of the fetal pituitary in the growth of the fetal adrenal glands.

MATERIAL AND METHODS

Pregnant female rats of the Fischer strain bearing a transplantable tumor (Bates, S. Milković, Garrison, 1962; K. Milković, Efendić, Paunović, Ronkulin, Dulibić, Milković, 1966; S. Milković, Milković, Efendić, 1968) have been used. This tumor produces and secretes large amounts of ACTH and causes a manifold increase and hypersecretion of the adrenal glands. During the second week of gestation adrenal weight of the tumor-bearing pregnant rat increased by 52%, and the thymus weight decreased slightly (30%). The last week was characterized by almost 4 times enlargement of the maternal adrenal glands and very pronounced thymolytic effect (S. Milković *et al.*, 1968). The females were placed with males for mating at 8 p.m. and the males were removed at 7 a.m. the following morning. The appearance of sperm in the vaginal smear was considered as the first day of pregnancy. Delivery took place early afternoon on the 22nd day. On the first day of pregnancy, or occasionally a few days earlier or later, the tumor was transplanted into the females as described elsewhere (K. Milković *et al.*, 1966). Operations were performed on day 14 of gestation for chronic adrenalectomy, and 24 hours before the animals were sacrificed for acute adrenalectomy. The females were sacrificed from days 17–22 of pregnancy under ether anesthesia by exsanguination through the vena cava. The fetuses were dried

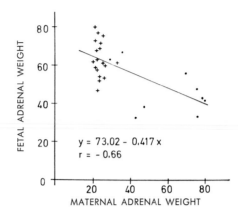

Fig. 1. Relationship between maternal and fetal adrenal weight on the 18th day of intrauterine development (+ normal intact females, · intact tumor-bearing rats). Data in Figs. 1–5 are expressed in mg/100 g body weight.

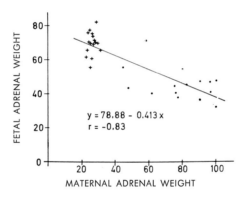

Fig. 2. Relationship between maternal and fetal adrenal weight on the 19th day of intrauterine development (+ normal intact females, · intact tumor-bearing rats).

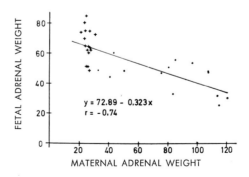

Fig. 3. Relationship between maternal and fetal adrenal weight on the 20th day of intrauterine development (+ normal intact females, · intact tumor-bearing rats).

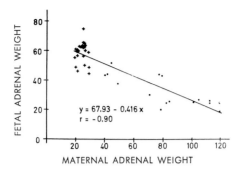

Fig. 4. Relationship between maternal and fetal adrenal weight on the 21st day of intrauterine development (+ normal intact females, · intact tumor-bearing rats).

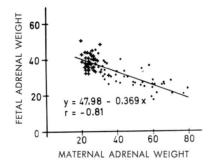

Fig. 5. Relationship between maternal and fetal adrenal weight on the 22nd day of intrauterine development (+ normal intact females, · intact tumor-bearing rats).

on filter paper and weighed on automatic analytical balance. The adrenal glands were dissected under lens of ten-fold magnification, dried quickly and carefully with strips of filter paper and weighed on automatic analytical balance. For corticosterone analyses blood was collected after decapitation of the mother and fetuses. Fetal plasma and adrenal glands were pooled and immediately analyzed for corticosterone content by the method of Zenker and Bernstein (1958).

RESULTS

Figs. 1 to 5 show a negative correlation between maternal and fetal adrenal weights from days 18 to 22 of the intrauterine development. The data include values of the adrenal weights of fetuses from normal intact mothers and those from the pregnant rats bearing ACTH-secreting tumor, thus the maternal adrenal size has a wide range. The maximal inhibition of fetal adrenal growth was found on day 18, 19, 20, 21 and 22 when the maternal adrenal weights were 80, 100, 120, 120, and 80 mg per 100 g of body weight, respectively. Beyond these limits of maternal adrenal enlargement the fetal adrenal weights were found to be constant and independent of further maternal adrenal hypertrophy.

References pp. 77–78

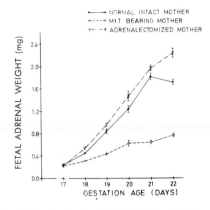

Fig. 6. Weights of one pair of adrenal glands of 17- to 22-day-old fetuses from normal intact mothers, normal adrenalectomized mothers and from pregnant tumor-bearing rats whose adrenal gland weight exceeded 110 mg/100 g body weight. Each point represents mean and standard error of 12–30 for control, 10–68 for tumor rats, and 10–22 for adrenalectomized mothers.

Adrenal weights of the fetuses increased from the 17th to 21st day of intrauterine development from 0.24 mg to 1.77 mg and were somewhat lighter on the last day (1.70 mg). Adrenal weights of the fetuses from ACTH-secreting tumor-bearing mother also increased, but only from 0.22 mg to 0.64 mg from day 17 to day 21, and 0.76 on the last day of pregnancy. The average daily increase of fetal adrenal weight in mothers with enlarged adrenals was 0.11 mg, which is less than 30% of the daily adrenal weight gain of the control fetuses (0.38 mg per day). Fig. 6 also shows that the daily adrenal weight increase of fetuses from adrenalectomized mothers (0.44 mg per day) was 16% more than in control fetuses, and four times more than in fetuses from tumor-bearing mothers. Further increase of the fetal adrenal weight was observed on the last day of intrauterine development in the group of fetuses from adrenalectomized females (0.17 mg).

Fig. 7 shows the fetal adrenal weight changes during 24 hours after adrenalectomy, in contrast to the above mentioned data obtained 3 or more days after adrenalectomy. In fetuses from normal adrenalectomized mothers acute adrenalectomy was followed by fetal adrenal hypertrophy only on the last day of pregnancy and it was 0.37 mg, but the same treatment applied to the tumor-bearing mother was followed by considerable enlargement of the adrenal size from day 19 to the end of gestation period: the values obtained were 0.36 mg, 0.47 mg, 0.90 mg and 0.76 mg on the last day of gestation period.

Table 1 shows that the stress of histamine injection into the fetuses of tumor-bearing females ex utero did not increase the adrenal and plasma corticosterone concentration on the 21st and 22nd day of intrauterine development.

DISCUSSION

Adrenal enlargement, to more than ten times normal size was produced in pregnant rats by ACTH-secreting tumors. This made it possible to observe the relationship

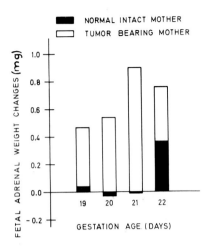

Fig. 7. Fetal adrenal weight changes during 24 hours after adrenalectomy of normal (black bar) and ACTH tumor-bearing mothers (white bar) on days 19, 20, 21 and 22 of intrauterine development.

TABLE 1

ADRENAL AND PLASMA CORTICOSTERONE CONCENTRATION BEFORE AND AFTER STRESS IN 21- AND 22-DAY-OLD FETUSES FROM MOTHERS BEARING ACTH-SECRETING TUMOR

Gestation age – days	Number of litters	Adrenal corticosterone $\mu g/g$		Plasma corticosterone $\mu g/g$	
		before stress	after stress	before stress	after stress
21	10	$23.8 \pm 2.05*$	20.9 ± 1.61	21.1 ± 1.85	22.3 ± 1.26
22	7	16.4 ± 1.01	16.1 ± 1.60	18.5 ± 1.23	15.2 ± 1.22
21–22**	10	—	—	21.8 ± 1.65	28.3 ± 1.72

* Mean $\pm$ S.E.
** Data from the paper of K. Milković and Milković (1963), *Endocrinology*, 73, 535–539.
 Normal intact mother.

between fetal and maternal adrenal size. The negative correlation between the relative weights of the maternal and fetal adrenal glands, from the 18th day of intrauterine development onward strongly indicates that inhibition of fetal adrenocorticotropic activity depends on the size of maternal adrenals. However, when the maternal adrenal weight exceeded 100 mg per 100 g body weight, this relationship no longer existed and the fetal adrenal weight was constant at the "atrophic" level. Complete blockade of the fetal adrenocorticotropic activity seems to have been reached at this degree of maternal adrenal enlargement. In tumor-bearing rats the hypersecretion of the maternal adrenal cortex resulted in a high corticosterone concentration in the fetal blood and caused a marked delay in fetal adrenal growth (Fig. 6, lower curve). On the other hand, adrenalectomy of the pregnant rat was followed by marked fetal adrenal enlargement due to the removal of the inhibitory action of maternal steroids (Fig. 6, upper curve). The most interesting fact is that the fetus distinguishes between excess and lack of maternal corticosteroids from day 18 of intrauterine development. The most plausible explanation of this phenomenon seems to be that in the fetus the target for maternal corticosteroids, *i.e.*, the adrenocorticotropic activity, did not exist until day 17. In other words, lack of fetal adrenal response to change in the concentration of maternal corticosteroids on the 17th day of intrauterine development is good evidence that, at this time, the fetal pituitary is not capable of secreting ACTH. After ACTH secretion appeared in the fetus, maternal corticoids could stimulate or depress it through the feedback mechanism known to exist at the end of pregnancy, and retard growth or cause hypertrophy of the fetal adrenal gland, depending on the levels of the circulating corticoids crossing the placenta.

The constant adrenal gland weights in fetuses from mothers with adrenal enlargement (more than 100 mg/100 g body weight) could be attributed to the total inhibition of fetal ACTH. This makes it possible to calculate the extent to which fetal adrenal growth is the result of self-differentiation (proliferation) and the extent to which it is due to the specific influence of the fetal pituitary gland (functional differentiation). These data allow us to conclude that between day 17 and 18 fetal ACTH participates in 60% of fetal adrenal growth, between day 18 and 19 in 65%, between day 19 and 20 in 55%. Its participation is the highest between day 20 and 21 when it accounts for 95% of fetal adrenal growth.

The fetal pituitary–adrenocortical system has been shown to be able to respond to stressful stimuli by adrenal ascorbic acid depletion and increase of plasma corticosterone concentration (K. Milković and Milković, 1958; S. Milković and Milković, 1961; K. Milković and Milković, 1962; Eguchi and Wells, 1965). The data in Table 1 show that the fetuses from tumor-bearing mothers cannot respond to injections of histamine on day 21 and 22, which indicates that fetal ACTH is blocked, as demonstrated by the morphological criteria. When ACTH is injected to the fetuses of tumor-bearing rats adrenal corticosterone is increased (unpublished data).

It is generally accepted that the corticoids operate in the feedback mechanisms through the hypothalamus. On the other hand, it is well known that the prehypophyseal neurovascular structures are not developed in rat until approximately one week after birth (Glydon, 1957; Campbell, 1966; Florsheim and Rudko, 1968). On the basis of the data presented in this paper direct action of corticoids on the pituitary should be supposed to exist during perinatal development. Recently, Dhariwall, Russel and Yates (1968) postulated that the adrenocortical system of the adult rat has a multi-stage feedback mechanism operating in sites of the anterior hypophysis as well as in several regions of the brain.

CONCLUSIONS

1. Fetal adrenocorticotropic activity begins between days 17 and 18 of intrauterine development.

2. Significant negative correlation between the relative maternal and fetal adrenal weights was found from day 18 to 22 of intrauterine development indicating partial inhibition of fetal ACTH.

3. When maternal adrenal weight was 100 mg/100 g body weight or more the correlation mentioned above disappeared and the fetal adrenal weight was constant at the "atrophic" level —indicating complete blockade of the fetal ACTH.

4. Acute adrenalectomy (24 hours) of normal pregnant rats was followed by fetal adrenal hypertrophy only on day 22 but not on day 19, 20 and 21 of intrauterine development, indicating maximal adrenocorticotrophic activity in normal fetuses on days 19, 20 and 21. Under the same circumstances fetuses of adrenalectomized mothers bearing ACTH-secreting tumors responded by significant adrenal enlargement from day 19 to the end of intrauterine development.

5. The pituitary–adrenocortical system of the fetuses from tumor-bearing mothers did not respond to histamine stress indicating, again, complete blockade of the fetal ACTH.

6. Direct action of corticoids on the hypophysis in the feedback control of the pituitary–adrenocortical system of rat fetuses must be assumed to exist, because the prehypophyseal neurovascular structures are not developed at that time.

REFERENCES

BATES, R. W., MILKOVIĆ, S. AND GARRISON, M. M., (1962) Concentration of prolactin, growth hormone and ACTH in blood and tumor of rats with transplantable mammotropic pituitary tumor. *Endocrinology*, **71**, 943–948.

CAMPBELL, H. J. (1966) The development of the primary portal plexus in the median eminence of the rabbit. *J. Anat.*, **100**, 381–387.

DHARIWALL, A. P. S., RUSSEL, S. AND YATES, F. E. (1968) Corticosteroid block of pituitary response to CRF in vivo. *Abst. Brief Communications, Third Intern. Congress Endocrinology, Mexico*, Excerpta Medica Foundation, Amsterdam, p. 80.

EGUCHI, Y. AND WELLS, L. J., (1965) Response of the hypothalamic-hypophyseal adrenal axis to stress: observation in fetal and caesarean newborn rats. *Proc. Soc. Exptl. Biol. Med.*, **120**, 675–678.

FLORSHEIM, W. H. AND RUDKO, P. (1968) The development of portal system in the rat. *Neuroendocrinology*, **3**, 89–98.

GLYDON, R. H. J. (1957) The development of the blood supply of the pituitary in the albino rat, with special reference to the portal vessels. *J. Anat.*, **91**, 237–244.

JOST, A. (1966) Problem of fetal endocrinology: the adrenal glands. *Recent Progr. Hormone Res.*, **22**, 541–569.

MILKOVIĆ, K. AND MILKOVIĆ, S. (1958) The reactivity of the fetal pituitary-adrenal system during the last days of pregnancy. *Arch. Intern. Physiol. Biochem.*, **66**, 534–539.

MILKOVIĆ, K. AND MILKOVIĆ, S. (1962) Studies of the pituitary-adrenocortical system in the fetal rat. *Endocrinology*, **71**, 799–802.

MILKOVIĆ, K. AND MILKOVIĆ. S. (1966) Adrenocorticotropic hormone secretion in the fetus and infant. In: *Neuroendocrinology*, Vol. I, L. MARTINI AND W. F. GANONG (Eds.), Academic Press, New York, pp. 371–405.

MILKOVIĆ, K., EFENDIĆ, S., PAUNOVIĆ, J., RONKULIN, J., DULIBIĆ, V. AND MILKOVIĆ, S. (1966) Effect of the autonomous transplantable pituitary mammotropic tumor on the pregnancy and the embryonic development in rat. *Bull. Sci. Yugosl. Acad.*, **11**, 107–108.

MILKOVIĆ, S. AND MILKOVIĆ, K. (1961) Reactiveness of fetal pituitary to stressful stimuli: Does the maternal ACTH cross the placenta? *Proc. Soc. Exptl. Biol. Med.*, **107**, 47–49.

MILKOVIĆ, S., MILKOVIĆ, K. AND EFENDIĆ, S. (1968) Significance of maternal corticosteroids in fetal adrenal development and organogenesis. *Gen. Compar. Endocrinol.*, **10**, 240–246.

MILKOVIĆ, S. AND MILKOVIĆ, K. (1969) Responsiveness of the pituitary-adrenocortical system during embryonic and early postnatal period of life. In: *Physiology and Pathology of Adaptation Mechanisms (International Series of Monographs in Pure and Applied Biology, Modern Trends in Physiological Sciences*, Vol. 27), E. BAJUSZ (Ed.), Pergamon Press, Oxford, pp. 28–47.

MILKOVIĆ, S. AND MILKOVIĆ, K. (1969) Development of response to stress. In: *Progress in Endocrinology, Proc. Third Intern. Congr. Endocrinology*, Excerpta Medica Foundation, Amsterdam (in press).

ZENKER, N. AND BERNSTEIN, D. E. (1958) The estimation of small amounts of corticosterone in rat plasma. *J. Biol. Chem.*, **231**, 695–701.

DISCUSSION

CLEGHORN: Did you observe any difference in the birth weight of the pups born to tumor-bearing mothers?

MILKOVIĆ: The course of pregnancy was completely normal, but spontaneous delivery did not occur. The pups were kept alive by cesarian section of the mothers; the weight was 7% lower than normal on day 22. We do not have data about pups from mothers with big tumors.

HENKIN: It is well known in cows and pigs, that exogenous cortisol will cause prematurity. In those animals that delivered spontaneously did you see any evidence of prematurity?

MILKOVIĆ: No we did not.

HENKIN: Some animals after adrenalectomy show a delay in parturition. Did you observe any delay in the rats that were adrenalectomized on day 22?

MILKOVIĆ: Sometimes we observed some delay, and we also noticed cannibalism. We do not really know the reason for the delay in parturition. Koren *et al.* (Am. J. Obst. Gynecol., 1965, 93, 411) reported that serotonin concentration in placenta is very high just before delivery, and MAO activity very low. We have been able to confirm their data. But we still do not see the reason for the delay in delivery.

LEVINE: The rat may differ from other animals on many points. We found that female rats, adrenalectomized prior to mating, show almost normal reproductive function.

The Pituitary—Adrenal System and the Developing Brain[*]

SEYMOUR LEVINE[**]

Stanford University School of Medicine, Stanford, Calif. 94305 (U.S.A.)

During recent years it has been demonstrated (Levine and Mullins, 1966) that gonadal hormones influence the central nervous system during critical periods of development and program subsequent neuroendocrine and reproductive activity. The basic hypothesis, developed by Harris (1964) and Young (1961), states that gonadal hormones acting on the central nervous system during fetal and neonatal life organize the sexually undifferentiated brain with regard to patterns of gonadotropin secretion and sexual behavior. Specifically, this hypothesis states, first, during critical periods early in development, androgens acting on the central nervous system are responsible for the programming of male patterns of gonadotropin secretion and sex behavior in much the same way that they determine the development of anatomical sexual characteristics. Second, during adult life, gonadal hormones activate the sexual differentiated brain and elicit the responses that were programmed earlier. Third, an additional component of the process of sexual differentiation is to render the tissues which are responsive to gonadal hormones differentially sensitive in the male and the female.

The purpose of this paper is to present evidence for the hypothesis that adrenal hormones may have a similar organizing effect on the developing central nervous system both with regard to neuroendocrine regulation of ACTH synthesis and release, and certain aspects of the behavior of adult organisms.

It has been generally accepted that the infant rat is incapable of an adrenal cortical response to stress within the first few days of life. Among the criteria used to evaluate the neonates' adrenal responses are changes in plasma corticosterone levels (Levine, 1965), adrenal corticosterone content (Schapiro, 1962, 1965; Schapiro, Geller, and Eiduson, 1962), and adrenal ascorbic acid depletion (Jailer, 1950; Levine, Alpert, and Lewis, 1958; Milković and Milković, 1959a and b). Schapiro *et al.* (1962) have referred to this period as the stress non-responsive period (SNR), and claim that the first several days of life is an absolute stress non-responsive period, and that there then ensues a relative non-responsive period during which the organism will respond to some stressful stimuli but not to others. Recently, a number of studies have been reported which raise questions concerning the validity of the concept of SNR. It has

---

[*] This study was supported by research grant NICH&HD 02881 from the National Institutes of Health and the Leslie Fund, Chicago.
[**] Supported by USPHS Research Scientist Award 1-K05-MH-19, 936-01 from the National Institute of Mental Health.

References pp. 84–85

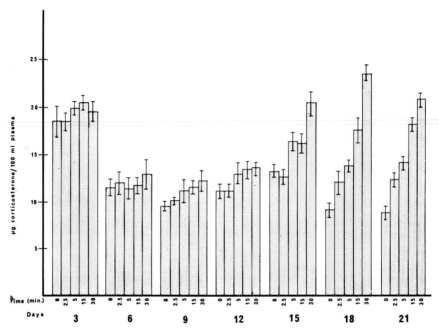

Fig. 1. Plasma corticosterone concentrations in various age groups of infant rats. The columns represent the mean values for control (0 min) and electrically shocked animals. The vertical lines on each column indicate the SE of the mean. The figures under the columns indicate the time following shock that each group was sacrificed.

been reported (Levine, 1968) that in the three-day-old rat, a significant increase in plasma corticosterone was seen if the animal had previously received infantile stimulation. Newborn rats also respond to heat with a significant elevation in both plasma and adrenal corticosterone (Haltmeyer, Denenberg, Thatcher and Zarrow, 1966). It has been shown (Milković and Milković, 1959b) that adrenalectomy of the mother prior to parturition or unilateral ligation of the fallopian tube prior to mating (Milković and Milković, 1959a) results in the offspring's being capable of giving an adrenal response to a severe stress as early as one to two days after parturition.

In view of these experimental data which were not compatible with the concept of an absolute SNR period in the newborn, a series of investigations was undertaken to systematically investigate some of the parameters of the maturation of the organism's capacity to respond as indicated by significant changes in both plasma and adrenal corticoids, as well as in plasma and pituitary ACTH. Our initial study revealed several interesting findings (Levine, Glick, and Nakane, 1967). The essence of these findings was that there is an extremely high level of adrenal activity in terms of both plasma and adrenal concentration of corticosterone in the newborn rat. There is also a clear and definitive response to administration of exogenous ACTH. However, following the initial period of high activity, there is a marked diminution of activity and the animal becomes unresponsive to ACTH and remains unresponsive until approximately 15 to 18 days of age. At that time the animal also becomes responsive to stress. Failure of the adrenal to respond to ACTH does not appear to be a defect

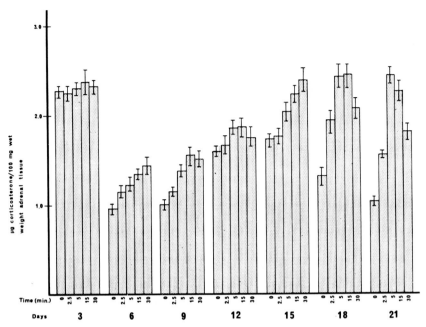

Fig. 2. Adrenal corticosterone content in various age groups of infant rats. The columns represent the mean values for control (0 min) and electrically shocked animals. The vertical lines on each column indicate the SE of the mean. The figures under the columns indicate the time following shock that each group was sacrificed.

in the adrenal per se, for studies by Zarrow and Denenberg (unpublished) have shown that if the newborn rat is primed with ACTH an active response to ACTH continues as long as the adrenal remains stimulated. What does appear to be happening is that the newborn pituitary–adrenal system behaves similarly to that of the hypophysectomized animal and that, if the adrenal is deprived of ACTH stimulation, it becomes insensitive to subsequent ACTH.

We have recently concluded* a large and extensive study on the development of the adrenal in terms of both plasma and adrenal corticosterone and pituitary and circulating ACTH. We felt that it was necessary to describe the total development of the system throughout the prenatal period. The essential data are shown in the figures. What can be seen is a fairly orderly sequence of events. During the very early prenatal period, there is a high concentration of corticosterone in the adrenal and, based on bioassay results obtained using a modification of the Rerup and Hedner (1963) procedure, there are also detectable levels of ACTH. However, there is a period of marked quiescence during which time the plasma and adrenal concentrations of corticosterone are reduced, and there is no ACTH detectable in the plasma, although there are detectable levels of ACTH in the pituitary. Pituitary ACTH increases markedly between six and nine days of age. Adrenal corticosterone concentrations and plasma ACTH again appear at approximately 12 days of age, and by

---

* Treiman and Levine, unpublished.

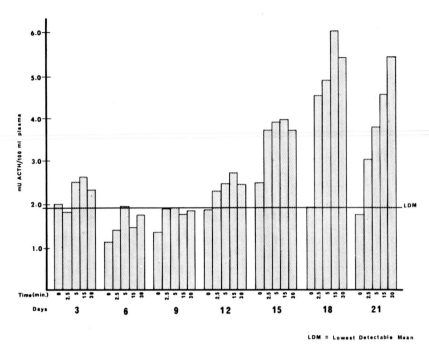

Fig. 3. Combined estimate of plasma adrenocorticotropin (ACTH) concentrations in various age groups of infant rats. The columns represent the mean values for control (0 min) and electrically shocked animals. The horizontal line represents an estimate of the lowest detectable mean concentration based on an average of all assays. The figures under the columns indicate the time following shock that each group was sacrificed.

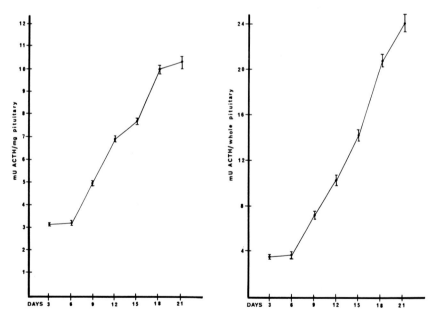

Fig. 4. The effect of age on pituitary ACTH concentration expressed as mU ACTH per mg tissue (left panel) and the effect of age on pituitary ACTH content expressed as mU ACTH per whole pituitary (right panel).

15 days of age the system appears to be totally active. What is interesting about this pattern is its resemblance to the developmental pattern of the male gonads. Examination of the development of the testes, as first described by Hooker (1948) and later by Niemi and Ikonen (1963), indicates that during the late prenatal periods, and for a brief period of time postnatally, the fetal and neonatal testes are exhibiting a high degree of activity. There is an active population of Leydig cells and recently, Resko, Feder, and Goy (1968) have clearly isolated both testosterone and andro- stenedione from the testes and in plasma of the newborn rat. However, following this brief period of activity, the testes become very quiescent, and there is very little Leydig cell production. Activity of the testes in terms of androgen production does not appear again until just prior to puberty.

The question then is what is the relevance of these particular high values of cir- culating corticosterone, both late prenatally and during the early postnatal period, for subsequent functioning of the organism? A number of years ago (1958) we in- vestigated the effects of a variety of early environmental influences on subsequent activity of the hypothalamic pituitary–adrenal system. It was found that the adrenal stress response in animals which had been handled as infants, is markedly different when compared to animals in which no such infantile treatment had been introduced. Recently (1968), we have shown that this very brief period of infantile handling, for as little as two days following birth, produces an organism which responds to stress at three days of age, whereas nontreated controls show no such response. Thus we can speculate that the process of early handling alters adrenocortical activity early in development, and that this alteration in adrenocortical activity is in part what produces the subsequent change in neuroendocrine processes in the adult. Further evidence for this hypothesis, that the effects of early handling are mediated via the changes in the adrenal, comes from a recent experiment by Denenberg and co-workers (1967) in which they observed that following early handling, there is an increase in circulating levels of adrenal corticosteroids.

There is also other evidence which suggests that changes in adrenocortical activity, during both prenatal and early postnatal life, can influence subsequent neuroendocrine activity in the adult organism. Newborn rats born of mothers adrenalectomized prior to conception, have hypertrophy of the adrenal and show higher plasma corticosterone concentrations than offspring of normal mothers (Thoman and Levine, in press). These animals also differ markedly in their response to stress in adulthood. The offspring of adrenalectomized mothers show significantly higher responses to stress than animals of nonadrenalectomized mothers. They also show marked differences in behavior in adulthood. Further, these effects are almost exclusively prenatal effects: Animals born of adrenalectomized mothers, but reared on normal animals, tended to show the effects of prenatal adrenalectomy whereas normal animals, reared on adrenalectomized mothers who do show deficiencies in lactation, still responded like normal animals reared on normal mothers.

Although there appear to be sufficient data to warrant the speculation that the hormones emanating from the fetal and newborn adrenal cortex act upon the central nervous system to organize and program the central nervous system with regard to subsequent neuroendocrine regulation of ACTH, the data are nowhere as clear as those presented for the action of gonadal hormones on the central nervous system during development. At least one reason for this is because present methods of experimentally manipulating the pituitary–adrenal system in the newborn animal may not produce unambiguous results. Removal of the newborn adrenals almost totally arrests growth. Injections of quantities of adrenal corticoids also produce profound physiological deficits. The animals fail to grow normally and are severely runted. However, it is hoped that in the very near future, newer methods can be developed whereby the influence of adrenal corticoids and ACTH on programming the central nervous system can be studied more directly. We believe that when such methods become available, it will be possible to show that like the gonadal hormones, adrenal hormones also have a profound effect upon central nervous system organization and influence a wide variety of adult functions, including neuroendocrine activity under conditions of stress, and behavioral responses which are associated with the neuroendocrine regulation of ACTH (Levine, 1969).

REFERENCES

DENENBERG, V. H., BRUMAGHIM, J. T., HALTMEYER, G. C., AND ZARROW, M. X. (1967) Increased adrenocortical activity in the neonatal rat following handling. *Endocrinology*, **81**, 1047–1052.

HALTMEYER, G. C., DENENBERG, V. H., THATCHER, JOAN AND ZARROW, M. X. (1966) Response of the adrenal cortex of the neonatal rat after subjection to stress. *Nature*, **212**, 1371–1373.

HARRIS, G. W. (1964) Sex hormones, brain development and brain function. *Endocrinology*, **75**, 627–648.

HOOKER, C. W. (1948) The biology of the interstitial cells of the testis. *Rec. Progr. Hormone Res.*, **3**, 173–195.

JAILER, J. W. (1950) The maturation of the pituitary–adrenal axis in the newborn rat. *Endocrinology*, **46**, 420–425.

LEVINE, S. (1965) Maturation of the neuroendocrine response to stress. *Excerpta Medica Intern. Congr. Ser.* No. 99.

LEVINE, S. (1968) Influence of infantile stimulation on the response to stress during preweaning development. *Developmental Psychobiology*, **1**, 67–70.

LEVINE, S. (1969) Hormones and conditioning. In: *Nebraska Symposium on Motivation*, W. J. ARNOLD (Ed.), University of Nebraska Press, Lincoln, Nebraska, pp. 85–101.

LEVINE, S., ALPERT, M. AND LEWIS, G. W. (1958) Differential maturation of an adrenal response to cold stress in rats manipulated in infancy. *J. Comp. Physiol. Psychol.*, **51**, 774–777.

LEVINE, S., GLICK, D. AND NAKANE, P. K. (1967) Adrenal and plasma corticosterone and vitamin A in rat adrenal glands during postnatal development. *Endocrinology*, **80**, 910–914.

LEVINE, S. AND MULLINS, R. F., JR. (1966) Hormonal influences on brain organization in infant rats. *Science*, **152**, 1585–1592.

LEVINE, S. AND THOMAN, E. B. (in press) Maternal factors influencing subsequent adrenocortical activity in the offspring. In: *Symposium on Postnatal Development of Phenotype, Liblice*, S. KAZDA AND V. H. DENENBERG (Eds.), Butterworths and Academic, New York, pp. 75–82.

MILKOVIČ, K. AND MILKOVIČ, S. (1959a) Reactiveness of the pituitary–adrenal system of the first postnatal period in some laboratory mammals. *Endokrinologie*, **37**, 301–310.

MILKOVIČ, K. AND MILKOVIČ, S. (1959b) The influence of adrenalectomy of pregnant rats on the reactiveness of the pituitary–adrenal system of newborn animals. *Arch. Intern. Physiol. Biochim.*, **67**, 24–28.

NIEMI, M. AND IKONEN, M. (1963) Histochemistry of the Leydig cells in the postnatal prepubertal testis of the rat. *Endocrinology*, **72**, 443–448.

RERUP, C. AND HEDNER, P. (1963) The assay of corticotrophin in mice. *Acta Endocrinol.*, **44**, 237–249.

RESKO, J. A., FEDER, H. H. AND GOY, R. W. (1968) Androgen concentrations in plasma and testis of developing rats. *J. Endocrinol.*, **40**, 485–491.

SCHAPIRO, S. (1962) Pituitary ACTH and compensatory adrenal hypertrophy in stress-non-responsive infant rats. *Endocrinology*, **71**, 986–989.

SCHAPIRO, S. (1965) Adrenal cortical hormones and resistance to histamine stress in the infant rat. *Acta Endocrinol.*, **48**, 249–252.

SCHAPIRO, S., GELLER, E. AND EIDUSON, S. (1962) Corticoid response to stress in the steroid-inhibited rat. *Proc. Soc. Exptl. Biol. Med.*, **109**, 935–937.

THOMAN, E. B. AND LEVINE, S. (in press) Influence of adrenalectomy in female rats on reproductive processes: effects on the foetus and offspring. *J. Endocrinol.*

YOUNG, W. C. (1961) The hormones and mating behavior. In: *Sex and Internal Secretions*, W. C. YOUNG (Ed.), Williams & Wilkins, Baltimore, pp. 1173–1239.

DISCUSSION

LARON: Is it possible to draw a parallel between the increased ACTH secretion in rats after birth and the increased somatotropic hormone (STH) secretion in the human newborn that lasts about 2 weeks? Would this increased secretion of hypothalamic–pituitary hormones represent a physiological reaction or would it be due to an immaturity of the pathways regulating secretion of the hormones?

LEVINE: I do not know the relationship between the growth hormone and ACTH at this age. The period of hyperactivity is presumably functional in terms of its activity on neural systems. After this period the system shifts over to its own homeostatic mechanism.

CLEGHORN: Could you elaborate on the last remark in your paper. I understand that certain circumstances in young rats led to a facilitation of the response to ACTH later in life. Is that so?

LEVINE: Many conditions, involving maternal factors or other early experience parameters can influence ACTH regulation in adulthood. Animals which have been given certain kinds of treatment in infancy have a more flexible modulating system. Without the treatment the animals tend to have a very inflexible system: an all or none response.

MILKOVIĆ: Several years ago, Bates and I (Bates *et al.* (1964) Endocrinology, 74, 714) found that in the presence of STH exogenous ACTH has only half of the effect on the adrenal gland relative to the effect of ACTH alone (adrenal weight, plasma corticosterone, adrenal ascorbic acid). On the other hand we know that STH content in the pituitary and in plasma is low at the end of the intra-uterine development and immediately after birth, at least in the rat. On day 10 following birth, STH is raised to values 10 to 15 times higher than on the first post-natal day. So it is possible that the lack of response to stress in this period is due to an antagonistic relationship between ACTH and STH.

LEVINE: But the adrenal also becomes non-responsive to exogenous ACTH. The adrenals lack sensitivity as in hypophysectomized animals. It has been shown that if you continue to give ACTH, the adrenal remains responsive to ACTH. Your explanation would hold if there was an inverse relationship between STH and ACTH. This may be one of the mechanisms by which ACTH is suppressed. The adrenal now deprived of ACTH, becomes relatively insensitive.

DE WIED: At 6 and 9 days of age, ACTH activity in the blood of the animals is low while ACTH content in the pituitary increases. Accordingly, ACTH synthesis is intact and only the release seems to be inhibited. This is a very interesting phenomenon, since synthesis and release seem to be dissociated under these conditions. The young animals might therefore be a good model to study the two phenomena.

LEVINE: This is indeed an interesting aspect of the whole development pattern. Before one can get release, apparently some sort of threshold concentration is needed. The increase in synthesis is very rapid, and it is not until the 12th day that you see any evidence for release in response to stress. Some neutral components might also need time to mature and to become integrated in the system.

MIRSKY: I was fascinated to note that it took between 12 and 18 days to obtain both an increase in responsiveness and in reactivity of the adrenal. It is very interesting that just at the same period there are concomitant changes in other systems, *e.g.* the blood–brain barrier develops at the same time. Compounds which would enter the brain very easily prior to 18 days, do not enter at all after 18 days.

LEVINE: If you look at the developmental pattern of some of the enzymes, of temperature regulation, etc., there is a remarkably uniform pattern to be seen. Development does not seem to go in a linear progression, but there is a critical period and inside 24 h sometimes the activity appears.

Effects of the Nervous System on Pituitary–Adrenal Activity

G. W. HARRIS

University of Oxford, Department of Human Anatomy, South Parks Road, Oxford (U.K.)

It has been a great pleasure to be invited to be Chairman of Section I of this symposium which deals with the effects of the nervous system on pituitary–adrenal activity, and to have the duty of attempting to sum up the papers and discussions we have heard in this section.

My own interest in the topic goes back more than twenty years. In 1948, when I was a young lecturer in the Department of Physiology under (then Professor) Lord Adrian, a guest worker from America, Dr. H. F. Colfer, and another from Holland, Dr. J. de Groot, joined me. At that time Dougherty and White (1944) had shown that administration of ACTH to rabbits resulted in acute lymphopenia and that this effect was mediated via adrenal cortical activation. These findings we confirmed in 1950, with Colfer and De Groot, and then used this simple, quick lymphopenic response as an indicator of increased secretion of ACTH. De Groot and I, in 1950, managed to show that electrical stimulation of various parts of the hypothalamus would elicit increased discharge of ACTH, whereas lesions placed in the hypothalamus would prevent such increased discharge following stressful stimuli. Evidence was also adduced that this hypothalamic influence over the anterior pituitary was mediated by the hypophyseal portal vessels. Shortly after these studies I made my first visit to the United States, where I had the pleasure and distinction of being able to meet workers who, with their colleagues, had put forward three different views of the mechanisms controlling ACTH secretion. First, in the University of Utah, Salt Lake City, I met Dr. George Sayers who had proposed that the rate of secretion of ACTH was primarily governed by the circulating blood level of adrenal steroids. Then in the University of Yale, New Haven, I met Dr. C. N. H. Long who believed that an increased secretion of adrenaline under conditions of stress, was a primary factor in mediating increased ACTH discharge. And thirdly, at Harvard, I met Dr. David Hume who, independently from De Groot and myself, had produced evidence from experiments in dogs that stimulation of the hypothalamus evoked ACTH secretion. For some time then, three views on the ACTH control mechanism were discussed—the feedback theory, adrenaline theory and the hypothalamic (CNS) control theory. A crucial experiment was then performed by Dr. Sayers, which was made possible by his development of a method of measuring an increase in concentration of the blood level of ACTH. It was shown that an increased blood concentration of ACTH followed a stress stimulus in *adrenalectom-*

ized animals. This simple and clear observation showed that a feedback mechanism of adrenal cortical steroids, or an adrenaline mechanism, played no essential part in the ACTH stress response, although leaving open the question of the part they might play under normal resting conditions. Since that time various data and ideas have been put forward, concerning such things as a hind-brain releasing factor and the inhibitory effect of cerebral cortical influences and so on, that have confused or amplified the general picture.

In Session I of this symposium we have been privileged to have up-to-date news of the effects of the nervous system on pituitary–adrenal activity. Dr. Schadé presented us with a fine account of the effects of the limbic system, acting through the "funnel" of the hypothalamus, on the secretion of ACTH. Present views on the role of the hypothalamus and adrenal steroid feedback in ACTH control were expounded by Dr. Hodges and by Professor Smelik. The adrenal steroid feedback problem gave rise, as it always has done, to very interesting discussions. Dr. Hodges put forward the theory that this feedback mechanism plays little part in ACTH control, under any circumstances. A number of us disagreed with this point of view. In thinking over our discussions it has occurred to me that little attention was paid to the protein-binding of adrenal steroids in the blood, and attention was mainly focussed on the total blood concentration of these steroids. If, for the sake of argument, we say the methods for measuring the total blood adrenal steroids are accurate to $\pm 5\%$, and of the total steroids only 10% are in the free and active form, then this free fraction could vary from $50–150\%$ of its initial value without any change in the total steroid concentration being detectable. Perhaps this possibility would explain some of the discrepancies that come to light in our deliberations.

The relatively new idea of the "short feedback loop", and the evidence concerning it, was presented to us by Professor Martini. The ingenious experiments and the data derived from them, concerning the possibility that an increased blood level of ACTH inhibits the secretion of ACTH from the pituitary, posed the question—(teleological in nature and therefore not really "proper") —of what possible purpose such a mechanism could play in the intact organism. No answer was forthcoming to this query. But perhaps it would be more effective not to concern ourselves with this aspect, but merely to collect more data as to whether "short feedback loops" exist, or do not exist.

The two papers of Dr. Mulder, and of Drs. Fuxe, Corrodi, Hökfelt and Jonsson, were concerned with aspects of the hypothalamic biochemistry of ACTH control. A fundamental question at the present time concerns the relationship between the electron-microscopic analysis of nerve terminals in the region of the median eminence of the tuber cinereum and the chemical and histochemical observations made on the same part of the brain. It seems clear that the median eminence nerve terminals are rich in two types of granules, synaptic vesicles and large electron-opaque granules— and this region of the brain is also rich in at least two chemical compounds, the so-called anterior pituitary releasing factors (probably peptide in nature) and monoamines (probably mainly dopamine). Here lies a provocative problem of trying to bring together the ultrastructural and chemical correlates.

The final papers in this session, of Professor Marks, Drs. Hall and Bhattacharya, and Professor Milković, Drs. Milković and Senčar, dealt with clinical, psychological effects of the hypothalamic–pituitary–adrenocortical system, and with its activity in the foetus. These fields of study are clearly of great importance, and exciting areas for further research were indicated by the presentations and subsequent discussions.

Professor De Wied, I should like to conclude by saying it was a privilege and pleasure to be present at this symposium.

NOTE OF THE EDITORS

In this book the contribution of Dr. LEVINE has been included in the first session; at the conference he presented his paper in session II.

SESSION II

Effects of ACTH and Adrenocortical Hormones on the Nervous System

Chairman: K. LISSÁK

Institute of Physiology, University Medical School, Rákóczi út 80, Pécs (Hungary)

Effects of Adrenocortical Hormones on the Electrical Activity of the Brain

SHAUL FELDMAN AND NACHUM DAFNY

Laboratory of Neurophysiology, Department of Neurology,
Hadassah University Hospital, Jerusalem (Israel)

There is considerable clinical and experimental evidence that the adrenocortical hormones affect, to a considerable degree, the function of the central nervous system. Most of this evidence comes from observations of psychiatric, neurological, and electroencephalographic disturbances in patients, and from brain excitability, metabolic and biochemical studies in animals with hypo-adrenalism or following adrenocortical therapy (Woodbury and Vernadakis, 1966). However, relatively little information exists on the electrophysiological changes accompanying altered states of adreno-cortical activity. It is, therefore, the purpose of this report to review our experiments on the effects of cortisol administration and adrenalectomy on the electrical activity of the brain.

EFFECTS OF CORTISOL

The effects of cortisol succinate on the electrical activity of the brain were investigated in rabbits with chronically implanted electrodes in the cortex, dorsal hippocampus, amygdala, septum, preoptic area, ventromedial hypothalamus, posterior hypothalamus and midbrain reticular formation. EEG activity, arousal thresholds and evoked potentials were studied. The intravenous injection of 10–25 mg of the hormone caused a generalized slowing in the electrical activity, up to 1/sec, fast activity (35–40/sec) in the amygdala, and spikes in the hippocampus, hypothalamus, amygdala and septum. Furthermore, convulsive electrical activity consisting of high amplitude spikes or delta waves was recorded in the ventromedial hypothalamus and septum, a half to one hour following hormone injection. These seizures either remained localized or spread to other brain areas. Cortisol had no effect on thresholds of arousal produced by reticular formation stimulation. An increase in the amplitude of the hypothalamic potentials evoked by reticular septal or photic stimulation occurred following cortisol administration. A similar phenomenon was observed in the septum and hippocampus following reticular formation stimulation (Fig. 1). Also, the hormone increased the neuronal recovery of the hypothalamic evoked potentials (Feldman and Davidson, 1966). No behavioral convulsions were observed in the rabbits, however in another series of experiments in cats (Feldman, 1966), when 4–6 mg/kg cortisol

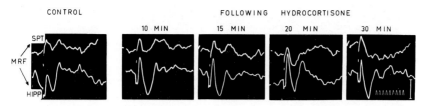

Fig. 1. Effects of 10 mg cortisol succinate on potentials evoked in the septum and dorsal hippocampus in a rabbit, following midbrain reticular formation stimulation. Calibration signal 10 msec and 100 μV.

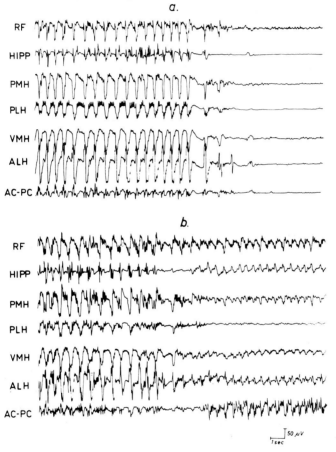

Fig. 2. Generalized seizure activity during two different attacks following the intraventricular administration of 4 mg/kg of cortisol succinate in a cat. RF—midbrain reticular formation; HIPP—dorsal hippocampus; PMH—posteromedian hypothalamus; PLH—posterolateral hypothalamus; VMH—ventromedial hypothalamus; ALH—anterolateral hypothalamus; AC—anterior cortex; PC—posterior cortex.

succinate was administered intraventricularly through a Feldberg cannula, both electrical and behavioral convulsions occurred within a few minutes (Fig. 2).

In acute experiments in cats, evoked potentials following sciatic nerve stimulation were recorded in the medial lemniscus, midbrain reticular formation, intralaminar

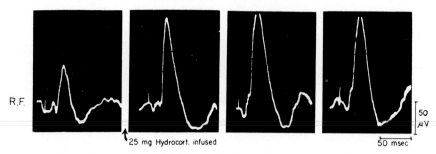

Fig. 3. Evoked potentials in the midbrain reticular formation following sciatic nerve stimulation before and 45, 120 and 180 min. following cortisol administration (Feldman *et al.*, 1961).

thalamic nuclei and the anterior hypothalamus. A few minutes after the intravenous administration of 25 mg cortisol succinate, an increase in the amplitude of the long latency reticular (Fig. 3), thalamic and hypothalamic evoked potentials was noted. Little change was observed in the amplitude of the initial positive wave of the lemniscal potential. The injection of adrenocortical extract had essentially the same effects as cortisol. The effects of cortisol were also examined in animals which were bilaterally adrenalectomized, and similar results were obtained. ACTH administration to intact cats caused also an increase in the long latency evoked potentials in the hypothalamus and reticular formation; this can be attributed to the secondary secretion of cortisol which is the main adrenocortical hormone in the cat (Feldman, Todt and Porter, 1961).

In view of the important role played by the hypothalamus in the regulation of adrenocortical secretion, and because there is considerable evidence that the corticoids, by a negative feedback, participate in this regulation (Mangili, Motta and Martini, 1966), the effects of cortisol succinate on single cell activity were studied in

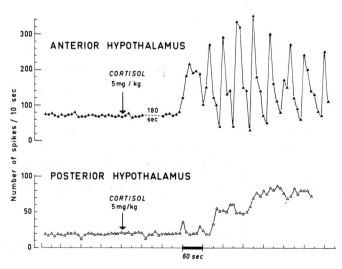

Fig. 4. Effect of cortisol succinate on the pattern of spontaneous firing of a single cell in the anterior and posterior hypothalamus respectively, in cats.

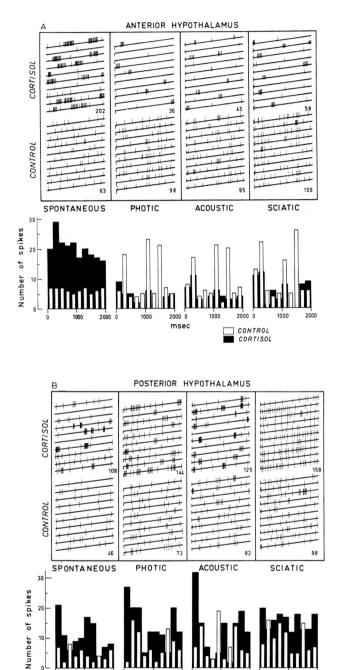

Fig. 5. Single cell recordings and their respective histograms of spontaneous activity and following sensory stimulation in cats, before and after cortisol succinate administration, in the anterior (A) and posterior (B) hypothalamus. Note that after cortisol the sensory stimulus produced in the anterior hypothalamus a decrease in firing, while in the posterior hypothalamus it caused an increase. The numbers indicate the total number of spikes in 20 sec.

the hypothalamus. In these experiments, conducted under light pentobarbital anesthesia, the electrical activity of one single cell was recorded extracellularly in each cat with stainless steel micro-electrodes in the medial anterior-tuberal (Feldman and Dafny, 1966) or posterior hypothalamus for more than one hour. In each cell the spontaneous activity and the responsiveness to single photic, acoustic and sciatic stimuli were studied, both before and following the intravenous administration of 5 mg/kg cortisol succinate. All spikes were counted from the films, for the whole period of the experiments, and the data were evaluated statistically using the critical ratio test $CR = (E - S)/(E + S)^{\frac{1}{2}}$ (where E and S signify evoked and spontaneous activity, respectively) to determine whether a significant increase or a decrease in the rate of firing had occurred. Following cortisol administration, the spontaneous discharge of the units was significantly increased in 11 out of 19, and in 12 out of 21 cells, in the anterior-tuberal and posterior hypothalamus, respectively. The onset of the increased spontaneous firing occurred earlier in the posterior hypothalamus and there were also differences in the pattern of firing in the two hypothalamic regions following cortisol administration (Fig. 4). The main difference was the responsiveness of the units to sensory stimulation: while the anterior-tuberal hypothalamus units, which were all facilitated by the three sensory modalities, were uniformly inhibited following hormone administration, the posterior hypothalamus units, which were facilitated by all the sensory modalities, responded uniformly by a further increase in the rate of firing following cortisol administration (Fig. 5A & B). The overall comparison of responsive units to the three sensory modalities indicates that while in the anterior-tuberal hypothalamus, before cortisol administration there were, out of 33 possible responses, 23 facilitatory and 9 inhibitory ones, following cortisol administration there were only 3 facilitatory and 29 inhibitory responses. On the other hand, in the posterior hypothalamus before cortisol administration there were, out of 42 possible responses, 18 facilitatory and 20 inhibitory ones, while following cortisol administration 32 responses were facilitatory and only one was inhibitory.

Because many of the neuroendocrine studies were done in rats, other experiments of single cell recording were performed on this species under urethane anesthesia. Extracellular single cell activity was recorded simultaneously with glass micro-pipettes in the anterior-tuberal and the posterior hypothalamus, near the midline, and the effects of 5 mg cortisol succinate introduced intraperitoneally were studied for a period of two hours and compared with non-treated animals. The unit activity was recorded on a magnetic tape recorder and evaluated by the computer of average transients (CAT 1000). The CAT provided outputs to an X–Y plotter, a printer and perforated tape. The paper tapes were subsequently translated and processed on a high speed digital computer (CDC 6400) for the determination of mean time intervals, modes and standard deviations, as well as mean rates of firing of the individual units. Statistical analysis was used to evaluate the changes in the average rate of firing following sensory stimulation in the same group of cells and comparisons made between rates of firing of different groups of units using the sign and the Mann–Whitney tests, respectively. Somatosensory stimulation produced in the anterior-tuberal hypothalamus in non-treated animals an increase in the rate of firing from 2.95 to

TABLE 1

RESPONSIVENESS OF UNITS TO SENSORY STIMULATION, IN PERCENT, IN NON-TREATED, CORTISOL TREATED AND ADRENALECTOMIZED RATS, IN ANTERIOR (AH) AND POSTERIOR (PH) HYPOTHALAMUS

		No. units	Responsive units	Increase in firing	Decrease in firing
AH	Non-treated	51	80.4	58.5	41.5
	Cortisol-treated	54	90.7	34.7	65.3 ($p < 0.03$)
	Adrenalectomized	46	87.0	47.5	52.5 (NS)
PH	Non-treated	46	80.4	54.1	45.9
	Cortisol-treated	44	88.6	66.7	33.3 (NS)
	Adrenalectomized	56	82.1	73.9	26.1 ($p < 0.04$)

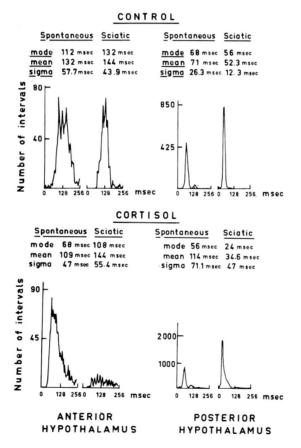

Fig. 6. Time interval histograms of the spontaneous activity and following sensory stimulation of single cells in the anterior and posterior hypothalamus, in non-treated (control) and cortisol treated rats, respectively.

References p. 100

3.61 spikes/sec ($p < 0.02$), while in the posterior hypothalamus a non-significant increase from 12.18 to 13.69 spikes/sec occurred. In the cortisol-treated rats, the average spontaneous firing rate in the anterior-tuberal hypothalamus was increased in relation to untreated animals to 6.06 spikes/sec ($p < 0.001$); however, the sensory stimulation reduced significantly the mean rate to 4.60 spikes/sec in relation to the spontaneous activity ($p < 0.02$). In the posterior hypothalamus, the hormone also increased the spontaneous average rate of firing to 16.34 ($p < 0.01$); however, sensory stimulation caused a further increase to 18.75 ($p < 0.05$). A statistical analysis of the responsiveness to sensory stimulation (CR test) of the individual units has demonstrated that, in the cortisol treated rats, the majority of cells in the anterior-tuberal hypothalamus responded by inhibition, while in the non-treated animals, there were more facilitatory units ($p < 0.03$) (Table I). In the posterior hypothalamus, the units in the treated rats responded mainly by facilitation and the difference in respect to the anterior hypothalamic responses was significant ($p < 0.003$). These differences in responsiveness of anterior-tuberal and posterior hypothalamic neurons were also demonstrated in the time interval histograms of the unit firing. Thus, in the anterior-tuberal hypothalamus in cortisol-treated rats, the spontaneous activity of which showed one mode, the height of the mode was reduced and it shifted to the right on the X axis, a finding which demonstrates a decrease in the rate of firing. On the other hand in the posterior hypothalamus, the sensory stimulation increased the amplitude of the mode and shifted it to the left, more than in non-treated rats (Fig. 6). Generally, in the anterior hypothalamus of the non-treated rats, the mean time intervals and their standard deviations were larger than in the posterior hypothalamus. In cortisol-treated rats these parameters became smaller in the posterior hypothalamus.

EFFECTS OF ADRENALECTOMY

Experiments were performed on rats with permanent bipolar electrodes implanted in the cortex and subcortical structures. After recovery, the electrical activity was recorded on an electroencephalograph for a number of days, bilateral adrenalectomy was performed and the recording continued daily for at least another week. As controls, sham-operated animals were subjected to the same procedure. While the sham operation produced an increase in the wave frequency both in the cortex and subcortical regions, the adrenalectomy caused a generalized slowing in the electrical activity of the brain. The slow activity in subcortical regions of 5–7/sec in intact animals shifted to 1.5–3/sec waves, following adrenalectomy. Furthermore, in adrenalectomized rats there appeared an increase in amplitude and bursts of high voltage activity (Fig. 7). Statistical analysis demonstrated that, while in the cortex and reticular formation no particular trend within the post-adrenalectomy period was found, in the hypothalamus a significant ($p < 0.001$) progressive decrease in wave frequency occurred (Feldman and Robinson, 1968).

Other experiments of single cell recording were performed on intact and adrenalectomized rats and the data evaluated as described above. The average spontaneous

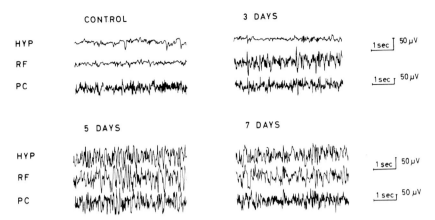

Fig. 7. Electrical activity of the brain before (control) and on different days following bilateral adrenalectomy. HYP—hypothalamus: RF—midbrain reticular formation; PC—posterior cortex (Feldman and Robinson, 1968).

firing rate of units in the anterior-tuberal hypothalamus was 3.06 spikes/sec. In another group of units, in rats one week after adrenalectomy, this was increased to 5.10 spikes/sec ($p < 0.05$). On the other hand comparisons of the spontaneous activity in the posterior hypothalamus of intact and adrenalectomized rats showed no differences. When the data were analyzed as to significant changes in the rate of firing, it was found that 80–87% of the units responded to sensory stimulation in intact and adrenalectomized animals, both in the anterior and posterior hypothalamus. As a result of adrenalectomy there was an increase in the percentage of units in the posterior hypothalamus, the rate of firing of which was increased by the sensory stimuli (Table I) and this difference was significant both in relation to the responsiveness of the posterior hypothalamic units in intact animals ($p < 0.04$), and of anterior hypothalamic units in adrenalectomized rats ($p < 0.01$).

Experiments using evoked potentials were concerned with changes in conduction, neuronal recovery and sensitivity to anesthesia in the brainstem and hypothalamus in adrenalectomized cats maintained on cortisol acetate for periods of one to four weeks. The stimulation of the contralateral sciatic nerve evoked potentials with latencies of about 5 and 7–10 msec in the oligosynaptic systems of the medial lemniscus and the posterolateral hypothalamus, respectively, with no differences between adrenalectomized and intact animals. On the other hand, the conduction in the multisynaptic systems was prolonged in the adrenalectomized cats, when compared with the intact animals. Thus, in the midbrain reticular formation and the ventromedial hypothalamus the mean latencies of the evoked potentials were in the two groups 22.8 and 14.6 msec ($p < 0.01$) and 38.9 and 29.3 ($p < 0.01$), respectively. There were no differences between intact and adrenalectomized cats in the neuronal recovery of the short latency responses in the medial lemniscus and the posterior hypothalamus. The recovery was prolonged in the reticular formation and particularly in the ventromedial hypothalamus (Fig. 8). The potentials evoked by sciatic nerve stimulation in the midbrain reticular formation and ventromedial hypothalamus in intact animals

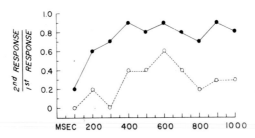

Fig. 8. Neuronal recovery in the ventromedial nucleus of the hypothalamus, following double stimulation of the sciatic nerve at varying intervals, in an adrenalectomized (open circles) and an intact (black circles) cat, respectively (Feldman, 1962).

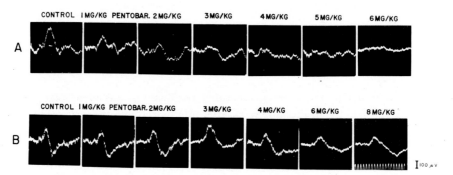

Fig. 9. Effects of small increments of pentobarbital on evoked potentials, following sciatic nerve stimulation, in the tegmentum of the midbrain reticular formation in an adrenalectomized (A) and an intact cat (B), respectively. Calibration signal 10 msec (Feldman, 1962).

are more sensitive to pentobarbital anesthesia in comparison to the responses recorded in the medial lemniscus. However, while in the adrenalectomized cats the lemniscal responses persisted under anesthesia, those in the reticular formation and the ventromedial hypothalamus were abolished with considerably smaller amounts than in intact cats (Fig. 9) (Feldman, 1962).

CONCLUSIONS

The present data indicate that cortisol has a considerable effect on the electrical activity of the brain. The described alterations in the rabbit and cat in the cortex and subcortical structures, as well as the convulsive phenomena, are related to an increase in brain excitability in experimental animals following the administration of the hormone (Woodbury and Vernadakis, 1966). Convulsive phenomena have also been reported in rats, cats and monkeys following the administration of compound S (Heuser and Eidelberg, 1961; Heuser, Ling and Buchwald, 1965). The increase in the amplitude of evoked potentials, which has been confirmed for visual cortical responses in the cat (Covian, Lico and Antunes-Rodrigues, 1963; Marcus, Watson and Goldman, 1966) and the increase in spontaneous unit discharge in the hypothalamus (Feldman and Dafny, 1966; Slusher, Hyde and Laufer, 1966) are further indications of increased brain excitability following cortisol administration. These changes are probably related to clinical observations of convulsions and EEG alterations, in the form of slow wave activity with paroxysmal bursts, in patients under adrenocortical therapy (Streifler and Feldman, 1953; Glaser, 1953). In addition to the general influences exerted by cortisol on brain excitability, it is evident from a number of observations that its effects may also be somewhat more specific. The differential effect of cortisol on the evoked potentials in the anterior hypothalamus and midbrain reticular formation, but not in the specific sensory pathways, which has been recently confirmed in the rat (Endroczi, Lissak, Koranyi and Nyakas, 1968) indicate that the hormone affects particularly the multisynaptic systems in the brainstem, which are known to play an important role in behavioral, visceral, endocrine and electrocortical regulation. The most prominent changes in the electrical activity in the rabbits were observed in the ventromedial hypothalamus and septum, and forebrain involvement was also manifest in cats following intraventricular injection of the hormone. Local implants of glucocorticoids in the median eminence and the anteromedian hypothalamus inhibit ACTH secretion (Davidson and Feldman, 1963; Mangili *et al.*, 1966), probably by their direct effect on steroid-sensitive cells in this region. As sensory stimuli normally increase ACTH secretion, it is of interest that following cortisol administration, sensory stimulation had a predominantly inhibitory effect on cell firing in this region, while in the posterior hypothalamus such stimuli had a facilitatory influence. This finding indicates that cortisol modifies the responsiveness of hypothalamic cells to incoming sensory impulses and demonstrates the interaction of neural and hormonal factors in the regulation of hypothalamic activity.

Animals which were subjected to adrenalectomy have also demonstrated electrophysiological changes. The slowing in the electrical activity of the brain and the appearance of paroxysmal high voltage activity, as well as the increase in unit discharge following adrenalectomy, are also probably related to an increase in central nervous system excitability in such preparations, as demonstrated by susceptibility to audiogenic seizures and a decrease in the electroshock seizure threshold, a few days after adrenalectomy (Woodbury, 1954). On the other hand, the progressive decrease in wave frequency found only in the hypothalamus may possibly be associated with neuroendocrine changes occurring in the hypothalamus following adrenalectomy. The demonstrated changes in conduction, neuronal excitability, and sensitivity to anesthesia in the polysynaptic systems in the brain, but not in the oligosynaptic pathways in the adrenalectomized cats, confirmed by Chambers, Freedman and Sawyer (1963), are additional indication that, normally, the adrenocortical hormones play an important role in synaptic transmission in the central nervous system. The clinical disturbances of mental alterations, convulsions, and EEG changes of slowing, bursts, and spike and wave activity in Addisonian patients, which are not necessarily associated with metabolic disturbances (Woodbury, 1958), are probably related to changes in brain excitability and to the neurophysiological alterations demonstrated in hypo-adrenalism.

ACKNOWLEDGEMENT

Part of these investigations has been aided by Agreement No. 4X5108 with the National Institutes of Health, Bethesda, Md. The technical assistance of Mr. N. Conforti is gratefully acknowledged.

REFERENCES

CHAMBERS, W. F., FREEDMAN, S. L. AND SAWYER, C. H. (1963) The effect of adrenal steroids on evoked reticular responses. *Exptl. Neurol.*, **8**, 458–469.
COVIAN, M. R., LICO, M. C. AND ANTUNES-RODRIGUES, J. (1963) Effects of adrenal corticoids on visual evoked cortical potentials in the cat. *Arch. Intern. Pharmacodyn.*, **146**, 81–92.
DAVIDSON, J. M. AND FELDMAN, S. (1963) Cerebral involvement in the inhibition of ACTH secretion by hydrocortisone. *Endocrinology*, **72**, 936–946.
ENDROCZI, E., LISSAK, K., KORANYI, L. AND NYAKAS, C. (1968) Influence of corticosteroids on the hypothalamic control of sciatic-evoked potentials in the brain stem reticular formation and the hypothalamus in the rat. *Acta Physiol. Acad. Sci. Hung.*, **33**, 375–382.
FELDMAN, S. (1962) Electrophysiological alterations in adrenalectomy. *Arch. Neurol.*, **7**, 460–470.
FELDMAN, S. (1966) Convulsive phenomena produced by intraventricular administration of hydrocortisone in cats. *Epilepsia*, **7**, 271–282.
FELDMAN, S. AND DAFNY, N. (1966) Effect of hydrocortisone on single cell activity in the anterior hypothalamus. *Israel J. Med. Sci.*, **2**, 621–623.
FELDMAN, S. AND DAVIDSON, J. M. (1966) Effect of hydrocortisone on electrical activity, arousal thresholds and evoked potentials in the brains of chronically implanted rabbits. *J. Neurol. Sci.*, **3**, 462–472.
FELDMAN, S. AND ROBINSON, S. (1968) Electrical activity of the brain in adrenalectomized rats with implanted electrodes. *J. Neurol. Sci.*, **6**, 1–8.
FELDMAN, S., TODT, J. C. AND PORTER, R. W. (1961) Effect of adrenocortical hormones on evoked potentials in the brain stem. *Neurology*, **11**, 109–115.
GLASER, G. H. (1953) On the relationship between adrenal cortical activity and the convulsive state. *Epilepsia*, **2**, 7–14.
HEUSER, G. AND EIDELBERG, E. (1961) Steroid-induced convulsions in experimental animals. *Endocrinology*, **69**, 915–924.
HEUSER, G., LING, G. M. AND BUCHWALD, N. A., (1965) Sedation or seizures as dose-dependent effects of steroids. *Arch. Neurol.*, **13**, 195–203.
MANGILI, G., MOTTA, M. AND MARTINI, L. (1966) Control of adrenocorticotropic hormone secretion. In: *Neuroendocrinology*, Vol. 1, L. MARTINI AND W. F. GANONG (Eds.), Academic Press, New York, pp. 297–370.
MARCUS, E. M., WATSON, C. D. AND GOLDMAN, P. L. (1966) Effects of steroids on cerebral electrical activity. *Arch. Neurol.*, **15**, 521–532.
SLUSHER, M. A., HYDE, J. E. AND LAUFER, M. (1966) Effect of intracerebral hydrocortisone on unit activity of diencephalon and midbrain in cats. *J. Neurophysiol.*, **29**, 157–169.
STREIFLER, M. AND FELDMAN, S. (1953) On the effect of cortisone on the electroencephalogram. *Confinia Neurol.*, **13**, 16–27.
WOODBURY, D. M. (1954) Effect of hormones on brain excitability and electrolytes. *Recent Progr. Hormone Res.*, **10**, 65–107.
WOODBURY, D. M. (1958) Relation between the adrenal cortex and the central nervous system. *Pharmacol. Rev.*, **10**, 275–357.
WOODBURY, D. M. AND VERNADAKIS, A. (1966) Effects of steroids on the central nervous system. *Methods Hormone Res.*, **5**, 1–57.

DISCUSSION

HENKIN: Taste and smell acuity are decreased in patients with Cushing's syndrome. Rabbits and cats treated with cortisol are essentially the same, with respect to sensory detection and recognition, as in patients with Cushing's syndrome.

ENDRÖCZI: How long was the time interval between cortisol administration and registration of unit activity in the anterior and posterior hypothalamus?

FELDMAN: In the cat each unit was observed for more than one hour and 100 stimuli were applied for each sensory modality. In the rat units were recorded for two hours following cortisol administration and 50 stimuli were given.

Effects of ACTH and Corticosteroids on Single Neurons in the Hypothalamus

FELIX A. STEINER

Department of Experimental Medicine, F. Hoffmann-La Roche & Co. Ltd., Basle, and Institute for Brain Research, University of Zurich, Zurich (Switzerland)

INTRODUCTION AND METHODS

In the past, effects of corticosteroids on the brain have been studied by a variety of experimental approaches. Overall effects—*e.g.*, EEG changes—have been described by Woodbury and Vernadakis (1967), and the effects of intravenously applied steroids on single units have been studied by Slusher, Hyde and Laufer (1966), and by Feldman and Dafny (1966). Experiments in which steroid crystals were implanted into various parts of the brain (*e.g.*, Endröczi, Lissák and Tekeres (1961); Smelik and Sawyer (1962); Chowers, Feldman and Davidson (1963)) have further defined the site of action of these steroids. However, none of these approaches has made it possible to study the *direct* effects of these substances on defined single neurons.

The use of micro-electrophoresis or iontophoresis (Curtis, 1964) is suited for this latter type of study. In this method, certain ionizable drugs may be applied through multibarrelled micropipettes to the extracellular environment of single neurons. The rate of delivery (or the retention) of these substances is accurately controlled by small electrical currents of opposite polarity. The outside diameter of the common tip of these micropipettes measures between 1–3 μ, and one of the barrels may therefore be used for the simultaneous recording of action potentials. Susceptible neurons change their rate of discharge in response to the applied drugs, and their accurate histological identification is possible through the ejection of dyes from one of the barrels according to the same principle. In this study, dexamethasone-21-phosphate has been applied micro-electrophoretically to single neurons in rat brain, and the following problems have been examined:

1) Localization of steroid-sensitive neurons in the hypothalamus and the midbrain,

2) sensitivity of these and other neurons to synthetic ACTH*,

3) responsiveness of steroid-sensitive single neurons to neurohumours (acetylcholine, noradrenaline, dopamine) which are normally present in the hypothalamus.

Preference was given to dexamethasone-21-phosphate (rather than corticosterone or cortisol) because of its ready water solubility. Methodological details and most of the results have been previously described (Steiner, Ruf and Akert, 1969; Steiner, Pieri and Kaufmann, 1968; Ruf and Steiner, 1967a; Ruf and Steiner, 1967b).

---

*1,24-beta-tetracosactide, Synacthen®.

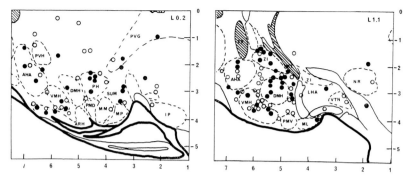

Fig. 1. Localization of single neurons inhibited (●) and not influenced (○) by dexamethasone phosphate on parasagittal sections according to De Groot (1959). Neurons in L 0 to L 0.5 are projected on L 0.2; neurons in L 0.6 to L 1.5 on L 1.1.

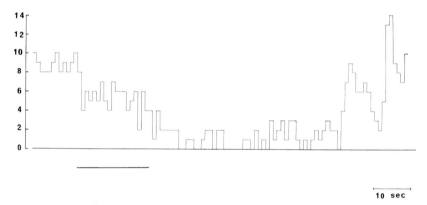

10 sec

Fig. 2. Frequency of discharge of a single neuron in the area hypothalamica anterior, plotted against time. Inhibition by micro-electrophoretically applied dexamethasone phosphate (20 nA). —— Duration of micro-electrophoresis.

RESULTS

Effects of dexamethasone

In 69 different experiments, the steroid sensitivity of 386 hypothalamic and mesencephalic neurons has been assessed. 66 of these neurons decreased their rate of discharge in response to micro-electrophoretic application of dexamethasone, whereas only 7 were activated. The anatomical distribution of these neurons (Fast Green technique, Thomas and Wilson, 1965) is shown in Fig. 1, and a typical example of the change in the rate of discharge is given in Fig. 2. No steroid-sensitive neurons were found in representative samplings in the cortex, the dorsal hippocampus or the thalamus.

Dexamethasone was applied by micro-electrophoresis for time periods ranging between 30–90 sec, and its effects, if present, were usually seen during this interval. In some cases, the effect was almost instantaneous, and neuronal inhibition persisted after the termination of micro-electrophoresis for 5–100 sec.

References p. 106

TABLE 1

RESPONSE OF DEXAMETHASONE PHOSPHATE-SENSITIVE NEURONS TO NEUROHUMOURS

	Activation	Inhibition	No effect	Total
Acetylcholine	16	2	12	30
Noradrenaline	4	13	10	27
Dopamine	0	7	2	9

TABLE 2

RESPONSE OF DEXAMETHASONE PHOSPHATE-SENSITIVE NEURONS
TO BOTH ACETYLCHOLINE AND NORADRENALINE

(↑ increase, ↓ decrease of the discharge rate, ø no effect.)

Acetylcholine	Noradrenaline		
12 ↑	3 ↑	7 ↓	2 ø
11 ø	0 ↑	5 ↓	6 ø

Effects of ACTH

ACTH was administered to 11 dexamethasone-sensitive neurons. It activated 8 of these and was without influence on one. The remaining 2 neurons showed a biphasic effect. Four further neurons, which had not changed their rate of discharge in response to dexamethasone, also remained uninfluenced by ACTH. 9 experiments were performed in this series.

Response of steroid-sensitive neurons to neurohumours

Acetylcholine, noradrenaline, and dopamine were locally administered to a number of dexamethasone-sensitive single neurons. In some cases, it was possible to test the responsiveness of a neuron to more than one neurohumour in consecutive applications. The following changes in the rate of discharge were observed, see Table 1.

It can be seen that acetylcholine had a tendency to activate these neurons, whereas noradrenaline, and especially dopamine, exerted a depressive effect. A similar tendency was observed in those steroid-sensitive neurons which were exposed to the influence of both acetylcholine and noradrenaline. These results are shown in Table 2.

DISCUSSION

These results demonstrate the existence of dexamethasone-sensitive neurons in rather extended areas of the hypothalamus and the midbrain. Most of these neurons are inhibited by dexamethasone, a few are activated. ACTH, in turn, activates certain of these neurons under the experimental conditions of the study. Neurohumours such as acetylcholine, noradrenaline and dopamine also influence the rate of discharge of steroid-sensitive neurons: acetylcholine predominantly in the sense of activation, noradrenaline and dopamine mainly in the sense of depression.

The technique of micro-electrophoresis offers the possibility of a direct assessment of steroid effects on single neurons which would not be obtainable by other techniques. In particular, this approach excludes the possibility of diffusion to neighbouring structures (Bogdanove, 1963), such as the pituitary. Micro-electrophoresis also circumvents diffusion problems caused by the "blood–brain barrier". However, certain questions inherent in this approach must also be considered. The method operates on a hit-or-miss basis and as such, may be subject to a sampling bias with regard to the cell population examined. Certain neurons may not be detectable due to their slow rate of discharge, whereas others may be picked up preferentially because of a particular size or abnormally high rate of discharge induced by stressful experimental conditions.

Nevertheless, the demonstration of selective steroid effects on certain neurons, which are part of a sizeable hypothalamic and mesencephalic population, may be of some physiological significance. It is conceivable that these neurons function as measuring devices for circulating steroids and thus play a role in the feedback control of corticotropin-releasing factor/ACTH secretion. This mode of action of dexamethasone phosphate could represent a negative feedback mechanism, while the ACTH effect may represent a positive (short) feedback mechanism (Sawyer, Kawakami, Meyerson, Whitmoyer and Lilley, 1968), both in the regulation of ACTH production. Some of these steroid-sensitive neurons may have other functions, *e.g.*, in the mediation of behavioural correlates of stress. The simultaneous identification of these neurons by other techniques (*e.g.*, peripheral activation of incoming pathways, experimental lowering of circulating steroids) would greatly facilitate the interpretation of these results.

It should be emphasized that the demonstration of steroid-sensitive neurons in the brain does not exclude feedback effects of corticosteroids in other organs, particularly the anterior pituitary (Kraicer, Milligan, Gosbee, Conrad and Branson, 1969).

SUMMARY

The effects of micro-electrophoretically applied dexamethasone phosphate on neuronal activity in the brain of rat anaesthetized with chloralose–urethane was studied. Dexamethasone phosphate-sensitive neurons were localized in the hypothalamus, and in the midbrain scattered over wide areas. Of these neurons, the large majority was clearly inhibited and a small number activated. No steroid-sensitive neurons were found in the cortex, the dorsal hippocampus, or in the thalamus. Locally delivered synthetic ACTH activated the steroid-sensitive neurons. Noradrenaline and dopamine inhibited, and acetylcholine activated dexamethasone-sensitive neurons. These results could indicate that specific nerve cells in the hypothalamus and midbrain are sensitive to both hormonal and neurohumoural factors.

REFERENCES

BOGDANOVE, E. M. (1963) Direct gonad-pituitary feedback: an analysis of effects of intracranial estrogenic depots on gonadotrophin secretion. *Endocrinology*, **73**, 696–712.

CHOWERS, J., FELDMAN, S. AND DAVIDSON, J. M. (1963) Effects of intrahypothalamic crystalline steroids on acute ACTH secretion. *Am. J. Physiol.*, **205**, 671–673.

CURTIS, D. R. (1964) Micro-electrophoresis. In *Physical Techniques in Biological Research*, vol. 5, Part A, W. L. NASTUK (Ed.), Academic Press, London, pp. 144–190.

ENDRÖCZI, E., LISSAK, K. AND TEKERES, M. (1961) Hormonal feedback regulation of pituitary adrenocortical activity. *Acta physiol. Acad. Sci. Hung.*, **18**, 291–299.

FELDMAN, S. AND DAFNY, N. (1966) Effect of hydrocortisone on single cell activity in the anterior hypothalamus. *Israel J. med. Sci.*, **2**, 621–623.

DE GROOT, J. (1959) The rat forebrain in stereotaxic coordinates. *Trans. Roy. Netherlands Acad. Sci.*, **52**, 1–40.

KRAICER, J., MILLIGAN, J. V., GOSBEE, J. L., CONRAD, R. G. AND BRANSON, C. M. (1969) Potassium, corticosterone, and adrenocorticotropic hormone release *in vitro*. *Science*, **164**, 426.

RUF, K. AND STEINER, F. A. (1967a) Steroid-sensitive single neurons in rat hypothalamus and midbrain: identification by micro-electrophoresis. *Science*, **156**, 667–669.

RUF, K. AND STEINER, F. A. (1967b) Feedback regulation of ACTH secretion. Suppression of single neurons in rat brain by dexamethasone micro-electrophoresis. *Acta Endocrinol.*, Suppl. 119, 38.

SAWYER, C. H., KAWAKAMI, M., MEYERSON, B., WHITMOYER, D. I. AND LILLEY, J. J. (1968) Effects of ACTH, dexamethasone and asphyxia on electrical activity of the rat hypothalamus. *Brain Res.*, **10**, 213–226.

SLUSHER, M. A., HYDE, J. E. AND LAUFER, M. (1966) Effect of intracerebral hydrocortisone on unit activity of diencephalon and midbrain in cats. *J. Neurophysiol.*, **29**, 157–169.

SMELIK, P. G. AND SAWYER, C. H. (1962) Effects of implantation of cortisol into the brain stem or pituitary gland on the adrenal response to stress in the rabbit. *Acta Endocrinol.*, **41**, 561–570.

STEINER, F. A., PIERI, L. AND KAUFMANN, L. (1968) Effects of dopamine and ACTH on steroid-sensitive single neurons in the basal hypothalamus. *Experientia*, **24**, 1133–1134.

STEINER, F. A., RUF, K. AND AKERT, K. (1969) Steroid-sensitive neurons in rat brain: anatomic localization and responses to neurohumours and ACTH. *Brain Res.*, **12**, 74–85.

THOMAS, R. C. AND WILSON, V. J. (1965) Precise localization of Renshaw cells with a new marking technique. *Nature*, **206**, 211–213.

WOODBURY, D. M. AND VERNADAKIS, A. (1967) Influence of hormones on brain activity. In: *Neuroendocrinology*, Vol. II, GANONG AND MARTINI (Eds.), Academic Press, New York and London, pp. 335–375.

DISCUSSION

FELDMAN: Is the density of steroid-sensitive neurons higher in any particular part of the hypothalamus?

STEINER: So far, we have restricted our investigations to neurons situated in or near the midsagittal plane. In these regions no conspicuous differences of density have been observed.

HENKIN: What percentage of the number of units measured was steroid sensitive?

STEINER: Sixteen per cent of spontaneously active neurons were depressed by microelectrophoretically applied dexamethasone phosphate.

KLEIN: Is it fair to state that all cells that did not respond were intrinsically different, *i.e.* "non steroid-responsive", or could this be a technical problem?

STEINER: We do think that technical reasons cannot account for this difference and therefore these non-responding neurons are probably different from the steroid-sensitive neurons.

LARON: Is it possible that the sensitive and the non-sensitive cells represent interchangeable states of the same kind of cells rather than that they represent two types of cells which permanently act differently.

STEINER: We cannot exclude the possibility that we are dealing with interchangeable states of the same kind of neuron, but we think that the two types of cells represent different populations.

FELDMAN: There are a number of neurons that are non-responsive to sensory stimulation and are also non-responsive to hormones. Maybe there exists some connection between these properties.

MARKS: In your model you propose that dexamethasone acts on the nerve cell membrane. How do you distinguish between pre- and post-synaptic effects?

STEINER: The technique of microelectrophoresis with extracellular recording of action potentials does not allow us to distinguish between pre- and post-synaptic effects.

McEWEN: Could you comment on the time course of the action of hormones? The cellular action of hormones may be distinguished on the basis of whether they act with a short lag period and for a short time (membrane effects) or with a longer lag period and for a longer time (protein synthesis, metabolic effects). Protein synthesis effects may involve a considerable lag period for production and transport of the protein to the site of action and may last for a long time until the proteins formed are used up.

STEINER: We have observed short term effects. Still, it is possible to divide these short term effects in two classes: 1, Effects with a very short latency, 2, Effects with a longer latency (several seconds). We have not been able to observe long term effects. Sawyer and co-workers have described short term (activation) and long term (inhibition) effects after ACTH.

BOHUS: Do you possess any evidence concerning steroid and ACTH sensitivity of thalamic and mesencephalic reticular neurons?

STEINER: We have not found steroid-sensitive cells in the thalamus. ACTH was not applied to thalamic neurons. In the mesencephalic area some steroid-sensitive cells were observed, but we have no data about ACTH.

SMELIK: It is tempting to conclude from your data that the steroid-sensitive cells are directly involved in the control of the pituitary–adrenal system. This need not be so, it is equally possible that these effects of dexamethasone are on cells belonging to other systems. The fact that application of much greater amounts of dexamethasone phosphate in this area inhibits the secretion of ACTH after a considerable delay of several hours, should caution us in interpreting your results, since in your experiments the effect on the rate of firing can be observed within a few seconds.

STEINER: I agree with you; the interpretation of these results is difficult and should be done with caution. We have discussed possibilities other than a direct action on the control of the pituitary–adrenal system in our papers.

Effects of ACTH and Related Polypeptides on Spinal Cord

WILLIAM A. KRIVOY

National Institute of Mental Health*, Addiction Research Center, P.O. Box 2000, Lexington, Kentucky (U.S.A.)

The fundamental hypothesis underlying this review is that certain polypeptides play a role in the nervous system as modulators of nervous activity. That is to say, they do not detonate nerve cells, but they alter the threshold for synaptic activation, as may occur in changes of central excitatory state. The evidence necessary to evaluate this hypothesis is not complete, but that which is available is compatible with it (Krivoy, Lane, and Kroeger, 1963). The melanotropic hormones, ACTH, α-MSH, and β-MSH are potential candidates for being modulator-transmitters for the following reasons. A substance with melanotropic activity has been found in the central nervous system (Mattei, 1928; Guillemin, Hearn, Cheek, and Householder, 1957; Mailhe-Voloss, 1958). Melanocytes are derived from the neural crest (Rawles, 1947). α-MSH and β-MSH are destroyed by an enzyme which is found in the brain (Long, Krivoy, and Guillemin, 1961). A number of pharmacological agents, such as chlorpromazine and caffeine, which are active on the nervous system, also alter dispersion of melanphores (Teague, Noojin, and Geiling, 1939; Scott and Nading, 1961). Finally, as will be considered in the following pages, ACTH and certain related peptides have an action on the nervous system.

The purpose of this review is to consider the actions of ACTH, and polypeptides similar to ACTH, on spinal cord. It should be emphasized that, although many of the studies cited permit conclusion related either to the spinal cord as a reflex pathway, or as an intercept between more peripherally and more centrally located tissues, the spinal cord can also be used as a model for studying those phenomena which also occur higher in the neuraxis. The reason for using spinal cord as a model is its relative simplicity, both anatomically, and in the fact that in spinal cord one can measure those phenomena which might be associated with the influence of "modulator-transmitters" (Krivoy, Lane, and Kroeger, 1963).

I. ACTIONS OF ACTH ON SPINAL CORD

a. Intact animals

Ferrari, Floris, and Paulesu (1955), Ferrari and Vargiu (1956a) and Ferrari, Gessa, and

* U.S. Department of Health, Education and Welfare, Public Health Service, Health Services and Mental Health Administration.

Vargiu (1963) reported that approximately 60 min after the intracisternal administration of ACTH (but not after somatotropin, thyrotropin, oxytocin, gonadotropin, insulin or bovine serum albumin) dogs began stretching repeatedly. The authors termed this a "stretching crisis". Additional symptoms which are at least mediated by way of the spinal cord include muscle tremors, scratching and vomiting. Similar phenomena were seen after intracisternal injection of ACTH in rabbits, rats, cats, and monkeys (Ferrari and Vargiu, 1956b; Ferrari, Gessa, and Vargiu, 1960). Symptoms such as sleep or behavioral changes were also reported, but are not the immediate province of this review. Given intrathecally in man, ACTH produces some stretching and vomiting. The latter symptom is thought due to impurities in the preparation (Floris, 1963).

The "stretching crisis" was evoked in dogs following the intracisternal injection of ACTH 0.006 IU/kg, whereas as much as one IU/kg given intravenously, or 10I U/kg given by intracarotid injection produced no obvious change in nervous activity (Ferrari, Floris, and Paulesu, 1957; Ferrari, 1958; Ferrari et al., 1963).

Later investigations with highly purified or synthetic ACTH yielded essentially the same results in lower animals as those reported in the preceding two paragraphs (Ferrari et al., 1960, 1963; Gessa, Vargiu, and Ferrari, 1966). That is, approximately 60 min after intracisternal injection into dogs, cats or monkeys, a "stretching crisis" ensued.

Adrenalectomy did not alter the production of the "stretching crisis" by ACTH, thereby demonstrating an extra-adrenal mechanism (Ferrari et al., 1957; Ferrari, 1958; Ferrari et al., 1963). Additional evidence for an extra-adrenal mechanism was the fact that boiling ACTH in NaOH causes disappearance of corticotropic activity, but no disappearance of neurotropic activity (Ferrari, Gessa, and Vargiu, 1959; Ferrari et al., 1963).

Nicolov (1967), using electrophysiological techniques, studied the actions of ACTH in dogs with electrodes chronically implanted in their spinal cords. His observations were in some respects similar to those related in the preceding paragraphs of this section, but dissimilar in others. In agreement, Nicolov found that, after a latent period, the electrical activity of the spinal cord increased. In disagreement, the latency was somewhat shorter, with demonstrable effects after 15 min. More importantly, Nicolov found that he could evoke the response by injecting the ACTH intramuscularly (2 U/kg). No attempt was made to separate the actions of ACTH directly on the nervous system from those mediated via the adrenal cortex. In fact, the author reported effects of hydrocortisone similar to those of ACTH.

b. Spinal cats

In contrast to the observations reported in the preceding section, Guillemin and Krivoy (1960) and Krivoy and Guillemin (1961) were unable to detect any action of highly purified ACTH on the ventral root potential evoked by stimulation of the dorsal root (the Lloyd preparation) at a frequency of 0.5 cps and using submaximal stimuli. Decerebrate cats with a low spinal section were used in this study. The dose of ACTH was 50 μg/kg and it was given intravenously.

II. RELATED PEPTIDES

a. Intact animals

Both highly purified and synthetic α-MSH and β-MSH also produce the "stretching crisis" when injected intracisternally into intact and adrenalectomized dogs, as well as intact dogs, rabbits, cats and monkeys (Ferrari and Vargiu, 1956b; Ferrari *et al.*, 1960, 1963; Ferrari, Gessa, and Vargiu, 1961; Gessa *et al.*, 1966). The minimal effective dose of α-MSH required to produce the "stretching crisis" was somewhat higher in the intact dog (40 μg/kg), than was the dose of β-MSH (10 μg/kg) when given by intracisternal injection. Neither drug evoked this response when given by intracarotid injection (Ferrari *et al.*, 1963).

Since boiling α-MSH, β-MSH, or ACTH in NaOH resulted in loss of their corticotropic activity without destroying their neurotropic activity, while boiling in HCl destroyed both actions, Ferrari *et al.* (1959, 1963) concluded that a polypeptide chain was necessary for the neurotropic activity, but that it was shorter than that required to maintain corticotropic activity. This led to a search for an active nucleus predicated upon similarities between ACTH, α-MSH and β-MSH. The amino acid sequence ACTH 4–10 (β-MSH 7–13), ACTH 5–10, and ACTH 6–10 were each increasingly less effective in evoking the "stretching crisis". These observations suggested that at least part of the ACTH molecule was necessary for neurotropic activity, and that the sequence ACTH 4–10 appears to be particularly important.

In all of the experiments related thus far in this section, there was a latent period of approximately one hour before the onset of the "stretching crisis".

Cotzias (1967), using patients with Parkinson's disease, observed muscle tremors after the intramuscular injection of β-MSH (20–40 mg IM). No statement was made regarding latency of this phenomenon.

b. Spinal cats

Using the Lloyd preparation under the same conditions described earlier (Ib), it was observed that within 4 min after the intravenous administration of β-MSH (2 μg/kg) there appeared a facilitation of the ventral root response to dorsal root stimulation (Guillemin and Krivoy, 1960; Krivoy and Guillemin, 1961). This action of β-MSH was seen after a latent period of approximately 5 min, reached a maximum after 15 to 20 min, and lasted in excess of one hour. α-MSH was found to be ineffective in doses up to 20 μg/kg given intravenously.

As will be described later, β-MSH was found to antagonize actions of bradykinin (Bk) on spinal cord dorsal root potentials. This suggested that similarities between Bk and β-MSH might account for their neurotropic activity (Krivoy, Bodanszky and Lande, 1963). Comparison of the sequence β-MSH 9–17 and of Bk (Fig. 1) reveals certain similarities. β-MSH 9 and 17 are basic amino acids, as are the terminal amino acids of Bk. Immediately adjacent to these basic amino acids are a Pro-Pro on the one hand, and a Phe on the other. Similarly, comparison of Bk with β-MSH 9–17 shows a Ser at Bk 6, in common with Ser at β-MSH 14. These similarities between β-MSH and

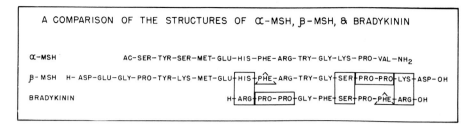

Fig. 1. The amino acid sequence of α-MSH, β-MSH, and of bradykinin, indicating points of similarity between β-MSH and bradykinin.

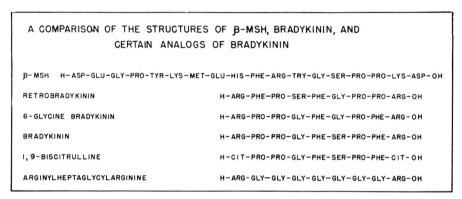

Fig. 2. The amino acid sequence of the peptides used to test the importance of those sequences which are common to bradykinin and to β-MSH.

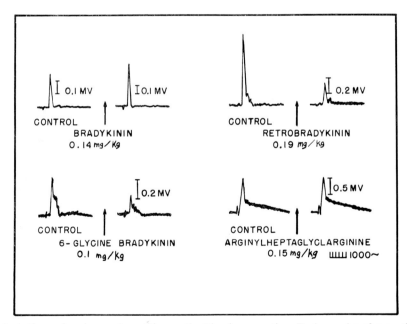

Fig. 3. Actions of various polypeptides on the Lloyd preparation. Each couplet of potentials was obtained from an experiment on a separate cat, and is typical of the pre- and post-drug record (control and experimental). The drugs used in each experiment are indicated.

References pp. 117–118

DRUG	ACTION ON RAT UTERUS	ACTION ON MEAN BLOOD PRESSURE OF THE CAT	ACTION ON CAT SPINAL CORD	ANTAGONISM BY β-MSH
BRADYKININ	↑	↘ DURATION: ABOUT 30 MIN. WITH 100 µg/kg	↗ ONSET: 2 MIN. TIME TO MAXIMUM: 10 MIN. DURATION: >120 MIN. MINIMAL DOSE:<0.08 mg/kg	
6-GLYCINE BRADYKININ	↑	↘ DURATION: ABOUT 30 MIN. WITH 200 µg/kg	↘ ONSET: IMMEDIATE TIME TO MAXIMUM: 5 MIN. DURATION: >55 MIN. MINIMAL DOSE:<0.05 mg/kg	+
1,9-BISCITRULLINE BRADYKININ	<1/4,000	○ DOSE TRIED: 200 µg/kg	○ DOSE TRIED:>0.14 mg/kg	
RETRO-BRADYKININ	<1/80,000	○ DOSE TRIED: 200 µg/kg	↘ ONSET: IMMEDIATE TIME TO MAXIMUM:>50 MIN. DURATION:>50 MIN. MINIMAL DOSE: 0.05 mg/kg	○
ARGINYLHEPTA-GLYCYLARGININE	<1/4,000	○ DOSE TRIED: 200 µg/kg	○ DOSE TRIED:>0.25 mg/kg	

↗ INCREASE   + − ANTAGONISM OBSERVED
↘ DECREASE   ○ − ANTAGONISM LOOKED FOR, BUT NOT OBSERVED

Fig. 4. Comparison of the actions of bradykinin and some of its analogues on rat uterus, cat blood pressure, and cat spinal cord.

Bk are not shared with α-MSH. However, these being unusual characteristics of β-MSH and Bk, it was of interest to test their contribution to the neurotropic activity of these peptides. To test the importance of the basic terminal amino acids, arginyl-heptaglycylarginine was synthesized. To test the importance of the basic amino acids relative to the rest of molecule 1,9-biscitrulline-Bk was synthesized. To test the importance of Ser at Bk 6, 6-glycine-Bk was synthesized. To test the importance of the position of Arg-Phe and Pro-Pro-Arg, retro-Bk was synthesized. These polypeptides, shown in Fig. 2, were synthesized by Dr. M. Bodanszky, and then tested electro-physiologically using the Lloyd preparation described in section 1b (Krivoy and Guillemin, 1961). After a control period lasting one hour, the peptides being investigated were injected intravenously. In Fig. 3, typical examples of the potentials recorded during the control period and during the post-drug period are presented for each of the drugs tested, with the exception of 1,9-biscitrulline-Bk. The latter drug, like arginyl-heptaglycylarginine, produced no change in the dorsal root potential. However, it may be seen that retro-Bk depressed spinal reflexes, as did 6-Gly-Bk. β-MSH was found capable of antagonizing 6-Gly-Bk, but not retro-Bk (Fig. 4). In the large doses used, Bk was found to be a stimulant of spinal cord (Figs. 3 and 4).

Comparing the actions of these polypeptides on rat uterus, cat blood pressure, and cat spinal cord (Fig. 4) the authors (Krivoy, Bodanszky and Lande, 1963) concluded that there is no obvious relation between the actions of these substances on these three test systems.

Because of the failure of 1,9-biscitrulline-Bk to exert an action, it was concluded that the terminal basic amino acids are important to the action of these peptides. These are not the only important components since arginylheptaglycylarginine was also without action. The positions of the Arg-Pro and of the Pro-Pro-Arg are also important as evidenced by the antagonism between β-MSH and retro-Bk. Similarly, the 6-Ser of Bk is important in that in these large doses Bk produced facilitation of spinal reflexes, whereas 6-Gly-Bk produced depression.

Also seen in Fig. 4 is the fact that there was a latent period associated with the actions of each of the peptides active on spinal cord.

III. INTERACTION WITH OTHER DRUGS

a. Intact animals

The "stretching crisis" induced by ACTH, β-MSH or α-MSH was found to be antagonized by chlorpromazine, atropine, scopolamine, and phenobarbital in un-anesthetized dogs. Melatonin, serotonin, and reserpine had no action. In anesthetized dogs the same authors found that morphine, chlorpromazine, diethazine and atropine were effective antagonists. Succinylcholine, mephenesin, reserpine, LSD, BrLSD, and GABA were practically inactive as antagonists (Ferrari *et al.*, 1963).

b. Spinal cats

Chlorpromazine has been found to depress the fifth dorsal root potential (DR V) of cat spinal cord (Krivoy and Kroeger, 1962). This potential arises from secondary neurons within the spinal cord (Lloyd and McIntyre, 1949). It is of long duration and associated with equally long periods of altered excitability of spinal neurons. β-MSH is able to antagonize this action of chlorpromazine (Krivoy and Guillemin, 1962). In addition, in the presence of chlorpromazine Bk depresses DR V, and this is antagonized by β-MSH (Krivoy, Lane and Kroeger, 1963).

IV. SITE OF ACTION

a. Intact animals

Gessa, Pisano, Vargiu, Crabai, and Ferrari (1967) attempted to gain insight into the site of action of ACTH. They did this by injecting synthetic ACTH into the brain of cats using chronically implanted cannulae. They demonstrated that the hypothalamic areas lining the third ventricle are the most sensitive parts of the brain to the neurotropic actions of ACTH, defined as production of the "stretching crisis".

Earlier in this review, citations were presented indicating that the phenomenon of the "stretching crisis" was extra-adrenal.

b. Spinal cats

By virtue of the fact that these preparations had a low spinal section, one must assume that the action was not superspinal in origin. However, the influence of the adrenal

References pp. 117–118

cortex was not directly evaluated. On the other hand, since neither ACTH nor α-MSH produced the enhancement of spinal transmission associated with β-MSH, it is not likely that the adrenal cortex was involved to any major extent.

DISCUSSION

In considering the observations presented, one must be mindful of the fact that although few laboratories have contributed information which is within the province of this review, each of the laboratories used a different preparation, measured a different phenomenon, and administered drugs by a different route. In fact, it was only recently that we could ascertain that most of the investigators were using the same drugs. Despite these problems, there is considerable agreement.

The majority of the investigations have supported the conclusion that in the intact animal, ACTH stimulates the spinal cord (Section 1a). It is not certain how much of this stimulation is due to a direct action on the spinal cord. At least part of it appears to be the consequence of stimulation at superspinal levels (Section IVa). One should recognize that the observations of Woodbury (1952), Torda and Wolff (1952), and DeSalva, Hendley, and Ercoli (1954) could also be due to an action of ACTH directly in the spinal cord, although this is unlikely.

The only reports in which a stimulant action of ACTH was not observed are those related in Section 1b, *i.e.*, where the preparation used was a cat with a low spinal section. It would therefore appear probable that ACTH has no action directly on the spinal cord below the level of L1, and that increased stretching and electrical activity of the spinal cord (Section 1a) originate at a higher level. Another explanation is that the quantity of ACTH which can get to active sites is less when the substance is given systemically than when it is given intracisternally. This explanation would seem inadequate in view of the findings of Nicolov (1967) that ACTH produces an increased electrical activity of dog spinal cord when the peptide is given intramuscularly. In the final analysis, it must be recognized that we are attempting to compare different preparations, and that they may be too different to permit valid comparison.

There is general agreement that β-MSH stimulates the nervous system if we can equate the "stretching crisis", the intramuscular administration of β-MSH in patients with Parkinson's disease (Section II a) and the observations based on electrophysiological techniques (section II b). The major disagreement here involves the effective route of administration. The "stretching crisis" was induced only when the peptides were given intracisternally, whereas the increased muscle tremors in patients with Parkinsonism were induced after intramuscular injection of β-MSH. This difference may be related to differences in the distribution of the β-MSH in each of the different experimental preparations used. It may be related to a different sensitivity of the experimental preparations, *i.e.*, it is possible that the patient with an extra-pyramidal lesion, and the Lloyd preparation with a low spinal lesion are more sensitive to β-MSH than the neuronal substrate responsible for the "stretching crisis". In this instance, the local application of β-MSH to nuclei associated with the "stretching crisis" would provide the local high concentration necessary to evoke the response, whereas larger

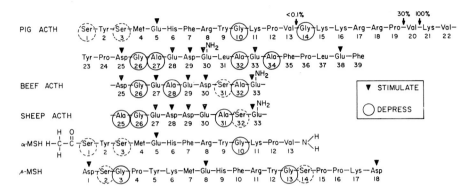

STRUCTURES AND BIOLOGICAL ACTIVITIES OF *ACTH* AND *MSH*

Fig. 5. The amino acid sequences of ACTH, α-MSH, and of β-MSH indicating those amino acids known to have stimulant or depressant activity. Arrows indicate residual corticotropic activity after degradation of the ACTH molecule.

amounts given peripherally would be diluted by the blood before they could get to the effective nuclei. The latter is not considered too likely an explanation by Ferrari *et al.*, (1963), who tried intracarotid administration and found it ineffective. Perhaps the most likely explanation of the divergence of observation is that the distribution of the peptide is different in each of the preparations used.

In contrast to the observations on β-MSH, those relating to α-MSH are in complete disagreement (Section II a and b). The "stretching crisis" could be induced by the intracisternal injection of α-MSH, but there was no alteration in the electrical signs of nervous activity in the Lloyd preparation following the intravenous administration of the same peptide. The explanations of this divergence follow our previous reasoning. First, it can be argued that the preparations were adequately similar to respond to β-MSH, but not to α-MSH. Secondly, the distribution of α-MSH may be different from that of β-MSH.

The observations reported in Section II were actually part of two separate attempts to learn more of the structure–activity relationships which might exist between neurotropic polypeptides. Therefore, some comments on structure–activity relationships are in order at this time.

Investigations into the structure–activity relationships of neurotropic polypeptides have generally been concerned with an active nucleus or sequence of amino acids. Although there is obvious merit in this approach, it is based upon indirect evidence. More direct evidence could be obtained by testing a solution of these amino acids which constitute ACTH or MSH, but in the same proportion that they normally occur.

It has been suggested that certain of the polypeptide venoms owe their activity to the fact that they are broken down and that the amino acid composition, or pool, determines the pharmacologic activity, as opposed to the sequence determining activity (Meldrum, 1965). In Fig. 5 are the sequences of ACTH and MSH with those amino acids identified which are known to stimulate or to depress the spinal cord (Curtis and

Watkins, 1965; Curtis, Hosli, and Johnston, 1968). It may be seen that the majority of active amino acids are in ACTH, the least neurotropically active of the three peptides. Therefore, this hypothesis would appear unlikely as it concerns the neurotropic polypeptides. However, we do not know the actions of the other amino acids on the spinal cord. Consequently the experiment proposed in the preceding paragraph is still in order.

It is conceivable that β-MSH owes parts of its neurotropic activity to terminal amino acids which have been found to be stimulant in spinal cord (Fig. 5). This might explain the difference observed between α-MSH and β-MSH in the Lloyd preparation. However, it is an unlikely explanation if one adheres to current theories of why amino acids act on neurons since they suppose the availability of an amino group and of a carboxyl group separated by a relatively short distance (Curtis and Watkins, 1965; Purpura, Girado, Smith, Callan, and Grundfest, 1959). On the other hand, peptides of the length being considered here could easily act by a different mechanism than do the amino acids. This concept has yet to be evaluated.

There seems to be general agreement that a long latent period precedes the action of these peptides. This could be ascribed to several causes. First, it is possible that the peptides do not act per se, but through an intermediate mechanism. One such mechanism might be the adrenal cortex. Since the peptides were found active after adrenalectomy, this explanation seems unlikely. Another explanation is that these substances alter the metabolism of the nervous system, and that this alteration requires time to become manifest. An alternative explanation is that the peptides do not act directly on receptors within the nervous system, but do so only after they have been further degraded or incorporated into larger or smaller peptides. These latter two explanations remain to be investigated. The latent period may be due simply to a failure of sufficiently rapid distribution of the drugs to active sites. These too remain to be investigated. The final attempt at explaining the long latency to maximal action resides in a postulated mechanism of action of β-MSH. It has been demonstrated that β-MSH alters the recovery period of nerve cells, causing these cells to remain in an hyperexcitable state for a longer period of time. It was further pointed out that with continuous input, these phenomena will summate with time (Krivoy, Lane, and Kroeger, 1963). It is possible that the latent period represents that amount of time required for suffcient summation to take place so that this hyperexcitability becomes manifest.

Evidence supporting the hypothesis that ACTH, α-MSH, or β-MSH are either neurohumors, or chemically related to neurohumors which subserve a modulator function, has already been presented in the introduction to this communication. This review has emphasized three additional pieces of evidence. First, not only do these three peptides act on spinal cord to alter synaptic transmission, but this alteration appears to be in the nature of a facilitation of normally active pathways, so that transmission through these pathways occurs more readily. Second, peptides similar to ACTH, α-MSH, or β-MSH also alter synaptic transmission. Third, drugs which have been found to antagonize the actions of ACTH, α-MSH, and β-MSH on the nervous system, also decrease the central excitatory state.

The preceding paragraph is an attempt at drawing together the little evidence we have to suggest that these peptides are associated with synaptic transmission, particularly in the spinal cord. A number of pieces of information are lacking and preclude serious conclusion. Thus, although there has been demonstration of an action on the nervous system, we have yet to have specific antagonists or potentiators of this action. We have yet to demonstrate the release of these substances from the nervous system in concert with nervous activity. Hopefully, when the evidence is fully assembled we will know whether ACTH, α-MSH, or β-MSH are active participants in synaptic transmission, whether they are similar to peptides which are active, or if peptides have a physiological role in synaptic transmission.

CONCLUSIONS

ACTH and related polypeptides are capable of altering transmission in the spinal cord under a variety of conditions. Although their action at this site supports the idea that they are active in synaptic transmission, and that they are able to modulate activity at this site, considerably more evidence is required before their importance or role can be ascertained.

REFERENCES

COTZIAS, G., VAN WOERT, M. AND SCHIFFER, L. (1967) Aromatic amino acids and modification of parkinsonism. *New Engl. J. Med.*, **276**, 374–380.

CURTIS, D., HOSLI, L., AND JOHNSTON, G. (1968) A pharmacological study of the depression of spinal neurones by glycine and related amino acids. *Exptl. Brain Res.*, **6**, 1–18.

CURTIS, D. AND WATKINS, J. (1965) The pharmacology of amino acids related to gamma-amino butyric acid. *Pharmacol. Rev.*, **17**, 347–392.

DESALVA, J., HENDLEY, C. AND ERCOLI, N. (1954) Acute effects of ACTH and cortisone on brain excitability. *Arch. Intern. Pharmacodyn.*, **100**, 35–48.

FERRARI, W. (1958) Influenza direttamente l'ipofisi l'attivata di alcuni centri nervosi. *Arch. ital. Sci. farmacol.*, **8**, 3–14.

FERRARI, W., FLORIS, E. AND PAULESU, F. (1955) Su di una particolare imponente sintomatologia prodotta nel cane dall'ACTH iniettato nella cisterna magna. *Boll. Soc. ital. Biol. sper.*, **31**, 862–864.

FERRARI, W., FLORIS, E. AND PAULESU, F. (1957) Su di una particolare imponente sintomatologia prodotta nel cane dall'ACTH iniettato nella "cisterna magna". *Arch. Intern. Pharmacodyn.*, **110**, 410–422.

FERRARI, W., GESSA, G. AND VARGIU, L. (1959) Sulle crisi di stiramento da iniezione endocisternale di ACTH. (VII) Prevalente importanza dell'attivita melanoforostimolante rispetto a quella adrenocorticotropica. *Boll. Soc. ital. Biol. Sper.*, **35**, 509–510.

FERRARI, W., GESSA, G. AND VARGIU, L. (1960) Sulle "crisi stiramento" da iniezione endocisternale, nel cane, di ACTH. (VIII) Attivita dell'intermedina. *Boll. Soc. ital. Biol. sper.*, **36**, 335–376.

FERRARI, W., GESSA, G. AND VARGIU, L. (1961) Stretching activity in dogs intracisternally injected with synthetic melanocyte stimulating hormone. *Experientia*, **17**, 90.

FERRARI, W., GESSA, G. AND VARGIU, L. (1963) Behavioral effects induced by intracisternally injected ACTH and MSH. *Ann. N.Y. Acad. Sci.*, **104**, 330–343.

FERRARI, W. AND VARGIU, L. (1956a) Sulle "crisi di stiramento" da iniezioni endocisternali di ACTH. III. Importanza dell'ormone melanoforostimolante. *Boll. Soc. ital. Biol. sper.*, **32**, 517–519.

FERRARI, W. AND VARGIU, L. (1956b) Effetti dell'introduzione endocisternale di intermedina in differenti specie animali. *Boll. Soc. ital. Biol. sper.*, **32**, 1368–1369.

FLORIS, E. (1963) Effetti dell'iniezione endorachnidea nell'uomo di ACTH. *Boll. Soc. ital. Biol. sper.*, **39**, 558–560.

GESSA, G., PISANO, M., VARGIU, F., CRABAI, F. AND FERRARI, W. (1967) Stretching and yawning movements after intracerebral injection of ACTH. *Rev. Canad. Biol.*, **26**, 229–236.

GESSA, G., VARGIU, L. AND FERRARI, W. (1966) Stretchings and yawnings induced by adrenocortico-tropic hormone. *Nature*, **211**, 426–427.

GUILLEMIN, R., HEARN, W., CHEEK, W. AND HOUSEHOLDER, D. (1957) Control of corticotropin release: further studies with *in vitro* methods. *Endocrinology*, **60**, 488–506.

GUILLEMIN, R. AND KRIVOY, W. (1960) L'hormone mélanophorétique β-MSH joue-t-elle un rôle dans les fonctions du système nerveux central chez les mammifères supérieurs. *Compt. Rend.*, **250**, 1117–1119.

KRIVOY, W., BODANSZKY, M. AND LANDE, S. (1963) Neurological and oxytocic actions of some no-napeptides related to bradykinin. *Biochem. Pharmacol.*, **12**, (Supp.), 179–180.

KRIVOY, W. AND GUILLEMIN, R. (1961) On a possible role of β-melanocyte stimulating hormone (β-MSH) in the central nervous system of the mammalia: an effect of β-MSH in the spinal cord of the cat. *Endocrinology*, **69**, 170–175.

KRIVOY, W. AND GUILLEMIN, R. (1962) Antagonism of chlorpromazine by β-melanocyte stimulating hormone (β-MSH). *Experientia*, **18**, 20–21.

KRIVOY, W. AND KROEGER, D. (1962) Chlorpromazine inhibition of the positive intermediary potential. *Proc. Soc. exptl. Biol. Med.*, **109**, 30–32.

KRIVOY, W., LANE, M. AND KROEGER, D. (1963) The actions of certain polypeptides on synaptic transmission. *Ann. N.Y. Acad. Sci.*, **104**, 312–329.

LLOYD, D. AND McINTYRE, A. (1949) On the origins of dorsal root potentials. *J. gen. Physiol.*, **32**, 409–443.

LONG, J., KRIVOY, W. AND GUILLEMIN, R. (1961) On a possible role of β-melanocyte stimulating hormone (β-MSH) in the central nervous system of mammalia: enzymatic inactivation *in vitro* of β-MSH by brain tissue. *Endocrinology*, **69**, 176–181.

MATTEI, P. DI (1928) Sopra l'espansione dei melanofori della rana come saggio biologico degli estratti ipofisori e sull'influenza che vi spiega il clorotone. *Arch. intern. Pharmacodyn.*, **34**, 309–330.

MELDRUM, B. S. (1965) The actions of snake venoms on nerve and muscle. The pharmacology of phospholipase A and of polypeptide toxins. *Pharmacol. Rev.*, **19**, 393–445.

MAILHE-VOLOSS, C. (1958) Activité corticotrope des extraits post-hypophysaires. *Acta Endocrinol.*, Supp. XXXV, 9–96.

NICOLOV, N. (1967) Effect of hydrocortisone and ACTH upon the bioelectric activity of spinal cord. *Folia med. (Plovdiv)*, **9**, 249–255.

PURPURA, D., GIRADO, T., SMITH, D., CALLAN, D. AND GRUNDFEST, H. (1959) Structure–activity determinants of pharmacological effects of amino acids and related compounds on central synapses. *J. Neurochem.*, **3**, 238–268.

RAWLES, M. E. (1947) Origin of pigment cells from the neural crest in the mouse. *Physiological Zoology*, **20**, 248–265.

SCOTT, G. AND NADING, L. (1961) Relative effectiveness of phenothiazine tranquilizing drugs causing release of MSH. *Proc. Soc. Exptl. Biol. Med.*, **106**, 88–90.

TEAGUE, R., NOOJIN, R. AND GEILING, E. (1939) The hypophysectomized frog (*Rana pipiens*) as a specific test object for melanophore hormone of the pituitary body. *J. Pharmacol. Exptl. Therap.*, **65**, 115–127.

TORDA, C. AND WOLFF, H. (1952) Effects of various concentrations of adrenocorticotrophic hormone on electrical activity of brain and on sensitivity to convulsion-inducing agents. *Am. J. Physiol.*, **168**, 406–413.

WOODBURY, D. (1952) Effect of adrenocortical steroids and adrenocorticotrophic hormone on electro-shock seizure threshold. *J. Pharmacol. Exptl. Therap.*, **105**, 27–36.

DISCUSSION

HENKIN: Do you have any information about excitatory or inhibitory effects on the spinal cord of thiol-containing amino acids such as methionine or cysteine? You are probably aware that Nach-manson feels that thiol-containing amino acids, or even thiols themselves, are critical for normal synaptic transmission.

KRIVOY: This is an important point, but we have not performed experiments using thiol-containing amino acids.

MARKS: Do these peptides actually get to the areas in the central nervous system that you have been discussing?

KRIVOY: We presume that if they act, they get to the effective site. In this preparation it is likely that the blood-brain barrier has been reduced so that penetration of these solutions into the central nervous system takes place.

MIRSKY: Is it possible that the different relative activities of the peptides are related to their ability to withstand degradation in passage through the different sites?

KRIVOY: This might explain the different potencies of these compounds.

DENTON: Have you tested the octapeptide angiotensin-II or the decapeptide angiotensin-I in this context?

KRIVOY: These compounds have not been tested.

Influence of Pituitary–Adrenocortical Hormones on Thalamo–Cortical and Brain Stem Limbic Circuits

L. KORÁNYI and E. ENDRÖCZI

Institute of Physiology, University Medical School, Rákóczi út 80, Pécs (Hungary)

It is well established that motivated behavioral processes are integrated at the brain stem and diencephalic level and are conditioned by humoral factors. The limbic system is also involved in these processes; however, its role is a modifying rather than an integrating one.

The main connections of the brain stem and basal forebrain structures playing a role in the organization of motivated behavioral reactions are shown in Fig. 1. The ascending activatory system, through multisynaptic and oligosynaptic pathways, influences the forebrain which is known to be involved in the organization of complex behavioral mechanisms and the regulation of pituitary functions. On the other hand, the descending inhibitory pathways of basal forebrain origin, terminating both at the thalamic and brain stem level, play an important role in the control of sensory input. In recent years, our attention has been focussed on the functions of the basal forebrain in relation to motivated behavioral processes. Experimental findings obtained in different experimental circumstances are summarized on the Table I. The main conclusion of these data is that the basal forebrain plays a basic role in the organization of sleep, reinforcement, and inhibition of brain stem and spinal reflexes (Hess, 1944; Nauta, 1945; Waldvogel, 1945; Adey *et al.*, 1957; Endröczi and Lissák, 1962; Endröczi *et al.*, 1964; Endröczi and Korányi, 1965, 1968; Hernandez-Peón *et al.*, 1963; Korányi and Endröczi, 1965; Korányi, 1965; Korányi *et al.*, 1963; Lissák and Endröczi, 1965, 1967; Clemente *et al.*, 1966).

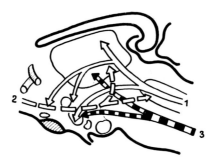

Fig. 1. The main connections of the brain stem and the forebrain which are involved in the organization of motivated behavioral processes and neuroendocrine responses. Ascending activatory (1) and the descending inhibitory (2) pathways and oligosynaptic connections (3) coming from specific projections.

TABLE I

EEG AND BEHAVIORAL CHANGES FOLLOWING BASAL FOREBRAIN STIMULATION

1. EEG synchronization
2. Inhibition of conditioned reflex activity and inter-trial responses
3. Inhibition of stress response
4. Inhibition of sensory input
5. Inhibition of mono- and polysynaptic reflex activity

Recent observations clearly show that corticosteroids, like other steroids of gonadal sources, can modify the central nervous system at two different levels and two different ways. Fig. 2 illustrates those routes which may be involved in corticosteroid action on the central nervous processes, and suggests priority of a neuronal excitability state which basically determines the behavioral resultant of hormonal influence. The hormones may exert both a facilitatory or an inhibitory effect, and the behavioral outcome can be facilitation or inhibition, depending on the site of action. According to this assumption, opposite behavioral effects of corticosteroids may explain changes in mood and emotionality in human beings, as well as diverse behavioral manifestations in different species, ambivalent reactions or rebound-like phenomena in the same individual.

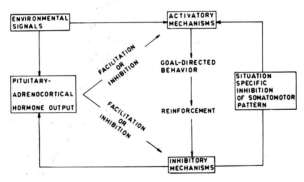

Fig. 2. For explanation see text.

A great number of data accumulated over recent years suggest that pituitary–adrenocortical hormones enhance different kinds of internal inhibition under conditioned reflex circumstances (Lissák *et al.*, 1957; Lissák and Endröczi, 1964; Endröczi and Lissák, 1962; Korányi and Endröczi, 1965/66, 1967; Bohus and Endröczi, 1965; Bohus and Korányi, 1969; Bohus and Lissák, 1968; De Wied, 1966; Levine, 1968).

From a neurophysiological point of view, internal inhibition and learning processes form an inseparable functional unit, and the participation of basal forebrain structures in these mechanisms has been suggested by several observations. This report deals with studies of the effect of corticosteroids on basal forebrain functions and on thalamic and forebrain connections.

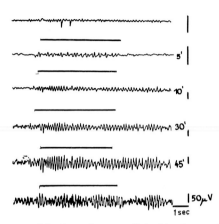

Fig. 3. Incremental responses of the frontal cortex elicited by 8 cps stimulation in the dorsomedial thalamic nuclei (3 V, 0.1 msec) before (upper record) and after 100 μg per 100 g hydrocortisone administration in the adrenalectomized rat. The time indicates the recordings after hydrocortisone injection. The last record shows the development of bursting theta rhythm in the hydrocortisone-treated animal.

Recruiting responses and spontaneous synchronization. Effect of corticosteroids on the "band-pass filtering" function of non-specific thalamic nuclei

Rats were immobilized with (±)-tubocurarine and the electrical activity of different parts of the central nervous system were recorded with a 12-channel EEG apparatus. Depending on stimulation parameters (frequency and intensity) bipolar electrical stimulation of non-specific thalamic nuclei may produce recruiting responses or desynchronization in the corticogram. Since the early observations of Dempsey and Morison (1942) and Morison and Dempsey (1942) the basic role of the non-specific dorsomedial and anterior thalamic nuclei in the organization of cortical augmenting responses evoked by low frequency stimulation of the ventrobasal complex of the thalamus or the brain stem reticular core, has been extensively studied and confirmed. In addition to the synchronizing function of the thalamic reticular system, the findings of Smirnov (1953) and Roitbak (1956) need to be recalled which pointed out that the cerebral cortex, in response to a train of stimuli, responds to every stimulus when the frequency is low. Increasing the frequency, the projection area fails to follow the rhythm of stimulation. According to the synaptological studies of Scheibel and Scheibel (1967) the nucleus reticularis thalami, as well as other non-specific thalamic nuclei, are functioning like "band-pass filters" and do not allow cell-firing toward the cortex because long-lasting (80 to 200 msec) inhibitory post-synaptic potentials in the diffuse thalamic reticular network determine the frequency specificity of triggered waves in the cortex (Purpura and Housepian, 1961; Purpura and Cohen, 1962; Purpura and Shofer, 1963).

In response to stimulation of non-specific thalamic nuclei, the development of incremental responses was markedly suppressed and the frequency-filtering capacity of the non-specific thalamic system was also impaired in adrenalectomized rats. Intravenous injection of hydrocortisone, 100 μg per 100 g body weight, led to normaliza-

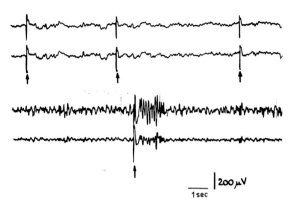

Fig. 4. Lack of spindling EEG after-discharges produced by single shocks in the dorsomedial thalamic nuclei in the adrenalectomized rat and its restoration after local injection of 5 μg hydrocortisone into the non-specific thalamic nuclei. Frontal records, suprathreshold stimulation intensity.

tion both of incremental responses and frequency-filtering capacity of the thalamo-cortical system within 30 to 45 min. The amplitude of the resting EEG activity became higher, however, spontaneous spindling activity did not appear but bursting slow waves in theta rhythm could be observed. The inappropriate post-synaptic inhibitory state at the thalamic neuronal network might be a possible interpretation for the lack of spontaneous thalamo–cortical synchronization and the impairment of recruiting responses in the adrenalectomized rats (Fig. 3). Local injection of 5 to 7 μg hydrocortisone in a volume of a few microliters of physiological saline solution into the dorsomedial complex of the thalamic nuclei resulted in augmentation of recruiting potentials and restored the filtering capacity of the system. Unilateral injection was effective on the thalamo–cortical circuit at ipsilateral side. Hydrocortisone injection into the preoptic region or basal and medial hypothalamus and the mammillary body area did not restore the recruiting responses in the adrenalectomized animals (Fig. 4).

The effect of corticosteroids on sensory afterdischarges following EEG arousal reaction

Bipolar electrical stimulation of the mesencephalic reticular formation (300 cps, 0.1 msec, 2.0 V) for 5 to 10 sec, results in EEG arousal lasting for 20 to 30 sec which is followed by bursting spindles as a rebound phenomenon of the forebrain synchronizing system in normal animals. This after-reaction was absent in adrenalectomized animals, namely, the EEG arousal was not followed by the typical low frequency, high amplitude pattern of synchronization characteristic to the intact animal. Intravenous injection of hydrocortisone or cortisone (dissolved in physiological saline solution) 100 μg per 100 g body weight, led to the normalization of this EEG phenomenon within 30 to 45 min. Aldosterone-treated adrenalectomized rats did not show signs of EEG after-reaction (Fig. 5).

Several investigators have reported the phenomenon of electro-encephalographic after-reaction, and its physiological properties have been analyzed in the course of sexual activity, conditioning and habituation (Sawyer and Kawakami, 1959; Hernan-

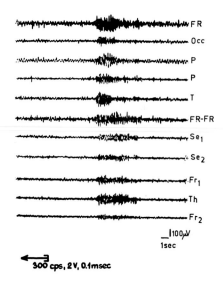

Fig. 5. Restoration of the EEG after-reaction by intravenous administration of 100 μg per 100 g body weight hydrocortisone in the adrenalectomized rat. The EEG arousal was elicited by high frequency stimulation of mesencephalic reticular formation 30 min after hydrocortisone injection. FR = frontal, Fr = Formatio reticularis mesencephali. Occ — occipital, P — parietal, Se — septal area. T — temporal, Th — nonspecific thalamic nuclei.

dez-Peón, 1960; Sadowski and Longo, 1962; Steiner, 1962; Clemente *et al.*, 1964, and others). It was concluded that it might be the expression of a type of internal inhibition (Magoun, 1962); but the mechanism and organization of this EEG phenomenon are not yet clearly understood.

It is known that the ablation of fronto-orbital cortex prevents the development of recruiting responses and spontaneous spindling in the thalamus and other parts of the cortex (Jouvet, 1961; Velasco and Lindsley, 1965). Recently, Endröczi, Korányi and Lissák (to be published) found that the removal of the basal forebrain area including the subcommissural preoptic region or bilateral lesions of the medial forebrain bundle at the anterior hypothalamic level prevented the development of the EEG after-reaction.

Intravenous injection of hydrocortisone, 100 μg per 100 g body weight, restored the EEG after-reaction in response to high frequency stimulation of the brain stem reticular formation. But local injection of hydrocortisone (5 to 7 μg), into the preoptic region led to normalization of the EEG after-reaction within 15 to 20 min after the corticosteroid had been injected into the thalamus of adrenalectomized rats. However, the local application of hydrocortisone into the thalamic reticular nuclei led to augmentation of recruitment in adrenalectomized animals. It was ineffective in restoring synchronized EEG after-reaction.

Concerning the action of corticosteroids and the mechanism of organization of recruiting responses, it is worth mentioning that the basal forebrain, namely, the orbito-frontal cortex and subcommissural preoptic region, play a basic role in the formation of incremental responses. Skinner and Lindsley (1967) reported that the cryo-blockade of subthalamic connections between non-specific thalamic nuclei and basal forebrain prevented the development of incremental responses elicited by the stimulation of the former nuclei. In recent studies we have observed that bilateral electrolytic lesions of the medial forebrain bundle, at the anterior hypothalamic level, led to the elimination of recruiting responses in rats. These observations indicated that the thalamo–cortical synchronization cannot be simply interpreted at the thalamic neuronal level only, and suggest that the basal forebrain structures are also deeply involved in this process.

The possibility of the extra-adrenal influence of ACTH on the central nervous processes

A number of data accumulated over the past years show that pituitary trophic hormones, in addition to their specific action on the target organs, exert a wide variety of extra-target effects. Concerning pituitary adrenocorticotropic hormone preparations, it is well known that crude pituitary extract, highly purified ACTH, or synthetic eicosapeptide-corticotrophin exert several extra-adrenal actions (Anselmino and Hoffmann, 1933; Dougherty and Berliner, 1958; Berliner *et al.*, 1961; Engel, 1961; Engel and Lebovitz, 1966; Kusama, 1963; Lebovitz, 1967; Trygstad, 1967). Recently we have reported (Korányi *et al.*, 1969a) that not only exogenous ACTH, but also endogenous ACTH liberated following systemic as well as psychic stress may induce hypoglycaemia. The modifying or mediating role of ACTH-induced insulin secretion and the resultant hypoglycaemia should be taken into account in the evaluation of changes of higher nervous activity, behavior and neural mechanisms of adrenalectomized or ACTH-treated animals.

The effects of ACTH on brain mechanisms have been studied in different laboratory animals (monkeys, dogs, cats, rabbits, rats and mice). Moiseev and Tonkikh (1940) were the first who suggested the involvement of pituitary hormones in the stimulation-induced internal inhibition. Borkovskaya and Fadeiva (1961) reported drowsiness following the administration of ACTH preceded by restlessness both in intact and adrenalectomized cats. These behavioral reactions could not be elicited by the administration of adrenocortical steroids.

In our earlier experiments, we observed that the intravenous injection of ACTH led to a suppression of conditioned avoidance reflex performance and to the elimination of sexual drive in male rabbits (Korányi *et al.*, 1965/66; Korányi and Endröczi, 1967). Contrary to these findings, ACTH appeared to be effective in inhibition of extinction of a conditioned avoidance response in rats (De Wied, 1966) and it exerts a biphasic effect depending on the doses of the hormone used, and on the type of the resting activity level of the central nervous system of mice (Korányi *et al.*, 1967). Furthermore, ACTH disinhibits the secondary phase of EEG habituation in humans (see Endröczi *et al.*, in this issue).

The conflicting data concerning behavioral reactions might be interpreted either by the presence of adrenals or by the different sensitivity of various species to the direct neural or other extra-adrenal effects of ACTH. It is plausible that other than neural extra-adrenal effects of ACTH: lipid mobilization, ketosis, hypoglycemia, hypocalce-

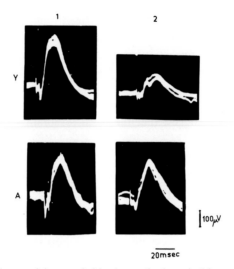

Fig. 6. Changes in evoked potentials recorded in the cerebral cortical layer of young chick (Y) and hen (A) before (1) and after (2) ACTH injection.

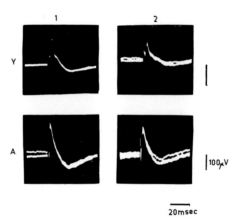

Fig. 7. Changes in evoked potentials recorded in the optic tectum of young chick (Y) and hen (A), before (1) and after (2) ACTH injection.

mia, hypotension, or changes in local cerebral circulation, probably contribute to its influence on central nervous events and behavior. Moreover, the influence of the blood–brain barrier may be of importance (Korányi et al., 1969b).

In young chicks, in which the blood–brain barriers' function is absent or poorly developed until the 4th to 5th week of life, 0.25 mg per kg body weight of ACTH (natural, synthetic) or of ACTH 1–10 analogue injected intravenously, resulted in a marked diminution of potentials in the cerebral corticoid layer evoked by stimulation of the reticular nuclei of the mesencephalon. The diminution of amplitude developed 5 to 10 min after the injection and lasted 40 to 60 min. A slight diminution of evoked potentials was also observed in the optic tectum elicited by electrical stimulation of the optic chiasm. No changes were found in evoked responses recorded from the cerebral

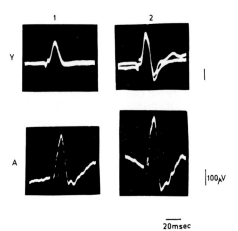

Fig. 8. Changes in evoked potentials recorded in the cerebral cortical layer of young chick (Y) and hen (A), before (1) and after (2) hydrocortisone injection.

corticoid layer or optic tectum in hens following ACTH injections (Figs. 6 and 7). However, hydrocortisone administration resulted in a prompt augmentation of the evoked responses, both in young and in adult animals (Fig. 8).

DISCUSSION

The existence of chemoreceptive fields for corticosteroids at thalamic, hypothalamic, and midbrain neuronal levels is suggested by several studies (Feldman *et al.*, 1961; Slusher, 1966; Slusher *et al.*, 1966; Ruf and Steiner, 1967; Sawyer *et al.*, 1968; Steiner *et al.*, 1969; Van Wimersma Greidanus and De Wied, 1969; Bohus, in this issue). However, it is difficult to interpret the participation of these structures unequivocally in the behavioral reactions. Nevertheless, the pre-optic steroid-sensitive neuronal network is closely related to both thalamo–cortical synchronization and internal inhibitory processes.

The involvement of thalamo–cortical synchronization and basal forebrain inhibition in learning and motivated behavior has been confirmed in recent years by a number of data (Endröczi *et al.*, 1964; Endröczi and Korányi, 1965; Korányi *et al.*, 1963; Korányi, 1965; Korányi and Endröczi, 1965; Lissák and Endröczi, 1965; Sterman and Wyrwicka, 1967).

The appearance of EEG after-reaction following the presentation of motivational stimuli or reinforcement in conditioned reflex situations is a characteristic phenomenon. The lack of EEG after-reaction as "reinforcing" synchronization in adrenalectomized animals fits well in the series of findings, namely, that rats with adrenocortical insufficiency show a slow rate of extinction as compared to intact animals, and that the administration of corticosteroids markedly facilitates the internal inhibition. The observations presented here support our hypothesis suggesting that the basal forebrain has a direct relationship to hormonally conditioned motivated behavior and is a site for corticosteroid action.

References pp. 128–130

REFERENCES

ADEY, W. R., SEGUNDO, I. P. AND LIVINGSTON, R. B. (1957) Corticofugal influences on intrinsic brain-stem conduction in cat and monkeys. *J. Neurophysiol.*, **20**, 1–16.

ANOKHIN, P. K. (1961) Electroencephalographic analysis of cortico-subcortical relations in positive and negative conditioned reactions. *Ann. N.Y. Acad. Sci.*, **92**, 899–938.

ANSELMINO, K. J. AND HOFFMANN, F. (1933) Die pankreatrope Substanz aus dem Hypophysenvorder-lappen. I. und II. *Klin. Wochschr.*, II, 1435–1436; 1436–1438.

BERLINER, D. L., KELLER, N. AND DOUGHERTY, T. F. (1961) Tissue retention of cortisol and meta-bolites induced by ACTH: An extra-adrenal effect. *Endocrinology*, **68**, 621–629.

BOHUS, B. AND ENDRÖCZI, E. (1965) The influence of pituitary-adrenocortical functions on the avoiding conditioned reflex activity. *Acta physiol. Acad. Sci. Hung.*, **26**, 183–189.

BOHUS, B. AND KORÁNYI, L. (1969) Hormonal conditioning of adaptive behavioral processes. In: *Recent Developments of Neurobiology in Hungary*, Vol. II, K. LISSÁK (Ed.), Akadémiai Kiadó, Budapest, pp. 50–76.

BOHUS, B. AND LISSÁK, K. (1968) Adrenocortical hormones and avoidance behaviour of rats. *Intern. J. Neuropharmacol.*, **7**, 301–306.

BORKOVSKAYA, YU. A. AND FADEIVA, O. N. (1961) Mechanism underlying the onset of sleep inhibition following adrenal administration. (In Russian). *Fiziol. Zh.*, **47**, 806–814.

CLEMENTE, C. D., STERMAN, M. B. AND WYRWICKA, W. (1964) Post-reinforcement EEG synchroniza-tion during alimentary behavior. *Electroenceph. clin. Neurophysiol.*, **16**, 355–365.

CLEMENTE, C. D., CHASE, M. A., KANUSS, T. K., SAUERLAND, E. K. AND STERMAN, M. B. (1966) Inhibition of a monosynaptic reflex by electrical stimulation of the basal forebrain or the orbital gyrus in the cat. *Experientia (Basel)*, **22**, 844–845.

DEMPSEY, E. W. AND MORISON, R. S. (1942) The production of rhythmically recurrent cortical poten-tials after localized thalamic stimulation. *Amer. J. Physiol.*, **135**, 293–300.

DE WIED, D. (1966) Antagonistic effect of ACTH and glucocorticoids on avoidance behaviour of rats. *2nd Intern. Congr. on Hormonal Steroids*, Excerpta Med. Intern. Congr. Series, **111**, 89.

DOUGHERTY, T. F. AND BERLINER, D. L. (1958) The effect of stress and ACTH on the metabolism of hydrocortisone in the liver. In: *Liver Function*, R. W. BRAUER (Ed.), Amer. Inst. Biol. Sci., Washing-ton, D.C. p. 416.

ENDRÖCZI, E. AND KORÁNYI, L. (1965) The effect of electrical stimulation of the limbic system on conditioned somatomotor patterns in double-choice conditioned reflex situation in cats. *Acta physiol. Acad. Sci. Hung.*, **28**, 327–337.

ENDRÖCZI, E. AND LISSÁK, K. (1962) Spontaneous goal-directed motor activity related to the alimen-tary conditioned reflex behaviour and its regulation by neural and humoral factors. *Acta physiol. Acad. Sci. Hung.*, **21**, 265–283.

ENDRÖCZI, E. AND KORÁNYI, L. (1968) Integration of emotional reactions in the brain-stem di-encephalic and limbic system. *Internat. Symposium on Aggressive Behavior, May 2–4, 1968, Milan, Italy*. In: *Aggressive Behavior*, S. GARATTINI AND E. B. SIGG (Eds.), Excerpta Med. Monograph, Amsterdam.

ENDRÖCZI, E., KORÁNYI, L., LISSÁK, K. AND HARTMANN, G. (1964) The role of mesodiencephalic activating mechanism in the habituation and avoiding conditioned reflex activity. *Acta physiol. Acad. Sci. Hung.*, **24**, 447–464.

ENGEL, F. L. (1961) Extra-adrenal action of adrenocorticotrophin. *Vitamins and Hormones*, **19**, 189–202.

ENGEL, F. L. AND LEBOVITZ, H. E. (1966) Extra-target organ actions of anterior pituitary hormones. In: *The Pituitary Gland*. Vol. II, G. W. HARRIS AND B. T. DONOVAN (Eds.), Butterworths, London, pp. 563–588.

FELDMAN, S., TODT, I. C. AND PORTER, R. W. (1961) Effect of adrenocortical hormones on evoked potentials in the brain stem. *Neurology*, **11**, 109–115.

HESS, W. R. (1944) Das Schlafsyndrom als Folge diencephaler Reizung. *Helv. physiol. pharmacol. Acta*, **2**, 305–344.

HERNANDEZ-PEÓN, R. (1960) Neurophysiological correlates of habituation and other manifestations of plastic inhibition. In: *Moscow Colloquium on EEG of Higher Nervous Activity*, H. H. JASPER, AND G. D. SMIRNOV (Eds.), *Electroenceph. clin. Neurophysiol.*, Suppl. 13, 101–114.

HERNANDEZ-PEÓN, R. AND CHÁVEZ IBARRA, G. (1963) Sleep induced by electrical and chemical stimulation of the forebrain. *Electroenceph. clin. Neurophysiol.*, **24**, 188–198.

JOUVET, M. (1961) Telencephalic and rhombencephalic sleep in the cat. In: *The Nature of Sleep*, G. E. W. WOLSTENHOLME AND M. O'CONNOR (Eds.), Little Brown, Boston, pp. 188–206.

KORÁNYI, L. (1965) The role of basal forebrain structures in the avoiding conditioned reflex activity in rats. Symposium on "*Early Manifestation of Conditioning*", Budapest, 1963, Acta physiol. Acad. Sci. Hung., **26**, 63–67.

KORÁNYI, L. AND ENDRÖCZI, E. (1965) The effect of electrical stimulation and lesions of the limbic structures on the development of conditioned somatomotor patterns in the albino rat. *Acta physiol. Acad. Sci. Hung.*, **28**, 339–347.

KORÁNYI, L., ENDRÖCZI, E. AND TÁRNOK, F. (1965/66) Sexual behaviour in the course of avoidance conditioning in male rabbits. *Neuroendocrinology*, **1**, 144–157.

KORÁNYI, L., ENDRÖCZI, E. AND LISSÁK, K. (1963) Somatomotor activity and avoidance conditioned reflex performance following forebrain lesions. *J. psychosom. Res.*, **7**, 159–164.

KORÁNYI, L., ENDRÖCZI, E., LISSÁK, K. AND SZEPES, É. (1967) The effect of ACTH on behavioural processes motivated by fear in mice. *Physiol. Behav.*, **2**, 439–445.

KORÁNYI, L. AND ENDRÖCZI, E. (1967) The effect of ACTH on nervous processes. *Neuroendocrinology*, **2**, 65–75.

KORÁNYI, L., ENDRÖCZI, E. AND TAMÁSY, V. (1969a) Pituitary-adrenocorticotrophic hormone (ACTH) induced hypoglycaemia. *Acta physiol. Acad. Sci. Hung.*, **35**, 41–46.

KORÁNYI, L., ENDRÖCZI, E. AND TAMÁSY, V. (1969b) Influence of pituitary-adrenocortical hormones on the central nervous system. Electrophysiological and behavioural studies on rats and chicks. *Acta physiol. Acad. Sci. Hung.*, (in press).

KUSAMA, M. (1963) Studies on the function of pituitary-adrenocortical and autonomic nervous system in neurosis. *J. Japan. Soc. Internal Med.*, **52**, 65–72.

LEBOVITZ, H. E. (1967) Some clinical implications of recent advances in the chemistry and physiology of protein hormones. In: *An Introduction to Clinical Neuroendocrinology*, E. BAJUSZ (Ed.), S. Karger, Basel, pp. 243–253.

LEVINE, S. (1968) *Hormones and conditioning. Nebraska symposium.*

LISSÁK, K. AND ENDRÖCZI, E. (1964) Neuroendocrine inter-relationships and behavioural processes. In: *Major Problems in Neuroendocrinology*, E. BAJUSZ AND G. JASMIN (Eds.), S. Karger, Basel, pp. 1–14.

LISSÁK, K. AND ENDRÖCZI, E. (1965) *The Neuroendocrine Control of Adaptation*, Pergamon Press, Oxford, p. 139.

LISSÁK, K. AND ENDRÖCZI, E. (1967) The role of the mesodiencephalic activating system in higher nervous activity: its role in habituation, learning mechanisms and conditioned reflex processes. In: *Brain Reflexes, Progress in Brain Research*, Vol. 22, E. A. ASRATYAN (Ed.), Elsevier, Amsterdam, pp. 298–311.

LISSÁK, K., ENDRÖCZI, E. AND MEDGYESI, P. (1957) Somatische Verhalten und Nebennierenrindentätigkeit, *Arch. ges. Physiol.*, **117**, 265–273.

MAGOUN, H. W. (1962) Brain mechanisms for internal inhibition. *Proc. 3rd World Congr. Psychiatry, Montreal, Canada*, **1**, 1–16.

MOISEEV, E. A. AND TONKIKH, A. V. (1940) The role of the hypophysis in the phenomena of sleep in the course of electrical stimulation of subcortical nuclei. (In Russian) *Fiziol. Zh. USSR*, **26**, 395–399.

MORISON, R. S. AND DEMPSEY, E. W. (1942) A study of thalamo-cortical relations. *Amer. J. Physiol.*, **135**, 281–292.

NAUTA, W. J. H. (1945) Hypothalamic regulation of sleep in rats. An experimental study. *J. Neurophysiol.*, **9**, 285–316.

PURPURA, D. P. AND COHEN, B. (1962) Intracellular recording from thalamic neurons during recruiting responses. *J. Neurophysiol.*, **25**, 621–635.

PURPURA, D. P. AND HOUSEPIAN, E. M. (1961) Alterations in corticospinal neuron activity associated with thalamocortical recruiting responses. *Electroenceph. clin. Neurophysiol.*, **13**, 365–381.

PURPURA, D. P. AND SHOFER, R. J. (1963) Intracellular recording from thalamic neurons during reticulocortical activation. *J. Neurophysiol.*, **26**, 494–505.

ROITBAK, A. I. (1956) *Cerebral Cortical Primary Responses of Normal Animals* (In Russian) Trudy Instituta Fiziologii im. I. C. Beritashvili, **10**, 131–137.

RUF, K. AND STEINER, F. A. (1967) Steroid-sensitive single neurons in rat hypothalamus and midbrain: identification by microelectrophoresis. *Science*, **156**, 667–669.

SADOWSKI, B. AND LONGO, V. C. (1962) Electroencephalographic and behavioral correlates of an instrumental reward conditioned response in rabbits. *Electroenceph. clin. Neurophysiol.*, **14**, 465–476.

SAWYER, C. H. AND KAWAKAMI, M. (1959) Characteristics of behavioural and electroencephalographic after-reactions to copulation and vaginal stimulation in the female rabbit. *Endocrinology*, **65**, 622–630.

SAWYER, C. H., KAWAKAMI, M., MEYERSON, B., WHITMOYER, D. I. AND LILLEY, J. I. (1968) Effects of ACTH, dexamethasone and asphyxia on electrical activity of the rat hypothalamus. *Brain Res.*, **10**, 213–226.

SCHEIBEL, M. E. AND SCHEIBEL, A. B. (1967) Structural organization of non-specific thalamic nuclei and their projection toward cortex. *Brain Res.*, **6**, 60–94.

SKINNER, M. AND LINDSLEY, D. B. (1967) Electrophysiological and behavioral effects of blockade of the non-specific thalamo-cortical system. *Brain Res.*, **6**, 95–118.

SLUSHER, M. A. (1966) Effects of cortical implants in the brain stem and neutral hippocampus on diurnal corticoid levels. *Exptl. Brain Res.*, **1**, 184–194.

SLUSHER, M. A., HYDE, I. E. AND LAUFER, M. (1966) Effect of intracerebral hydrocortisone on unit activity of diencephalon and midbrain in cats. *J. Neurophysiol.*, **29**, 159–169.

SMIRNOV, G. D. (1953) Lability of central nervous processes in the central and peripheral areas of the visual analyzer. (In Russian) *Pavlov J. Higher Nervous Activity*, **3**, 941–951.

STEINER, W. G. (1962) Electrical activity of rat brain as a correlate of primary drive. *Electroenceph. clin. Neurophysiol.*, **14**, 233–243.

STEINER, F. A., RUF, K. AND AKERT, K. (1969) Steroid-sensitive neurones in rat brain: anatomical localization and responses to neurohumors and ACTH. *Brain Res.*, **12**, 74–85.

STERMAN, M. B. AND WYRWICKA, W. (1967) EEG correlates of sleep; evidence for separate forebrain substrates. *Brain Res.*, **6**, 143–163.

TRYGSTAD, O. (1967) The lipid-mobilizing effect of some pituitary gland preparations. I. Evidence for a lipotrophic contamination with rabbit serum calcium-lowering effect in adrenocorticotrophin and human growth hormone preparations. *Acta Endocrinol.*, **56**, 626–648.

VELASCO, M. AND LINDSLEY, D. B. (1965) Role of orbital cortex in regulation of thalamocortical electrical activity. *Science*, **149**, 1375–1377.

WALDVOGEL, W. (1945) Gähnen als diencephal ausgelöstes Reizsymptom. *Helv. physiol. pharmacol. Acta*, **3**, 329–334.

WIMERSMA GREIDANUS, TJ. B. VAN AND WIED, D. DE (1969) Effects of intracerebral implantation of corticosteroids on extinction of an avoidance response in rats. *Physiol. Behav.*, **4**, 365–370.

DISCUSSION

LARON: How can you be sure that the effect obtained with ACTH and ACTH-(1-10) is a specific effect and not a non-specific one?

KORÁNYI: ACTH-(11-24), in a dose of 0.25 mg/kg body weight did not result in any changes of the evoked potentials.

FELDMAN: You have shown that the altered recruiting response in adrenalectomized rats was corrected by cortisone. But what happens to the recruiting response of intact animals under influence of cortisone?

KORÁNYI: In intact animals no marked change in the threshold of recruitment could be observed.

Pituitary–Adrenal Axis and Salt Appetite[*]

D. A. DENTON AND J. F. NELSON

Howard Florey Laboratories of Experimental Physiology, University of Melbourne, Parkville, 3052, Victoria (Australia)

The question which logically presents from the title suggested for this talk is whether pituitary and adrenal hormones have a physiological role in the causation of salt appetite analogous to that of sexual hormones in the genesis of sexual behaviour.

First, it is established that mineralocorticoids do affect salt appetite. The mechanism of this effect is unexplained and the significance is controversial.

Richter's (1936) early finding was that adrenalectomized rats showed a greatly increased intake of NaCl, and ingested enough to keep themselves alive and free from symptoms of insufficiency. When treated with DOCA the increased appetite for salt disappeared. Rice and Richter (1943) and then Braun-Menendez and Brandt (1952) made the unexpected finding that in normal rats DOCA produced the opposite effect —an increase in salt appetite.

Subsequently, Wolf (1964a) showed that aldosterone (0.5 mg/day) elicited a sodium appetite when administered to rats. Wolf and Handal (1966) then showed that if sodium appetite was studied by a method which avoided any accumulation of sodium in the body, a significant increase of sodium intake was caused by doses of aldosterone which were probably in the range of adrenal output in rats with severe sodium deficiency. They also showed the appetite was specific for sodium ion. Fregly and Waters (1965) have also suggested that the blood level of aldosterone is the causal vector of salt appetite. Wolf (1964b) found that lesions in the dorsolateral hypothalamus severely disrupt the potentiation of saline intake by DOCA in rats.

Discussion of this data by our laboratories (Denton, Nelson, Orchard and Weller, 1969) has placed emphasis on the question whether effects on appetite are seen at levels of dosage related to physiological output in the rat under sodium-deficient conditions. Attention has been drawn to the fact that many of the measurements of adrenal output upon which deductions have been based were made on anaesthetized traumatized animals incurring additional blood loss in the course of collecting the specimens for analysis. Considerable light on this issue has come from Bojeson's (1966) estimations of secretion rate in the conscious rat by peripheral blood concentration measurement and concurrent determination of metabolic clearance rate. He finds a sodium-

* This work was supported by research grants from the National Health and Medical Research Council of Australia, and from the National Institutes of Health in Washington — HE 11580-01 (GMB), the Rural Credits Fund of the Reserve Bank of Australia and the Wool Research Fund of the Commonwealth.

References pp. 139–140

replete output of about 2 μg/day—a figure consistent with the results of other workers in relation to aldosterone requirement for maintenance of adrenalectomized rats in good health. He finds a large rise of secretion rate with sodium deficiency—up to 60 μg/day—which is the order of the lowest doses found by Wolf and Handal (1966) to induce sodium appetite. So it is possible that with severe salt deficiency, aldosterone may play a contributory role in the causation of salt appetite.

Thus far, we have discussed the domesticated laboratory rat. To consider other species, we have described the avid specific appetite for sodium salt exhibited by wild rabbits in the Alps of Australia (Blair-West, Coghlan, Denton, Nelson, Orchard, Scoggins, Wright, Myers and Junqueira, 1968). This behaviour is seen mainly in the spring and early summer—the salt impregnated sticks being largely ignored in the autumn. Concurrent metabolic studies show that at this season, sodium is virtually a trace element in grass (less than 0.5 mequiv/kg wet wt.) and urine sodium is negligible and renal renin is greatly increased. Peripheral blood aldosterone is also found to be very high—whereas in autumn it is much lower, and at this time, there is little evidence of appetite. Desert rabbits which excrete a large amount of sodium and have peripheral blood aldosterone concentrations in the normal range do not exhibit salt appetite.

We have brought young wild rabbits from the Alps, and studied their intake under laboratory conditions when they have been offered a variety of mineral solutions—and then the influence of DOCA on this intake (Denton et al., 1969). The diet which was of constant composition throughout, had a substantial sodium content—5 mequiv/day.

The data from experiments with 150 mequiv/l solutions shows that under control conditions the mean need free intake of NaCl was very small, but it was increased eightfold by 2 mg DOCA/day and twentyfold by 5 mg DOCA/day. There was a larger intake of divalent cations which was not influenced by DOCA.

During the initial control period the mean intakes of the four electrolyte solutions presented (NaCl, KCl, $MgCl_2$ and $CaCl_2$) were 0.16, 0.6, 1.0 and 5.2 mequiv/day. Following treatment with 2 mg DOCA/day these values were 1.3, 0.6, 1.4 and 5.4 mequiv/day whilst when the dose of DOCA was increased to 5 mg/day the amounts drunk were 3.5, 0.9, 1.6 and 5.1 mequiv/day.

A similar group of experiments was conducted with 500 mequiv/l electrolyte solutions. The mean initial daily intake of NaCl was 0.4 mequiv. This was increased with daily DOCA doses of 2 mg to 4.3 mequiv/day and with 5 mg DOCA daily to 9.5 mequiv/day. Each of these DOCA doses increased $CaCl_2$ consumption to 10.5 mequiv/day from a base level of 6.5 mequiv/day. KCl intake increased with the lower dose from 1.0 to 2.2 mequiv/day but with the higher dose the change was not significant, the intake being 1.3 mequiv/day. The larger amount of DOCA depressed $MgCl_2$ appetite from 1.6 mequiv/day to 0.2 mequiv/day but the smaller dose had no significant effect, the intake being 1.4 mequiv/day during treatment. The injection of 1 mg DOCA/day had no effect on the appetite for any of these electrolyte solutions.

The effect of DOCA on salt appetite in the rabbit, though statistically significant, is much smaller than in the rat. The 250 g rat with ca. 8 mequiv of E.C.F. sodium drinks ca. 10 mequiv of sodium/day with 1 mg/day DOCA—*i.e.*, they turn over their total E.C.F. sodium per day. The rabbits which are 5 times heavier with a 40 mequiv of E.C.F. sodium do not usually take in more than 10 mequiv when given 5 mg DOCA/ day—which is equivalent dosage on a body weight basis. Also, whereas Rice *et al.* (1943) and Fregly *et al.* (1965) do not record any deleterious effects in the rat with 5 mg/day, in the rabbit though 5 times larger, loss of appetite occurred, general decline in condition, and four of the 10 animals in the series died. It seems unlikely that any physiological significance could attach to effects of dosage above 2 mg/day. Recently we have also made a preliminary study with rabbits when 250 μg/day of (+)-aldo-sterone in oil was administered. Though this dose is equivalent to the daily aldosterone secretion during sodium deficiency of the sheep (an animal 15 times larger) there was no effect on voluntary sodium intake of the rabbit.

With man salt hunger or analogous behaviour is not seen as a presenting feature of Conn's syndrome where high levels of circulating aldosterone occur (Conn—personal communication).

Under laboratory conditions, many but not all sheep show an intake of hypertonic NaCl solution (300 mequiv/l) which is not metabolically determined in that their food contains adequate sodium (60 mequiv/day). This is under the experimental conditions where the hypertonic salt solution is continuously avi.lable concurrently with water. We have found that when such animals were given 5 mg DOCA/day there was little or no influence on voluntary intake.

With 20 mg/day—which is a high dose for the sheep—hypokalaemic alkalosis developed, and, after an initial rise, body weight fell because of anorexia. Of the 4 animals in an experiment, one died at the end of 6 days dosage and it showed a small increase of sodium intake. With two others, intake declined. Other approaches to the problem have included study as to whether DOCA increases salt appetite of the mildly depleted animal. No effect was seen.

It does not appear that mineralocorticoid affects salt appetite in the sheep and man in the way it does in the rat. An effect occurs in the rabbit but there is general deterioration with doses sufficient to produce a physiologically significant increase of intake. However it must be considered that in sodium deficiency the metabolic context of action of aldosterone will be different, and, thus, this data does not eliminate entirely the possibility that the sodium-deplete animal may be more sensitive to aldosterone and it acts as a contributory cause of the behaviour in these circumstances.

A major difficulty in the hypothesis that the contemporary level of aldosterone in blood is determinant of salt appetite is that salt appetite is exhibited by adrenal-ectomized sodium-deficient animals. In Epstein and Stellar's (1955) study on the rat, external sodium balances were not done, but the data suggest that appetite is related to extent of deficit.

An investigation which was conducted with external sodium balances shows that in both adrenal intact and adrenalectomized sheep with a parotid fistula, salt appetite was commensurately related to state of sodium balance (Denton *et al.*, 1969; Denton, Orchard and Weller, 1969).

The experimental conditions with normal sheep with a parotid fistula were that access to sodium solution was permitted for 15 min after it had been withheld for 24, 48 or 72 hours. Also on some occasions the animals were kept near replete by returning salivary loss to the animal via rumen tube over the 24 h preceding presentation of the solution for 15 min. The solution presented was 300 mequiv/l NaHCO₃. It was found that the voluntary $NaHCO_3$ intake was related to external sodium loss at the various levels of body deficit thus contrived.

The same experimental procedure was carried out on adrenalectomized sheep. The appetite test was made 24 h after the last dose of maintenance mineralocorticoid hormone (5 mg DOCA, 25 mg cortisone), at which time the effect of injected DOCA had disappeared as shown by a normal potassium concentration in the saliva. A commensurate relation between voluntary intake and extent of body deficit was found, and the same result obtained if the test was made 48 h after the last injection of maintenance hormone. The results of these experiments in sheep indicate that salt appetite may be generated commensurately with body deficit independently of the contemporary level of aldosterone in circulating blood.

Wolf and Stricker (1967) have proposed that salt appetite may be determined by the concurrent effect of blood aldosterone level and plasma sodium concentration. However they found in adrenalectomized rats concurrently depleted of water as well as salt, so that a fall of plasma sodium was largely obviated, that sodium appetite was exhibited. We have summarized elsewhere the data from experiments on sheep indicative that appetite is not simply and directly related to the concentration of sodium in circulating blood (Denton, 1967).

We have put forward the following hypothesis in relation to the salt appetite generating effects of mineralocorticoid. Whereas aldosterone may possibly be a contributory cause of salt appetite in some species with severe depletion, the principal basis of effect is that it causes chemical changes in the neural areas controlling appetite analogous to changes which do occur in sodium deficiency, and which are normally responsible for the evocation of appetite.

There has been very little systematic investigation of the influence of hypophysectomy on salt appetite. However, we have observed in hypophysectomized sheep with parotid fistulae that the animals will maintain themselves in normal sodium balance if permitted access to 300 mequiv/l NaHCO₃ solution.

An area of investigation of great potential importance in relation to hormones and appetite is the effect of pregnancy and lactation. Some twenty years ago, Richter and Barelare (1938) observed that rats on a salt-free diet, showed an increase in NaCl intake very early in pregnancy and that this was maintained until the end of the lactation period but returned to normal after weaning. They did not find any change in calcium lactate or sodium phosphate intake during pregnancy. Both, however, were increased during lactation. Very little work has been done in this field in the interim.

Since with our studies in the Alps, the period of maximum environmental salt deficiency corresponded to the reproductive period, we decided to study the effect of pregnancy and lactation on mineral appetite of wild rabbits under metabolic balance conditions.

For two months prior to mating, the animals were offered solutions of 500 mequiv/l

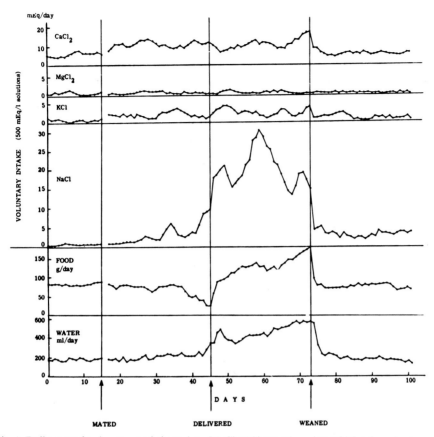

Fig. 1. Daily mean food, water and electrolyte (NaCl, KCl, MgCl₂ and CaCl₂) intake prior to mating, during pregnancy and lactation, and following weaning of the litters.

CaCl₂, MgCl₂, KCl and NaCl and water. The food contained 80 mequiv/kg of sodium so that the mean intake of sodium was about 6 mequiv/day. Measurement of food, water and electrolyte intake and urine output were made daily, and Fig. 1 here represents the mean findings with 7 animals. All animals including litters were weighed at weekly intervals during each phase of the test.

Following an initial control period of 15 days the animals were mated. During pregnancy there was a significant increase in mean NaCl intake after 10 days. The peak value was 9.5 mequiv/day just before parturition.

The mean intake of both KCl and CaCl₂ solution was significantly increased by pregnancy, and the rise occurred within 2–3 days of mating. Following parturition the amount of NaCl solution drunk was greatly increased—the mean intake on the 14th day of lactation was 31 mequiv. This represents turnover of a major portion of extracellular sodium each day.

The mean daily consumption of KCl and CaCl₂ during lactation was approximately the same as that observed during pregnancy. On the 22nd day of lactation small amounts of faeces from the baby rabbits were found in the metabolism area of several

TABLE 1

MEAN DAILY FOOD, ELECTROLYTE SOLUTION, AND TOTAL ELECTROLYTE (Na^+, K^+, Mg^{++} and Ca^{++}) INTAKE PRIOR TO MATING, DURING PREGNANCY AND LACTATION, AND FOLLOWING WEANING OF THE LITTERS

mequiv/day	Control	Pregnancy	Lactation	Post-weaning
Food				
Weight	82.5 ± 2.9	66.7 ± 16.8	117.2 ± 21.0	79.0 ± 7.2
Na^+	6.6 ± 0.22	5.35 ± 1.34	8.8 ± 1.7	6.3 ± 0.58
K^+	11.9 ± 0.39	9.7 ± 2.4	16.0 ± 3.0	11.5 ± 1.10
Mg^{++}	0.83 ± 0.03	0.67 ± 0.17	1.10 ± 0.21	0.79 ± 0.07
Ca^{++}	25.5 ± 0.81	20.6 ± 5.2	34.0 ± 6.6	24.2 ± 2.2
Solution				
Na^+	0.89 ± 0.17	3.30 ± 0.63	22.0 ± 4.4	3.4 ± 0.7
K^+	0.51 ± 0.10	1.95 ± 0.70	2.69 ± 0.81	1.85 ± 0.67
Mg^{++}	0.67 ± 0.42	0.82 ± 0.32	0.81 ± 0.33	0.48 ± 0.23
Ca^{++}	5.72 ± 0.95	10.7 ± 1.31	10.0 ± 1.6	8.6 ± 1.6
Total				
Na^+	7.5 ± 0.28	8.7 ± 1.60	30.8 ± 4.8	9.7 ± 0.89
K^+	12.4 ± 0.40	11.7 ± 2.51	18.7 ± 3.3	13.4 ± 1.37
Mg^{++}	1.51 ± 0.42	1.39 ± 0.36	1.91 ± 0.39	1.27 ± 0.24
Ca^{++}	31.2 ± 0.25	31.3 ± 1.41	44.0 ± 6.8	32.8 ± 2.8
Water				
ml/day	175 ± 12	210 ± 36	428 ± 30	180 ± 14

TABLE 2

MEAN LITTER WEIGHT AND MEAN BODY WEIGHT OF MOTHERS AT WEEKLY INTERVALS

	Control			Pregnancy				Lactation					Post-weaning			
Weeks	0	1	2	1	2	3	4	0	1	2	3	4	1	2	3	4
Mothers	1710	1709	1726	1757	1810	1892	1975	1735	1771	1741	1750	1756	1731	1728	1737	1722
Litters	–	–	–	–	–	–	–	205	310	552	811	1290	–	–	–	–

cages, and from then on a number of the young were seen in the body of the cage and were seen to eat and drink. They contributed to direct food and water intake after this time, and may conceivably have contributed to the secondary peak of NaCl intake, though the outlets of these containers were probably well above their reach.

The changes in electrolyte, food, and water intake reversed rapidly after weaning. In two of the seven animals, the intake of electrolyte solutions remained elevated, and it is due to their contributions that the mean values are higher than the initial control levels.

Other aspects of the experimental findings were as follows:

(1) After the 25th day of pregnancy each rabbit was allowed access to a rectangular

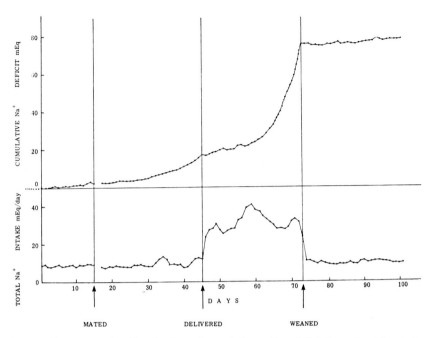

Fig. 2. Daily mean total sodium intake and cumulative sodium deficit throughout the study.

plastic box attached to the back of the cage in such a fashion that any excreta in the box could be collected in the metabolism cage. The box was lined with well washed hessian. After 21 days post partum this was removed and thoroughly washed and the washings analysed for sodium and potassium. At no stage did the nest contain any obvious faeces or urine, nor did the hessian have any significant amounts of sodium or potassium.

(2) The mean weight of the animals rose 250 g over pregnancy (Table 2). Within 24 h the weight had returned to near the original. Of 31 young born, 30 survived till after weaning.

(3) Sodium balance during the test is shown in Fig. 2, The average total sodium intake during the 15-day control period was 112 mequiv/rabbit or 7.5 mequiv/rabbit/day. Of this intake 98 % was recovered in the urine, the deficit representing faecal and other loss. During the 30 days of pregnancy the mean total sodium intake was 250 mequiv (8.7 mequiv/day), with 235 mequiv excreted in the urine. The difference in sodium deficit in these phases of the study of approximately 10 mequiv/rabbit would be largely accounted for by sodium accumulation in the young and the other products of conception—as judged by maternal weight increase. It is important to note that the increased voluntary intake of NaCl—as high as 9 mequiv/day at the end of pregnancy—is far greater than that required to satisfy the sodium demand consequent on the small extent of sodium sequestration.

During lactation there was a mean total sodium intake of 860 mequiv and a deficit of 60 mequiv not accounted for by urine loss. The mean gain in litter weight was 1085 g, so that about 40–45 mequiv of sodium were accounted for by accumulation during

References pp. 139–140

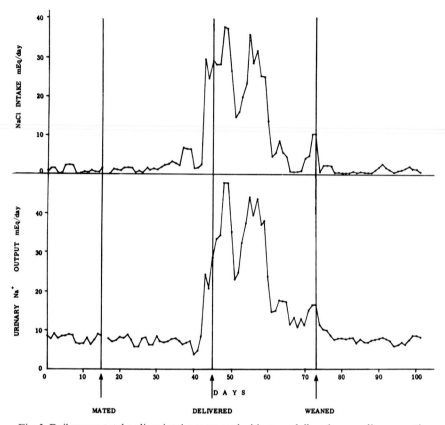

Fig. 3. Daily mean total sodium intake compared with mean daily urinary sodium excretion.

litter growth. If, as during the control period, about 2 % of the total sodium intake was lost in faeces or otherwise not collected, the remaining 15–20 mequiv of this sodium deficit can also be accounted for. Again the great disparity between sodium sequestration in the young and daily mean voluntary intake—on several occasions as high as 30 mequiv/day—is emphasized.

In examination of the individual animals, mean daily sodium intake during lactation was clearly related to litter size. The maximum daily intake in a doe with 7 young was 92 mequiv/day—with a litter of 2, 10 mequiv/day. The sodium content of the milk of two of the rabbits was measured on the 15th day of lactation, *i.e.*, when voluntary sodium intake was near its peak. The concentrations in the two samples were 32 and 38 mequiv/l. Cross's (1955) figure for the maximum milk output of any of a group of 4-kg rabbits (twice as large as these) was 240 ml/day. Even if this figure were accepted as the mean daily milk production of our rabbits, sodium loss in milk could not have accounted for more than 1/3 of the voluntary salt intake.

(4) The relation of voluntary sodium intake and sodium output in urine is shown in Fig. 3. The principal point is that the large rise in voluntary sodium intake in pregnancy, late pregnancy or lactation is not related to any sudden preceding drop in urinary

sodium excretion indicative of body deficit, or relative deficit, associated with the metabolic demands of pregnancy or lactation.

(5) The data, by virtue of the observations on urine and the external sodium balance, raise a whole new set of considerations in relation to the genesis of mineral appetite in animals.

Brain-Menendez (1952) showed that neither oestradiol, progesterone or stilboestrol will enhance sodium appetite of rats, but the question of combinations of hormones may have to be considered. For complete mammary development prior to birth and for continued efficient lactation both prolactin and somatotrophin appear essential (Cotes, Crighton, Folley and Young, 1949; Lyons, Li, Cole and Johnson, 1953) so that either or both of these hormones might be implicated in the sharp rise of NaCl intake at the end of pregnancy and during lactation. These are only a few of the possibilities presenting in a fascinating new field for dissection of the mechanism of salt appetite. The sharp cut-off of high intake with weaning also raises questions of sensory induction of the centrally directed drive.

REFERENCES

BLAIR-WEST, J. R., COGHLAN, J. P., DENTON, D. A., NELSON, J. F., ORCHARD, E., SCOGGINS, B. A., WRIGHT, R. D., MYERS, K. AND JUNQUEIRA, C. L. (1968) Physiological, morphological and behavioural adaptation to a sodium deficient environment by wild native Australian and introduced species of animals. *Nature*, **217**, 922–928.

BOJESON, E. (1966) Concentrations of aldosterone and corticosterone in peripheral plasma of rats. The effects of salt depletion, and intravenous injections of renin and angiotensin II. *European J. Steroids*, **1**, 145–169.

BRAUN-MENENDEZ, E. (1952) Aumento del apetito especifico para la sal provocado por la desoxy-corticosterona: substancias que potentian o inhiben esta accion. *Rev. Soc. Arg. Biol.*, **28**, 23–32.

BRAUN-MENENDEZ, E. AND BRANDT, P. (1952) Aumento del apetito especifico para la sal provocado por la desoxycorticosterona: caracteristicas. *Rev. Soc. Arg. Biol.*, **28**, 15–23.

COTES, P. M., CRIGHTON, J. A., FOLLEY, S. J. AND YOUNG, F. G. (1949) Galactapoietic activity of purified anterior pituitary growth hormone. *Nature*, **164**, 992–993.

CROSS, B. A. (1955) Neurohormonal mechanisms of emotional inhibition of milk ejection. *J. Endocrinol.*, **12**, 29–37.

DENTON, D. A. (1967) Salt appetite. Chapter 31. In: *Handbook of Physiology, Section 6: Alimentary Canal*, Am. Physiol. Soc. Washington, Vol. 1, pp. 433–459.

DENTON, D. A., NELSON, J. F., ORCHARD, E. AND WELLER, S. (1969) The role of adrenocortical hormone secretion in salt appetite. *Proc. 3rd Intern. Symposium on "Olfaction and Taste"*, C. PFAFFMAN (Ed.), The Rockefeller University Press, in the press.

DENTON, D. A., ORCHARD, E. AND WELLER, S. (1969) The relation between voluntary sodium intake and body sodium balance in normal and adrenalectomized sheep. *Communications in Behavioural Biology*, in the press.

EPSTEIN, A. N. AND STELLAR, E. (1955) The control of salt preference in the adrenalectomized rat. *J. Comp. Physiol. Psychol.*, **48**, 167–172.

FREGLY, M. J. AND WATERS, I. W. (1965) Effects of mineralocorticoids on spontaneous sodium chloride appetite of adrenalectomized rats. *Physiology and Behaviour*, Pergamon Press, London, 1–65.

LYONS, W. R., LI, C. H., COLE, R. D. AND JOHNSON, R. E. (1953) Some of the hormones required by the mammary gland in its development and function. *J. Clin. Endocrinol. Metabl.*, **13**, 836–837.

RICE, K. K. AND RICHTER, C. P. (1943) Increased sodium chloride and water intake of normal rats treated with desoxycorticosterone acetate. *Endocrinology*, **33**, 106–115.

RICHTER, C. P. (1936) Increased salt appetite in adrenalectomized rats. *An.. J. Physiol.*, **115**, 155–161.

RICHTER, C. P. AND BARELARE, JR., B. (1938) Nutritional requirements of pregnant and lactating rats studied by the self selection method. *Endocrinology*, **23**, 15–24.

WOLF, G. (1964a) Sodium appetite elicited by aldosterone. *Psychonomic Science*, **1**, 211–212.

WOLF, G. (1964b) Effects of dorsolateral hypothalamic lesions on sodium appetite elicited by desoxy-corticosterone and by acute hyponatremia. *J. Comp. Physiol. Psychol.*, **58**, 396–402.

WOLF, G. AND HANDAL, P. J. (1966) Aldosterone induced sodium appetite: Dose response and specificity. *Endocrinology*, **78**, 1120–1124.

WOLF, G. AND STRICKER, E. M. (1967) Sodium appetite elicited by hypovolemia in adrenalectomized rats: Reevaluation of the "Reservoir" hypothesis. *J. Comp. Physiol. Psychol.*, **63/2**, 252–257.

DISCUSSION

MILKOVIĆ: Recently, at Dr. Levine's laboratory (Stanford) and at Dr. K. Milković' laboratory (Zagreb), it was found that rats bearing ACTH-secreting tumors preferred to drink saline rather than water when the tumors were well developed. The water/saline ratio at the beginning of the experiment was approximately 15. Within 3–4 weeks this ratio had dropped to 0.5 or less. Pharmacological doses of dexamethasone or DOC caused a reduction of water and sodium intake; however, no marked changes in the water/saline ratio were observed.

DENTON: Due to high peripheral blood concentrations of ACTH in tumor-bearing rats the aldosterone secretion might be stimulated, with the typical effect on saline ingestion.

LARON: Have you any information concerning the effect of androgens and growth hormone on salt appetite? We know that in man, androgens and growth hormone cause a water and NaCl retention; this cannot be explained by an increased aldosterone secretion. In your lactating rabbits, prolactin might have a similar effect to that of growth hormone.

DENTON: Braun-Menendez tested the effect of sex hormones on salt appetite and found no response. We are going to examine the effect of growth hormone and prolactin on salt appetite of female and male rabbits.

Effects of ACTH and Corticosteroids in the Regulation of Food and Water Intake

JAMES A. F. STEVENSON AND CLAIRE FRANKLIN
with the assistance of J. A. GEDDES

Department of Physiology, University of Western Ontario, London, Ontario (Canada)

The adrenal cortex has long been known to influence food and water intake. Addison's disease involves an increased appetite for salt but eventually a decrease in general appetite, anorexia, and body weight loss; Cushing's syndrome is often characterized by the development of a rather specific obesity, enhanced by the retention of salt and water. The specific influences of ACTH and the adrenocortical hormones on food and water intake, however, remain unexplained. Clinical studies have often reported an increase in food intake of patients treated with adrenocortical hormones, but here the issue has been clouded by the fact that the patients were frequently underweight to begin with, and the effect of the hormone on food intake was probably secondary to its effect on the general health and sense of well-being of the patient. In most, if not all, of the experimental studies of the effect of the adrenocortical hormones on food intake and/or body weight changes in the intact animal, the administration of the exogenous hormone has inhibited weight gain or induced its loss. In the few quantitative experimental studies that have been made of the effect of the various glucocorticoids on food intake the conclusion has been that these hormones when administered exogenously, if anything, depress food intake.

EXPERIMENTAL

During the past year, our group has carried out further quantitative studies cf the effect of various adrenocortical hormones on food intake in the rat. For these studies adult male Wistar rats, weighing 200–400 g at the beginning of the experiment, were kept in individual cages in a room at a constant temperature of $22 \pm 1°C$, with 12 hours light and 12 hours dark each day. Five rats were used in each experimental group and in any one experiment the groups were of similar age and weight. Water and food were provided ad libitum. The diet consisted of ground Purina Lab Chow except in the cortisone experiment when a diet was used consisting of casein, sucrose and corn oil, with adequate supplements of a salt mixture and a vitamin mixture, which provided 4.11 calories per gram. Food and water consumptions were measured daily at approximately the same time each day and the 24-hour intakes recorded. The administration of the various adrenocortical hormones and ACTH used is described with the individual experiment. The controls were given sham injections of saline or of the vehicle

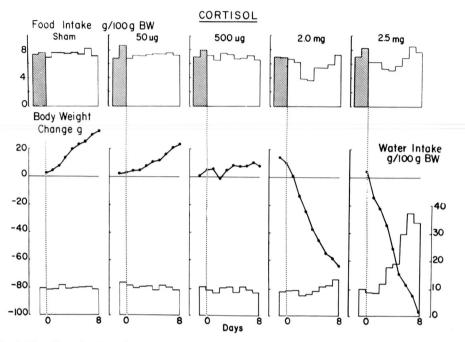

Fig. 1. The effect of various doses of cortisol, given subcutaneously each day for eight days, on food intake, body weight and water intake (lower columnar graph). The values to the left of the vertical dotted line indicate the values on the control days preceding treatment. The controls (Sham) received injections of the vehicle only.

each time the experimental animals received an injection of hormone. On certain occasions a 24-hour collection of urine from the individual animals was made in the usual rat metabolism cage. Urine glucose was measured using an automated microchemical procedure (Technicon Method N-9a) and sometimes was estimated using the Ames Clinistix. Adrenalectomized animals were prepared by removal of the adrenals through paravertebral incisions under trichlorethylene anesthesia and all were maintained on 1 % saline throughout the experiment.

In our first experiment, a suspension of cortisol and carboxymethyl cellulose in normal saline was administered subcutaneously daily for eight days to rats at each of the following levels: 50 μg, 500 μg, 2.0 mg, and 2.5 mg per 100 g of body weight. Fig. 1 shows the effect on food and water intake and on body weight compared to controls sham-injected with the vehicle. The two lowest doses did not affect food or water intake significantly but appeared to reduce body weight gain some 30 and 75 % to 23 and 8 g respectively *vs.* 33 g for the controls. The two highest doses reduced food intake significantly during the first four days of treatment but the animals showed an increasing escape from this effect during the last four days and food intake was within normal limits by day 8. Nevertheless, there was a significant body weight loss throughout the experiment and this was greatest with the highest dose. This pronounced catabolism required a marked increase in water turnover. Urine output and water intake ran parallel in all experiments and, therefore, only the latter is shown in the

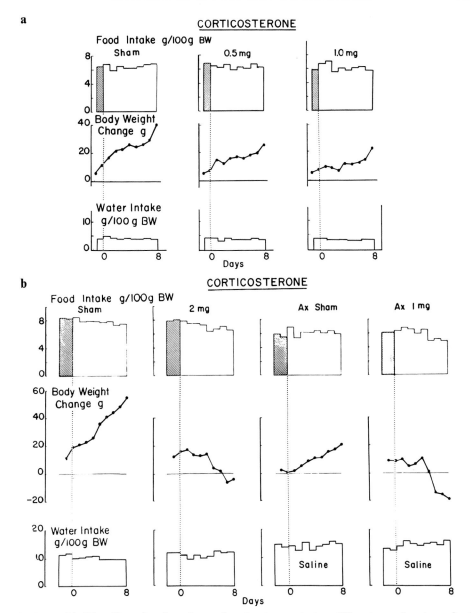

Fig. 2 a and b. The effect of various doses of corticosterone, in two different experiments on food intake, body weight and water intake, described as in Fig. 1. The adrenalectomized rats (Ax) were maintained on saline.

figures. The ratio of water/food intake also rose from a normal of around 1.3 to 3.0–4.0 as more water was required for excretion of the greatly increased load of solutes derived from the enhanced catabolism.

One group of adrenalectomized rats, maintained on saline, was treated with cortisol 2.0 mg for eight days. At this high dose there was a slight temporary reduction of food intake and a body weight loss similar to that seen in the intact animals.

References pp. 150–151

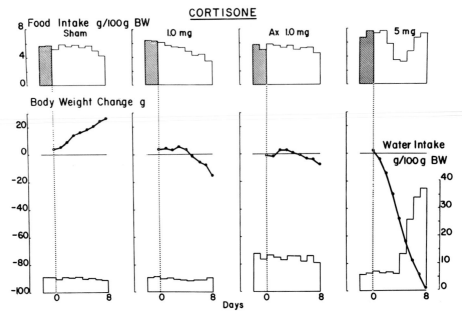

Fig. 3. The effect of various doses of cortisone, given subcutaneously each day for eight days, on food intake, body weight and water intake, described as in Fig. 1. The adrenalectomized rats (Ax) were maintained on saline.

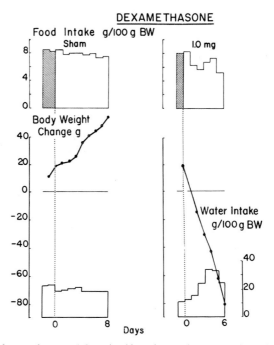

Fig. 4. The effect of dexamethasone, 1.0 mg/rat/day given subcutaneously each day for eight days, described as in Fig. 1.

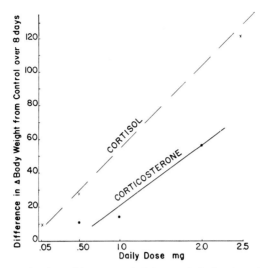

Fig. 5. The relation between the dose of hormone administered daily for eight days and the difference in the weight change between the sham controls and the treated animals from Day 1 to 8.

Corticosterone, also as a suspension, was administered subcutaneously at doses of 0.5, 1.0, and 2.0 mg per 100 g body weight daily for eight days. The effects on food and water intake as seen in Fig. 2 a and b were similar but less, for the same dose of hormone, to those seen with cortisol. For example, at a dose of 2.0 mg corticosterone much less catabolism and loss of body weight occurred, so that the demands on water turnover for excretion of the metabolites were almost negligible. In view of the effect in the intact animal, the marked loss of body weight in the adrenalectomized animal is surprising. Cortisone appeared to be somewhat more potent both in its depression of food intake and in its catabolic effect (Fig. 3).

In another experiment, the effect of dexamethasone 1 mg daily for six days was determined. As shown in Fig. 4, this agent caused the usual depression of food intake with some indication of later escape, but it was particularly potent as a catabolic agent, as seen in the rapid fall in body weight and increase in water turnover.

The effects of these adrenocortical hormones on food and water intake were qualitatively similar though varying in degree: an early, and apparently temporary, moderate depression of food intake but a continuing increase in tissue catabolism, as reflected in the body weight, which required a parallel increase in water turnover to excrete the products. The effect of body weight change was approximately in linear relation to dose (Fig. 5).

The effects of exogenous adrenocorticotrophic hormone and its stimulation of endogenous adrenocortical hormone production on food and water intake were next examined. ACTH at 1.5 units per day for eight days had no significant effect on food and water intake or on weight gain in the intact animal (Fig. 6a). In the adrenalectomized animal it may have improved slightly the reduced food intake and weight gain. At 3.0 units per day, ACTH again caused no change of intakes or weight gain but apparently improved the weight gain of the adrenalectomized aniamls (Fig. 6b).

References pp. 150–151

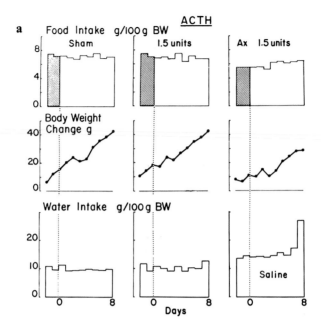

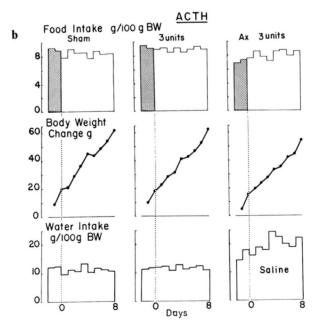

Fig. 6 a and b. The effect of ACTH, 1.5 or 3.0 units given subcutaneously each day for eight days on food intake, body weight and water intake in intact and adrenalectomized (Ax) rats, described as in Fig. 1.

The changes in endocrine and other organ weights obtained on autopsy under anesthesia at the end of the eight-day experiments were typical of the particular hormonal treatment.

DISCUSSION

Although clinical reports have emphasized the increase in food intake in patients treated with adrenocortical hormones, (Van Putten, Van Bekkum, and Querido, 1953), neither this or the few previous experimental studies (Bellamy, 1964; Bodansky and Money, 1964; Cannon, Frazier, and Hughes, 1956; Grossie and Turner, 1965; Johannessen, Davidovitch, and Blackey, 1966; Winter, Silber, and Stoerk, 1950) confirm this effect in the normal animal given exogenous adrenocortical hormone. The present investigation might be criticised for the brevity of the treatment period, but the earlier studies of Bodansky and Money (1954), in which cortisone at about 1 mg/ 100 g/day was given for 43 days and that of Cannon, Frazier, and Hughes (1956) in which cortisone (5 mg/rat/day) was given for 24 days to rats previously depleted of protein, indicate that the effect of body weight seen in the present experiment continues for these much longer periods of time. The most impressive phenomenon in the present and these two previous investigations is this continuing catabolism and marked loss of weight without any compensating increase in food intake. The increase of appetite seen clinically when patients suffering various illnesses are treated with adrenocortical preparations would appear to be due to a non-specific effect of the hormone improving general health and a sense of well-being. The present study has dealt only with the glucocorticoid hormones. The influence of the mineralocorticoids on the intake of water and other fluids has been investigated by the Halls (Hall and Hall, 1965a and b, 1969) and by Denton (1969), and the controls for water intake have been recently reviewed (Stevenson, 1967).

From the point of view of the control of food intake it is interesting to speculate on the mechanisms involved in, first, the early depression of food intake on treatment with adrenocortical hormones and, second, in the failure of intake to increase later to compensate for the loss of energy to the body caused by the catabolic effect of these hormones. There are, at present, three major mechanisms postulated for the evocation of feeding in response to bodily energy needs. These are: the glucostatic (Mayer, 1965), the lipostatic (Kennedy, 1969), and the thermostatic (Brobeck, 1960). All postulate systems with receptor cells specific to some particular parameter in the internal environment and/or cells. Electrophysiological evidence has been reported for glucoreceptor cells in the hypothalamus (Anand, 1967) and the liver (Niijima, 1969) which change their discharge rate in relation to the level of circulating glucose and its rate of entry into the cell. Similar receptors have been postulated for some circulating metabolite of fat, the level of which could reflect the level of the fat depots. Both cutaneous and hypothalamic thermosensitive neurons are well known and it has been hypothesized (Stevenson, 1964, 1969) that information from both of these, when integrated centrally, could reflect the rate of heat loss giving information about insulation (fat) as well as the more immediate state of energy exchange. It would not be

References pp. 150–151

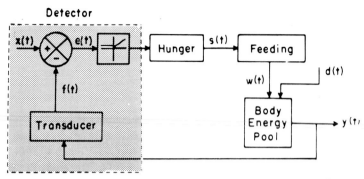

Fig. 7. Simple model of a hypothetical control system for food intake. The parts of the system inside the square (−−−) could all be functions of a single receptor cell. Some characteristic of energy flow, y(t), activates a transducer which supplies a feedback signal, f(t), which is compared at the summing point to some reference value, x(t). As a result an appropriate error signal, e(t), when it is positive, activates those cell-assemblies responsible for the subjective impression of energy hunger. These provide a steering signal, s(t), to the part of the overall system responsible for selecting the most appropriate response at the moment and, if feeding is appropriate, the necessary somato-sensory and somato-motor systems are activated. Depending on the rate of feeding, w(t), the body energy pool is returned to the resting or optimal state and the feeding behavior is no longer evoked. A similar model could represent satiety and cessation of feeding.

surprising if several such control systems were involved in an activity as important as energy intake.

A major focus for the central control systems for feeding and drinking appears to be situated in the mid-hypothalamus with a predominance of facilitatory (feeding) elements in the lateral hypothalamus and of inhibitory (satiety) elements in the ventromedial region (Stevenson, 1969). Nevertheless, it is now recognized that there are important ramifications of these systems throughout the limbic system and also in the lower brain, with receptors situated both centrally and in the periphery.

Fig. 7 gives a general outline of a possible control system for food intake. The detector or receptor cell could serve as a transducer of chemical or thermal information to nerve impulses, comparing this to some reference level determined, say its own metabolism. It can also serve as a pass gate, only firing when the measured item moves above (or below) the reference level to evoked activity in those systems, with which is associated the subjective sensation of hunger and the operation of feeding, or the sensation of satiety and the absence of feeding.

The depression of food intake initially by excessive adrenocortical hormones may be due to a continuous and plentiful supply of glucose to the cells, obviating any activation of a feeding receptor or providing continuing stimulation of a satiety detector. The return to normal food intake could be due to adaptation of such receptors or to increasing activity of receptors for other aspects of the internal environment not so influenced by the adrenocortical hormones. In view of the fact that food intake is increased in response to the enhanced energy loss induced by excess thyroid hormone, it is surprising that food intake eventually fails to increase to provide a similar compensation for the increased energy loss from excess adrenocortical hormone. This could be due to confusion of the control system because the level of a circulating metabolite

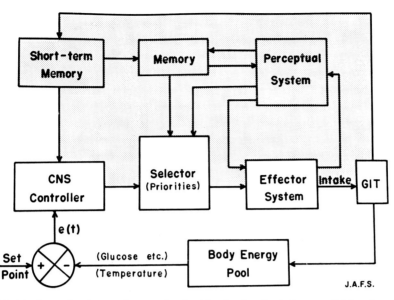

Fig. 8. Model of postulated control system for food intake showing influence of higher functions on fundamental system.

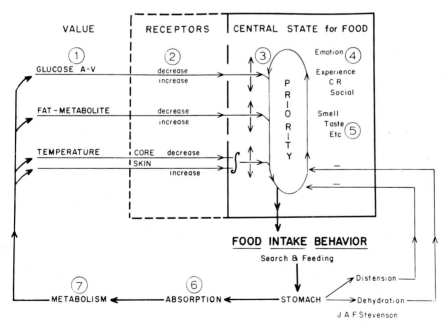

Fig. 9. Diagram of postulated receptors and control systems for food intake. See text for explanation of numbers. Modified from Stevenson, 1969.

References pp. 150–151

like glucose no longer bears its usual relation to the overall store of energy.

Fig. 8 gives a more comprehensive view of the mechanisms involved in the central control of food intake. Those systems showing in the shaded area are situated in cortical and limbic regions. The adrenocortical hormones could affect the neurons subserving any of these systems either directly or through their influence on some aspect of the internal environment.

In Fig. 9, which is a summary of the postulated controls of food intake, the possible sites of influence of the adrenocortical hormones and their effects are suggested. (1) The influence on the level of glucose has already been discussed. Some adrenocortical hormones may also increase the level of lipid metabolites (Barrett, 1966). On the several occasions when colonic temperature was measured, we found no significant differences to suggest an influence through this receptor system. (2) The function of the receptors themselves could be affected either in terms of their inherent reference value or their efficiency of function. (3,4) The function of the neurons subserving the higher systems could also be influenced for it is known that adrenocortical hormones affect mood and emotional behavior in man. (5) Similarly, the neuronal systems for the special senses involved in food intake might be affected. (6) Absorption is apparently not significantly impaired by excess adrenocortical hormone. (7) Metabolism is markedly influenced; the effects on the control systems have already been mentioned.

The mechanism by which excess adrenocortical hormones influence intake remains undetermined because of the complexity of the control systems involved but we are now much nearer to useful hypotheses that can be submitted to experimental test.

ACKNOWLEDGEMENTS

The assistance of Miss Blanche Box, B.Sc., is gratefully acknowledged. Mrs. P. Lucas and Mrs. R. Speigel, B. Sc., gave help in preparing the illustrations.

Supported by Grant M339 from the Medical Research Council of Canada.

REFERENCES

ANAND, B. K. (1967) Central chemosensitive mechanisms related to feeding. In: *Handbook of Physiology, Alimentary Canal, Sect. 6*, Vol. 1, *Control of Food and Water*, American Physiological Soc., 249–263.

BARRETT, A. M. (1966) The role of plasma free fatty acids in the elevation of plasma cholesterol and phospholipids produced by adrenaline. *J. Endocrinol.*, **36**, 301–316.

BELLAMY, D. (1964) Effect of cortisol on growth and food intake in rats. *J. Endocrinol.*, **31**, 83–84.

BODANSKY, O. AND MONEY, W. L. (1954) Rates of development and regression of changes during and after prolonged cortisone administration in rats. *Endocrinology*, **55**, 173–185.

BROBECK, J. R. (1960) Food and temperature. *Recent Progr. Hormone Res.*, **16**, 439–466.

CANNON, P., FRAZIER, L. E. AND HUGHES, R. H. (1956) The influence of cortisone upon protein metabolism. *Arch. Pathol.*, **61**, 271–279.

DENTON, D. A. AND NELSON, J. F. (1970) Pituitary–adrenal axis and salt appetite. *Progr. Brain Res.*, this volume, pp. 131–140.

GROSSIE, J. AND TURNER, C. W. (1965) Effect of thyroxine, hydrocortisone and growth hormone on food intake in rats. *Proc. Soc. Exptl. Biol. Med.*, **118**, 28–30.

HALL, C. E. AND HALL, O. (1969) Interaction between desoxycorticosterone treatment, fluid intake, sodium consumption, blood pressure, and organ changes in rats drinking water, saline, or sucrose solution. *Can. J. Physiol. Pharmacol.*, **47**, 81–86.

HALL, C. E. AND HALL, O. (1965a) Hypertension and hypersalimentation. 1. Aldosterone hypertension. *Lab. Invest.*, **14**, 285–294.

HALL, C. E. AND HALL, O. (1965b) Hypertension and hypersalimentation. 2. Deoxycorticosterone hypertension. *Lab. Invest.*, **14**, 1727–1735.

JOHANNESSEN, L. B., DAVIDOVITCH, Z. AND BLACKEY, W. E. (1966) Effects of cortisone and calorie restriction on skeletogenesis in immature rats. *Arch. Oral Biol.*, **11**, 31–39.

KENNEDY, G. C. (1969) Interaction between feeding behavior and hormones during growth. *Ann. N. Y. Acad. Sci.*, **157**, 1049–1061.

MAYER, J. (1965) Regulation of energy intake and the body weight. The glucostatic theory and the lipostatic hypothesis. *Ann. N. Y. Acad. Sci.*, **63**, 15–42.

NIIJIMA, A. (1969) Afferent impulse discharges from gluco-receptors in the liver of the guinea pig. *Ann. N. Y. Acad. Sci.*, **157**, 690–700.

STEVENSON, J. A. F. (1964) The hypothalamus in the regulation of energy and water balance. *Physiologist*, **7**, 305–318.

STEVENSON, J. A. F. (1967) Central mechanisms controlling water intake. In: *Handbook of Physiology. Alimentary Canal*, W. HEIDEL (Ed.), Am. Physiol. Soc. Washington, D.C., *Sect. 6*, Vol. 1, pp. 173–190.

STEVENSON, J. A. F. (1969) Mechanisms in the control of food and water intake. *Ann. N. Y. Aacd. Sci.*, **157**, 1069–1083.

VAN PUTTEN, L. M., VAN BEKKUM, D. W. AND QUERIDO, A. (1953) Influence of cortisone and ACTH on appetite. *Acta Endocrinol.*, **12**, 159–166.

WINTER, C. A., SILBER, R. H. AND STOERK, H. C. (1950) Production of reversible hyperadrenocortinism in rats by prolonged administration of cortisone. *Endocrinology*, **47**, 60–72.

DISCUSSION

HODGES: We have recently been administering betamethasone to rats in their drinking water. This reduces their growth rate, without having much effect on food intake and causing only a slight increase in water intake; results which are not very different from yours.

I would like to ask you about the mode of action of amphetamine on food intake according to your control system?

STEVENSON: It has been considered, on the basis of the finding of Andersson and his group that frontal lobotomy in the dog obviated the reduction of water intake caused by amphetamine, that this drug activates inhibitory systems in the frontal regions which influence food and water intake systems in the hypothalamus and limbic system. On the other hand, as shown by Mogenson, amphetamine increases lever pressing, but decreases intake in rats with chronic electrodes in the lateral hypothalamus through which self-stimulation which also evokes intake is normally obtained.

MISHER: Just a comment regarding the effects of amphetamine. Rats which are made hyperphagic by bilateral ventromedial lesions are hypersensitive to the anoretic effects of amphetamine. Doses less than 0.5 mg/kg orally give you very pronounced effects.

JONES: Dr. Imms and myself have carried out some balance studies in the rat. We have found that small doses of corticosterone (100–200 μg) to adrenalectomized rats cause an increase in food intake. A large dose of corticosterone of 2 mg certainly causes a loss in body weight, but these animals are very active; indeed it is sometimes difficult to get them out of the cage. What part, do you think, does increased activity play in the weight loss? It is interesting that the small dose of corticosterone prevents the increased excretion of noradrenaline which follows adrenalectomy, but the 2-mg dose causes a very large increase in noradrenaline excretion.

STEVENSON: The adrenalectomized animal shows a reduced food intake and replacement doses of hormone restore this to normal. As you and we have found, high doses of glycocorticoids cause excessive catabolism in the adrenalectomized animal as they do in the intact one. We are now carrying out experiments to determine the role of metabolic rate and activity in the loss of body weight observed on administration of excessive glycocorticoids. If large doses of glycocorticoids increase circulating levels, as well as excretion of noradrenaline, this may be an important factor in enhancing the effect of thyroid hormone and perhaps of the adrenocortical hormones in the catabolism of peripheral tissues.

DE WIED: What kind of ACTH did you use? And would you care to comment on the interesting effect of ACTH on body weight gain in adrenalectomized rats?

STEVENSON: The ACTH used was obtained from Sigma Chemical Co., St. Louis, as Corticotrophin A. It was dissolved in normal saline just before injection. We have no explanation (other than that it may be an extra-adrenal effect) of the improvement in weight gain of the adrenalectomized rats treated with ACTH at 3 units/day. These results need to be confirmed and, if they are, perhaps you will explain them for us.

McEWEN: Does ACTH secretion accompany hunger or thirst in normal or extreme deprivation? Such a secretion, if it occurs, may be very important for the question of arousal, especially with regard to appetitive conditioning for food or water reward.

STEVENSON: I do not know of any evidence on the circulating level of ACTH, related to evocation of intake, in food or water deprivation. Both deprivations are stressful and starvation results in an early increased activity of the pituitary–adrenal axis which in turn produces the necessary glyconeogenesis.

Dehydration, of course, releases antidiuretic hormone (ADH), which might influence the anterior pituitary. The present study would not suggest that ACTH has any direct effect on food intake.

MILKOVIĆ: You found unchanged food intake after dexamethasone application, and body weight went down because of the inadequate balance between food intake and metabolic processes in such a situation. We gave to our rats with ACTH-secreting tumor three times the normal amount of food by stomach tube in the phase of tumor growth when rats started to lose body weight, but this forced feeding did not help these rats much in maintaining their body weight. This indicates that food intake in such a situation is not the main factor.

STEVENSON: Dr. Milković' observation is most interesting and is reminiscent of the catabolic phase that follows damage in man or animal. During this phase, when adrenocortical activity and secretion are markedly increased, a forced increase of protein and caloric intake by mouth or vein neither improves nitrogen balance nor maintenance of body weight. This is in contradiction to the marked ability to retain protein, nitrogen, and calories in the later anabolic phase when adrenocortical function has returned to resting levels. Presumably, a similar catabolic set in our animals receiving excess glycocorticoids might well have negated any increase in food intake, had this been the response.

MIRSKY: Whereas hyperthyroidism induces a tremendous increase in peripheral utilization of glucose, free fatty acids, etc., hypercorticalism produces no effect on this peripheral utilization. There seems to be an entirely different mechanism. Maybe that is why animals do not compensate for weight loss by increased food uptake.

STEVENSON: I agree with Dr. Mirksy that the peripheral aspects of the catabolism caused by excessive adrenocortical hormones and excessive thyroid hormone are entirely different; as I suggested, it may be in this difference that we will find a clue as to why the body increases food intake in the latter but not in the former instance of what can be a fatal loss of energy and substance.

Effects of ACTH and Adrenocortical Hormones on the Nervous System

K. LISSÁK

Institute of Physiology, University Medical School, Rákóczi út 80, Pécs (Hungary)

I think that all of the experimental findings which have been presented in this section under my chairmanship favour the concept that pituitary–adrenocortical hormones exert their influence on the central nervous system at different levels; and that their effects appear on those structures which are also deeply involved in the organization of motivated and conditioned behavioural reactions. This data indicates that these hormones can influence both the facilitatory and the inhibitory processes of the central nervous system as well as control sensory input, at least at the brain stem and diencephalic levels.

More than 50 years ago, Kraepelin initiated a new scientific approach called "endocrine psychopathia". Although our knowledge of the hormones at this time was rather scanty, this approach was directed towards the brain and behaviour relationships. In connection with the effect of the pituitary–adrenocortical hormones upon brain mechanisms, the first experimental reports were published by Liddel *et al.* in 1935. After the introduction of both ACTH and corticosteroids into routine clinical use and animal experimentation, the number of data suggesting diverse effects of ACTH and corticosteroids on the central nervous system has been accumulating in the recent literature. Many attempts have been made to understand the mechanisms of action of these hormones; and the papers presented in the first section of the conference provided a great deal of recent information in this field.

The electrophysiological techniques have produced a revolutionary development in many branches of physiological sciences; and the papers of this section, I think, just confirmed this statement. The analysis of hormonal effects with micro-electrode recordings, and the use of chemical stimulation of single cells by use of the iontophoretic technique, indicate a real progress in the area of neuroendocrine research. According to these studies, a broad area within the diencephalon and the rostral brain stem shows chemosensitivity to corticosteroids. It is well known from neurophysiological studies that these structures are deeply involved in the organization of complex motivated behavioural reactions; and that they also act as neuroanatomical substrates for the establishment of temporary connections.

Generally speaking, the hormonal effects upon brain mechanisms can be regarded as conditioning influences; furthermore, they appear in threshold changes of central nervous processes. The papers presented in this section reveal that the presence of corticosteroids is necessary for the development of thalamocortical incremental responses and EEG after-reaction following activation of the forebrain structures. In addition to this, it was found that administration of corticosteroids elicits firing responses in the cells of the posterior hypothalamus, while suppressing the unit activity in the anterior diencephalon. These observations indicate a dynamic chemoreceptive field for corticosteroids in the hypothalamus; and suggest that the central role of this cell system lies in relation to both the neuroendocrine feedback action as well as to brain behaviour.

An action of ACTH, distinct from that of corticosteroids, on the central nervous processes had been suggested by many authors in the early 1950's. They observed differential effects of ACTH and corticosteroids on the mood and emotional status of human beings. In this section, one of the papers related to this topic has been presented and provides data of the extra-adrenal action of ACTH on the nervous system. The effects of the ACTH peptide on nervous functions seem to be very promising; although we are still far from understanding the role of extra-adrenal ACTH action in the homeostatic function of the organism.

New information is presented by using peptides of different chemical structure. These peptides were well tested on the spinal cord. This approach to the action of peptides upon nervous processes seems to be a useful study method for the near future.

An ontogenetical approach to the relationships existing between these hormones and the brain is one of the most fascinating and hopeful aspects, both in the field of neurobiology and neuroendocrinology. Data presented in this section's program clearly show that early experience during the first post-natal days, decisively influences the maturation of adaptive functions as well as determining adult behaviour.

It is interesting to note that the papers of this section, and even of the entire symposium, pay much attention to the effects of ACTH and corticosteroids upon brain mechanisms which are more related to organization of complex behavioural reactions than to the feedback regulation of the pituitary–adrenal system. This trend is in keeping with the general tendency of the neurobiological field in that it requires a multidisciplinary approach to the brain and behaviour functions, since it includes the methods of biochemistry, electrophysiology, and experimental psychology.

The data presented in this section clearly show that the understanding of hormonal influence on the central nervous processes on the basis of a "compartmentalized view" is not possible. Thus, the pituitary–adrenocortical hormones can determine both facilitatory and inhibitory processes; and their effect is exerted at different levels of the neuronal hierarchy.

I wish to express thanks to all the speakers who contributed to the success of this section. All the speakers provided a great amount of information regarding the relationships between the pituitary–adrenocortical system and the central nervous functions.

NOTE OF THE EDITORS

In this book the contributions of Drs. DENTON and STEVENSON have been included in the second session. At the conference they presented their papers in session III.

Dr. LEVINE's paper, originally presented in session II, has been included in the first session.

SESSION III

Effects of ACTH and Corticosteroids on Animal Behavior

Chairman: I. A. MIRSKY

Laboratory of Clinical Sciences, University of Pittsburgh, School of Medicine, 3811 O'Hara Street, Pittsburgh, Penna. 15213, U.S.A.

Specific Functions of a Medial Thalamic Structure in Avoidance Conditioning in the Rat

JEAN DELACOUR

Centre d'Etudes de Physiologie nerveuse, Département de Psychophysiologie du Comportement,
4, Avenue Gordon-Bennett, Paris 16ème (France)

Previous investigations have analyzed the role of the Centrum-Medianum-Para-fascicularis complex (CM-Pf) of the thalamus in defensive conditioning. Lesions of this structure clearly impair the retention and the acquisition of active avoidance responses in the two-way shuttle-box (Cardo, 1961; Delacour and Libouban, 1964). On the other hand, this lesion does not hinder the acquisition of a vegetative defensive reaction (change in cardiac rhythm) in a classical conditioning situation (Delacour and Santacana, 1967). Acquisition of a passive avoidance response and the retention of the active avoidance response conditioned in the one-way shuttle-box is spared as well (Delacour and Alexinsky, 1968). On the other hand, the role of the CM-Pf complex in positively reinforced conditioning has not been studied precisely: preliminary data were obtained from tests which were not comparable to those used in aversive situations (Delacour, Albe-Fessard and Libouban, 1966). In order to clarify the functions of the CM-Pf complex according to the type of the reinforcement, we have studied the effects of lesions on both defensive and appetitive responses, of similar characteristics.

Four experiments (I, II, III, IV) were performed. These experiments were matched by pairs: in each pair, one experiment was based on a defensive test, and the other, on a food-reinforced test. In the first two experiments, operant conditioning was used: Sidman test (I) and fixed-interval test (II). In both these cases, the subjects had to adapt their behavior to some temporal relationship between the response and the reinforcement without a discriminative conditioned stimulus. On the other hand, in the two other experiments, a discriminative visual CS was used. By responding to this CS, the subjects could avoid an electric shock (Exp. III) or obtain a food-pellet (Exp. IV). In all four tests, the response to be conditioned was a bar-press and the general conditions and procedures were identical.

GENERAL METHOD

The subjects were 71 male albino rats of the Wistar strain, 3 to 6 months old. The general procedure was the following: experimental groups were submitted to bilateral electrolytic lesions in the CM-Pf complex (CM groups). Control groups (Ccm) were submitted to the same surgical procedure, with the exception that no lesion was made. Operations were performed under Penthotal anesthesia (70–80 mg/kg i.p.). A d.c. current (1 to 2 mA) was passed through a steel electrode for 20 to 30 seconds; the electrode was connected to the cathode of the generator. Lesions were stereotactically placed according to the atlas of Albe-Fessard, Stutinsky and Libouban (1966). Letter A will designate an antero-posterior localization; letter L, a lateral distance from the midline of the brain; letter H, a localization on the vertical axis. Lesions were produced by one electrode penetration on each side of the midline, according to the following coordinates: A — 4.0 to 4.5; L — 0.5 to 1.0; H — 4.5. A minimum of 6 days was allowed for recovery. The rats were housed in individual cages. They were submitted to a regular cycle of artificial illumination with the light phase between 6 a.m. and 8 p.m. The test room was sound proof and dimly illuminated. Programming and recording devices were located in an adjacent room from which animals were observed through a closed circuit TV.

Routine observations were taken on alimentary behavior, spontaneous activity, emotional responses, and sensory-motor capacities. Data from systematic observations have been reported previously (Delacour *et al.*, 1966, 1967).

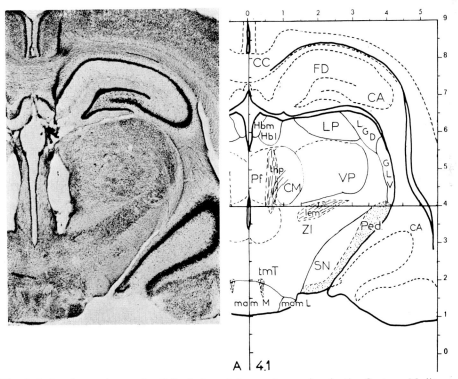

Fig. 1. Left, photo-micrograph of the lesion at its maximum size, in the Centrum-Medianum-Parafascicularis (CM-Pf). On right, the corresponding scheme taken from the atlas of Albe-Fessard *et al.* (1966). Abbreviations: CC: corpus callosum; CA: hippocampus; LP: nucleus lateralis posterior thalami; VP: nucleus ventralis posterior; LG: nucleus genicularis lateralis; Ped: pedunculus cerebri; SN: substantia nigra; ZI: zona incerta; lem: lemniscus medialis; Hb: nucleus habenularis; tmT: tractus mammillo-thalamicus; mam: corpus mammillare.

At the end of the experiments, each rat was sacrificed by an overdose of Penthotal. The brain was perfused, fixed in 10% formalin and stored in the fixative for 1–2 weeks. Frozen serial sections 100 microns thick were made. All the sections containing the lesion were stained with thionin and examined under a 10 × magnification.

Two-tailed parametric and non-parametric statistical tests were employed (Mc Nemar, 1955; Siegel, 1956).

RESULTS

Histological control

Lesions of CM-Pf complex (Fig. 1) accepted as correct were located between A — 3.5 to A — 4.8 and extended from 0.5 to 1.2 mm on the anterio-posterior axis. At the point of their maximal size, they extended 0.5 to 1.2 mm in the lateral direction between L—0 and L—1.5; and from 1.2 to 2.2 mm on the vertical axis, between H—3.5 and H—6.0. The adjacent structures which were most frequently touched were the habenulo-peduncular tract, Habenula and Zona Incerta.

General effect of the lesions

Previous observations (Delacour et al., 1966, 1967) have shown that lesions of the CM-Pf complex have no effect on sensory-motor capacities, spontaneous activity, alimentary or emotional behavior. An important point to be noted is that these lesions do not modify the threshold of the flinch or escape responses elicited by electric shock. Routine observations made during the present experiments were also negative.

Experiments I and II

Experiment I

Forty rats were tamed by daily handling for a period of 10 days. They were then trained on the Sidman avoidance schedule. The interior dimensions of the box were 30 × 30 × 40 cm (height). The bar, 5 × 5 cm, was located 6 cm above the floor; a 10-g pressure was necessary to close the contact. The original procedure of Sidman was somewhat modified: the duration of the shock (0.8 to 1.0 mA) was not fixed; its maximum duration was 10 sec but it could be terminated by the bar-press response. The S–S interval was 30 sec and the R–S, 20 sec. These parameters have been chosen in order to compare the results of this experiment with those of our previous experiments using the shuttle-box technique. Probably because of the long duration of the S–S interval, 16 rats failed to reach the criterion which was 15 or less shocks per session for 5 consecutive sessions. The sessions were 20 min long. The first 5 min were considered as a warming-up period, and scores were taken only during the last 15 min. The rats who reached the criterion were divided in two comparable groups for operation: a CM group ($n = 13$) and a control group Ccm ($n = 11$). Two control rats and one experimental died shortly after operation. The remainder were allowed

TABLE 1

MEAN POST-OP PERFORMANCES IN TEST I (SIDMAN)

Groups	n	Responses		Shocks	
		Mean	Range	Mean	Range
CM	10	66.8	43.8 – 108	16.5*	6.8 – 24.8
Ccm	9	72.6	44.6 – 96.2	10.7	3.2 – 19.6

* $p < 0.01$.

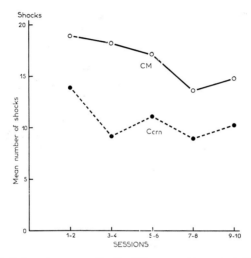

Fig. 2. Relearning curves for the Sidman avoidance test (Exp. I).

7 days for recovery and then were given ten retraining sessions. After histological control, data from two experimental rats were discarded.

Results

Table 1 and Fig. 2 show the mean post-op performance of the two groups: lesions produced significant ($p < 0.01$) deficits in avoidance behavior since the experimental group received more shocks than the control. This effect was not accompanied by a decrease in the frequency of response: scores of the two groups were comparable in this respect. Therefore we can assume that the deficit of the experimental group was not due to some motor impairment but rather, that it affected the adjustment of the responses to the temporal parameters of the situation, *i.e.* the S–S and R–S intervals. In the Sidman test, given the over-all frequency of responding, the number of shocks avoided depends on the inter-response time (IRT) patterns. These patterns were probably less adapted to the program of reinforcement in the experimental group than in the control. Unfortunately no IRT histograms were available to check this hypothesis directly.

Experiment II

The general conditions were very similar to those of experiment I. The same test apparatus was used. After taming, 25 rats learned to bar-press in order to receive food-pellets (45 mg each, Noyes). They were given first thirteen 5-min sessions on a continuous reinforcement schedule, one session a day. At the end of this period, each rat displayed a high and fairly steady rate of responding. Then a fixed interval schedule of reinforcement was introduced: for the first four sessions, the interval was 20 sec long; after this, it was 60 sec. The limited hold condition was not used. A maximum of 30 pellets could be obtained in each session. The rats were given 30 sessions (one session a day) on the FI-60 sec program. The 60-sec interval was divided into four 15-sec long sub-intervals (I, II, III, IV); responses given during each sub-interval were recorded independently on four electro-mechanical counters. Fig. 3 shows the mean percentage of responses given in each sub-interval during the first 5 sessions and during the last 5 sessions (26th to 30th session) for 18 selected rats. Seven rats who failed to display clear and reliable improvement of performance were discarded. Rats were selected according to the percentage of responses given in the subinterval IV: the criterion being that 40% or more of the total number of responses, for five consecutive sessions, occur during this period. From the selected rats, two groups were formed: a CM-Pf group ($n = 10$) and a control (Ccm) group ($n = 8$). After recovery (7 days), the two groups were submitted to 7 retraining sessions. Scores of two experimental rats were discarded after histological control.

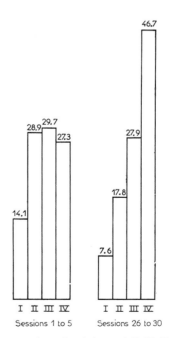

Fig. 3. Evolution of the response rate in each sub-interval (I, II, III, IV) in the fixed interval (FI) test (Exp. II) during pre-operative training.

TABLE 2

MEAN PERCENTAGES OF RESPONSES IN EACH SUBINTERVAL IN TEST II (FI)

Groups	n	Subintervals			
		I	II	III	IV
CM	8	7.5	20.3	27.8	44.4
Ccm	8	4.7	19.4	30.8	45.1

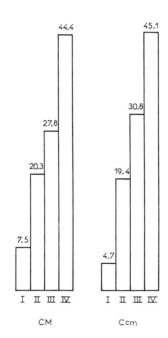

Fig. 4. Response rate in each sub-interval (I, II, III, IV) in the FI test (Exp. II) during the post-operative retraining.

Results

Table 2 and Fig. 4 show the mean percentage of responses in each sub-interval for the two groups; the two distributions do not differ significantly according to the chi-square test. The over-all frequency was slightly increased in the CM group after operation (*cf.* Table 3) but this increase was not significant.

Unlike the preceding experiment, the CM-Pf lesions seem to have no effect on the temporal adjustment of the instrumental responses, in the FI situation.

Experiments III and IV

The general conditions were very similar to those of the preceding ones; the test apparatus was identical. The only systematic difference was that a discriminative

References pp. 169–170

TABLE 3

MEAN FREQUENCY OF RESPONSE IN TEST II (FI)

Groups	n	Pre-op		Post-op	
		Mean	Range	Mean	Range
CM	8	132.1	90.7—161.3	158.6	99.3—190.4
Ccm	8	124.7	102.2—158.1	135.5	95.7—177.0

visual stimulus was used. This CS was delivered by a 15-W lamp located at the top of the box, above the bar.

Experiment III

The US was an electric shock (0.8 to 1.0 mA) delivered through the floor and the walls by a scrambler generator. By pressing the bar during the CS–US interval, rats were able to stop the CS and avoid the shock (conditioned avoidance response, CAR); during the US, they could also escape the shock by pressing the bar. The CS overlapped the US and the two stimuli were always stopped simultaneously. After a series of training steps, the subjects were submitted to the following schedule: 60 trials a day; mean inter-trial interval = 32 sec (20 to 44); CS–US interval = 6 sec; maximum duration of the US = 4 sec. Twenty-three rats were selected who had reached a 60% CAR level during two successive sessions. This rather low criterion was due to the difficulties, frequently reported by others (Meyer, Cho and Weseman, 1960; Hoffman, Fleshler and Chorny, 1961) encountered in training a bar-press avoidance response. These 23 rats were divided into two comparable groups and operated upon: CM-group ($n = 14$) and Ccm-group (control, $n = 9$). After recovery (7 days), the rats were submitted to five retraining sessions. One experimental rat died shortly after operation; data from three others were discarded after histological control.

Results

Table 4 shows pre-op and post-op percentage of CAR. Analysis of co-variance yielded highly significant differences between post-op performances of the two groups

TABLE 4

MEAN PERCENTAGE OF CAR (TEST III)

Groups	n	Pre-op		Post-op	
		Mean	Range	Mean	Range
CM	10	83.5	72.1—93.5	48.3*	5.3—82.0
Ccm	9	79.5	65.8—90.0	84.7	70.0—97.0

* $p < 0.001$.

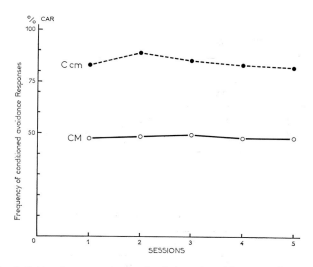

Fig. 5. Relearning curves in the discriminated avoidance test (Exp. III).

TABLE 5

MEAN FREQUENCY OF BAR-PRESSING (TEST III)

Groups	n	Pre-op		Post-op	
		Mean	Range	Mean	Range
CM	10	90.7	64.0—123.0	90.6	69.8—124.6
Ccm	9	85.1	71.0— 97.7	78.8	70.0— 89.4

($p < 0.001$) and between pre- and post-op performances within the CM-group ($p <$ 0.001). Fig. 5 shows the evolution of performances during retraining: the deficit shown by the CM-group appears to be poorly reversible as was the deficit demonstrated in the two-way shuttle box (Delacour *et al.*, 1966). The lesions had no effect on the overall frequency of response (*cf.* Table 5).

Experiment IV

The principle of the test used in this experiment was the following: the reinforcement was a 45-mg food-pellet. When no response was given in the presence of the CS, no reinforcement was delivered and the CS had a fixed duration of 3 sec. The first response in the presence of the CS was immediately reinforced and it prolonged the CS by a supplementary interval of 2 sec. The responses given during the supplementary interval were not reinforced. Twenty-two rats were trained on a continuous reinforcement schedule during at least 12 five-min sessions. At this stage, the box was permanently lighted by a 15-W lamp. When the rats reached a high and rather steady level of bar-pressing, they were submitted to the second stage of the procedure: the test-box was only lit by the CS, and the responses reinforced according to the

TABLE 6

MEAN PERCENTAGE OF PELLETS OBTAINED PER SESSION (TEST IV)

Groups	n	Pre-op		Post-op	
		Mean	Range	Mean	Range
CM	9	78.7	73.3—95.0	82.8	74.0—92.0
Ccm	8	79.9	76.6—96.6	83.6	81.0—94.0

TABLE 7

MEAN FREQUENCY OF BAR-PRESSING (TEST IV)

Groups	n	Pre-op		Post-op	
		Mean	Range	Mean	Range
CM	9	73.9	47.6—139.3	76.1	61.8—101.4
Ccm	8	69.3	37.3—103.0	60.7	26.6— 85.0

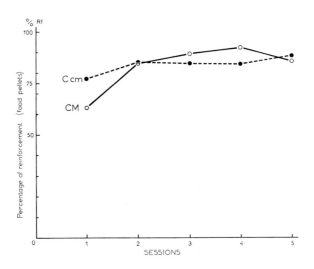

Fig. 6. Relearning curves for the alimentary bar-press responses (Exp. IV).

above-mentioned conditions. During each daily session, the CS was presented 20 times with a mean interval of 32 sec (20 to 44). The criterion was reached when a rat obtained 14 or more pellets (*i.e.* 70% of the maximum number) during three consecutive sessions. All the 22 rats fulfilled this condition; they were then divided into two groups for operation, a CM-group ($n = 13$) and a Ccm-group ($n = 9$). Two experimental rats and a control died shortly after the operation. The remainder were allowed 6 days for recovery and then submitted to five retraining sessions. Scores from two experimental rats were discarded after histological control.

Results

Table 6 gives the mean number of pellets obtained by session during the last three sessions before operation and the five post-op sessions; this number is expressed as percentage of the maximum number of pellets available by session (*i.e.* 20). Fig. 6 shows the retraining curves of the two groups. It appears clearly that lesions of the CM had no effect on the retention of the conditioned response, unlike in the preceding experiment. Moreover, the over-all frequency of responding is not greatly affected (Table 7): analysis of co-variance shows no significant differences between the response rates of the two groups or between the number of food pellets received.

DISCUSSION

1. — Of the four conditioned responses studied in these experiments, only the two defensive ones were impaired by the lesion of the CM-Pf complex. These deficits confirm those produced by the same lesion in other defensive tasks (Cardo, 1961; Thompson, 1963; Delacour and Libouban, 1964), especially in the shuttle-box situation (Delacour *et al.*, 1966; 1967). Negative results found by others in acquisition of a defensive task (Bohus and De Wied, 1967 a and b) can (perhaps) be explained by:

— Differences in the size of the lesions: those made by Bohus seem to be restricted to the Pf part of the CM-Pf complex. Our routine observations indicate that efficient lesions destroyed more than 40% of the whole complex on the average.

— Differences in the location of the lesions: the respective role of the Pf and the CM in the deficits produced by the lesion of the CM-Pf complex have not been studied. On the other hand, recent experiments show that the critical location of medial thalamic lesions is fairly precise on the antero-posterior axis: neither the lesions of the pretectal area or the dorsomedial nucleus produce comparable effects to those found after CM-Pf lesions. (Alexinsky, Etchevarria and Delacour, 1969, to be published). More lateral lesions located in the ventral posterior lateral nucleus produced no deficit (Delacour *et al.*, 1966).

— Differences in the characteristics of the task: In the present experiments, we used bar-press conditioning, which was very different from the shuttle-box test used by Bohus *et al.* In our previous experiments, we used a strictly two-way shuttle-box: the CS was simultaneously delivered in the two compartments which were identical; no directional cue was in operation during the test. Directional cues could have given some characteristics of a one-way situation to the shuttle-box used in the experiments of Bohus. The CAR trained in the two-way shuttle-box seems to be controlled by different factors than the response trained in the one-way shuttle-box (Theios and Dunaway, 1964; Moyer and Korn, 1964, 1966). In our experiments we found (Delacour and Alexinsky, 1968) that lesions in the CM-Pf complex produced no deficit in the retention or in the acquisition of a one-way avoidance response.

2. — The deficits produced by the CM-Pf lesions in defensive conditioning contrast sharply with the lack of effect of this same lesion on positively reinforced conditioning. This differential action has already been reported (Delacour *et al.*, 1965, 1966) but in our previous experiments aversive and appetitive situations were not comparable. In the present experiment, we tried to fulfill this condition: the general procedure, the test apparatus and the response to be conditioned were identical. In the two first experiments, the conditioning procedure resulted in the adaptation of the subjects to a temporal relationship between the response and the reinforcement, with no discriminative CS. In experiments III and IV, the bar-press response was conditioned to the same discriminative CS with the same inter-trial interval. Differences in the training procedure due to the characteristics of each test were probably not critical. The time allowed for a correct response in the last experiment (IV) was reduced, thus making the task more difficult. Despite this fact, there was no deficit in alimentary conditioning. In so far as the essential features of both aversive and appetitive situations were comparable, it appears that the CM-Pf complex can play a rather specific role in some mechanisms of instrumental defensive responses.

3. — Several interpretations of this role have already been discussed: it is not completely specific to avoidance responses since lesions of the CM-Pf complex produced significant (although reversible) deficits in the acquisition and retention of complex food–reinforced tasks as well (Delacour *et al.*, 1966). This role cannot be attributed to some general factor such as memory, level of arousal or central control of "voluntary" movement since these same factors are probably present in positively reinforced conditioning which is spared by the lesion. Moreover, direct evidence opposes these hypotheses since recordings of the EEG failed to reveal significant effects of the lesion on the relative duration and gross characteristics of electrophysiological patterns of sleep and wakefulness (Delacour and Santacana, 1967). Numerous observations on sensory-motor reactivity and spontaneous activity were also negative. Rates of responding were not affected in any of the situations described here, even in the defensive tasks. This fact precludes the interpretation of the role of the CM-Pf complex as some starting mechanism of "voluntary" movement (Vanderwolf, 1967).

More specific factors have to be investigated:

— The US in defensive conditioning is a nociceptive stimulus; on the other hand, physiological data showed that the CM-Pf complex receives some part of the spino-thalamic afferents (Albe-Fessard and Fessard, 1963). But experimental evidence has so far failed to correlate these two facts since lesions did not raise the threshold of flinch or escape responses elicited by electric shocks used as US in our experiments. Still, because of the complexity of central pain mechanisms (Albe-Fessard and Delacour, 1968), this hypothesis cannot be completely abandoned.

— Defensive motivation (conditioned "fear") seemed not to be decreased by the lesion. Lesions do not impair the acquisition of a vegetative defensive reaction (change in cardiac rhythm) in a classical conditioning situation (Delacour and Santacana, 1967) nor a passive avoidance response or an active one-way avoidance response in the shuttle-box (Delacour and Alexinsky, 1968). Behavioral manifestations of conditioned "fear" clearly appeared in the experimental as well in the control animals in the aversive situations. The role of the CM-Pf complex seems to be restricted to *some* instrumental defensive responses such as those trained in the two-way shuttle-box, on the Sidman schedule or in a bar-press discriminative avoidance situation. This specificity does not preclude entirely the motivation hypothesis (Bohus and De Wied, 1967 a and b). The role of the CM-Pf complex could concern the interaction between defensive motivation and some mechanism of avoidance responding. Studies on the behavioral action of ACTH, alpha-MSH and beta-MSH (Murphy and Miller, 1955; Levine and Brush, 1967; De Wied, 1965; Bohus and Endröczi, 1965) are already promising and will probably be fruitful.

REFERENCES

ALBE-FESSARD, D. AND FESSARD, A. (1963) Thalamic integrations and their consequences at the telencephalic level. In *Progress in Brain Research*, Vol. I, MORUZZI, G., FESSARD, A. AND JASPER H. H. (Eds.), Elsevier, Amsterdam, pp. 115–148.

ALBE-FESSARD, D., STUTINSKY, F. AND LIBOUBAN, S. (1966) *Atlas Stéréotaxique du Diencéphale du Rat Blanc*. Editions du Centre National de la Recherche Scientifique, Paris.

ALBE-FESSARD, D. AND DELACOUR, J. (1968) Notions anatomophysiologiques sur les voies et les centres d'intégration des messages douloureux. *J. Psychol. Norm. Pathol.*, **65**, 1–44.

BOHUS, B. AND ENDRÖCZI, E. (1965) The influence of pituitary-adrenocortical function on the avoiding conditioned reflex activity in rats. *Acta Physiol. Acad. Sci. Hung.*, **26**, 183–189.

BOHUS, B. AND DE WIED, D., (1967a) Failure of α-MSH to delay extinction of conditioned avoidance behavior in rats with lesions in the parafascicular nuclei of the thalamus. *Physiol. Behav.*, **2**, 221–223.

BOHUS, B. AND DE WIED, D. (1967b) Avoidance and escape behavior following medial thalamic lesions in rats. *J. Comp. Physiol. Psychol.*, **64**, 26–29.

CARDO, B. (1961) *Rapports entre le Niveau de Vigilance et le Conditionnement chez l'Animal*, Masson, Paris.

DELACOUR, J. AND LIBOUBAN, S. (1964) Action différentielle de diverses lésions de noyaux-relais thalamiques sur des conditionnements instrumentaux. *J. Physiol.*, **56**, 555.

DELACOUR, J., LIBOUBAN, S. AND MARTINEZ, M. P. (1965) Effets de lésions thalamiques sur deux types de conditionnement instrumental. *J. Physiol.*, **57**, 238.

DELACOUR, J., ALBE-FESSARD, D. AND LIBOUBAN, S. (1966) Rôle chez le Rat de deux noyaux thalamiques dans le conditionnement instrumental. *Neuropsychologia*, **4**, 101–112.

DELACOUR, J. AND SANTACANA DE MARTINEZ, M. P. (1967) Rôle du thalamus médian dans l'établissement et la rétention de conditionnements défensifs, classiques et instrumentaux. *Neuropsychologia*, **5**, 237–252.

DELACOUR, J. AND ALEXINSKY, T. (1968) Analyse par les méthodes de conditionnement instrumental des effets de lésions thalamiques médianes. *J. Physiol.*, Paris, **60**, 235.

DE WIED, D. (1965) The influence of the posterior and intermediate lobe of the pituitary and pituitary peptides on the maintenance of a conditioned avoidance response in rats. *Intern. J. Neuropharmacol.*, **4**, 157–167.

HOFFMAN, H. S., FLESHLER, M. AND CHORNY, H. (1961) Discriminated bar press avoidance. *J. Exptl. Anal. Behav.*, **4**, 309–316.

LEVINE, S. AND BRUSH, F. R. (1967) Adrenocortical activity and avoidance learning as a function of time after avoidance training. *Physiol. Behav.*, **3**, 385–388.

MC NEMAR, Q. (1955) *Psychological Statistics*, Wiley, New York.

MEYER, D. R., CHO, C. AND WESEMANN, A. F. (1960) On problems of conditioning discriminated lever press avoidance responses. *Psychol. Rev.*, **67**, 224–228.

MOYER, K. E., AND KORN, J. H., (1964) Effect of UCS intensity on the acquisition and extinction of an avoidance response. *J. Exptl. Psychol.*, **67**, 352–359.

MOYER, K. E. AND KORN, J. H., (1966) Effect of UCS intensity on the acquisition and extinction of a one-way avoidance response. *Psychonomic Sci.*, **4**, 121–122.

MURPHY, J. V. AND MILLER, R. E. (1955) The effect of adrenocorticotrophic hormone (ACTH) on avoidance conditioning in the rat. *J. Comp. Physiol. Psychol.*, **48**, 47–49.

SIEGEL, S. (1956) *Non-parametric Statistics for the Behavioral Sciences*, Mc Graw-Hill, New York.

THEIOS, J. AND DUNAWAY, J. E., (1964) One-way versus shuttle-box avoidance conditioning. *Psychonomic Sci.*, **1**, 251–252.

THOMPSON, R. (1963) Thalamic structures critical for retention of an avoidance conditioned response in rats. *J. Comp. Physiol. Psychol.*, **56**, 261–267.

VANDERWOLF, C. H. (1967) Medial thalamic functions in voluntary behavior. *Canad. J. Psychol.*, **16**, 318–330.

DISCUSSION

BOHUS: With what anatomical structure of the brain is the centromedial-parafascicular area (CM-Pf) mainly connected; with the mesencephalic reticular formation or with the forebrain?

DELACOUR: The anatomical definition of the CM-Pf is still a subject of controversy. This structure receives afferents from the bulbar reticular formation; it also receives afferents from the pallidum, from cortical areas, such as the motor and pre-motor cortices in the monkey, and perhaps from the brachium conjunctivum. Direct afferents of the CM-Pf to the cortex are still under discussion. Those to the striatum are generally accepted.

Central Nervous Structures and the Effect of ACTH and Corticosteroids on Avoidance Behaviour: A study with Intracerebral Implantation of Corticosteroids in the Rat

B. BOHUS

Institute of Physiology, University Medical School, Rákóczi út 80, Pécs (Hungary)

It is a well established fact that adaptive reactions elicited by environmental stimuli consist of both behavioural and viscero-endocrine events. From the behavioural point of view, among the various responses, the conditioned behaviour is the highest form of adaptive neural processes. From an endocrine point of view, it has been well established that the pituitary–adrenal system plays an essential role in the adaptation to environmental changes and it is well known that adaptive pituitary–adrenal responses are controlled by the central nervous system.

Experimental data indicate close relationships between behavioural and pituitary–adrenal responses during conditioning in several species (Mason *et al.*, 1957; Endröczi *et al.*, 1957; Bohus *et al.*, 1963; Wertheim *et al.*, 1969). Besides numerous reports indicating the occurrence of reversible mental aberrations in patients on corticosteroid therapy, there has been abundant evidence of the influence of pituitary–adrenal hormones on animal behaviour. Profound effects of ACTH, ACTH-like peptides, and corticosteroids on acquisition, extinction, and inhibition of conditioned responses have been reported by several groups (Lissák and Endröczi, 1964; 1965; De Wied, 1967; De Wied *et al.*, 1968; Levine and Jones, 1965; Bohus and Korányi, 1969). It is of interest that the effect of ACTH and corticosteroids may be different or even opposite (De Wied, 1967; Bohus *et al.*, 1968a; Bohus and Lissák, 1968).

Recent attempts to study the mechanisms of action of pituitary–adrenocortical hormones on the conditioned avoidance behaviour of rats was met with the problem of localization of hormonal influences in the central nervous system. Are there special loci in the central nervous system where hormones are acting, or is the whole CNS hormonally conditioned?

Evidence in favour of a generalized hormonal influence on the CNS has been presented by Woodbury *et al.* (1957); they demonstrated that administration of various corticosteroids or adrenalectomy resulted in changes of cerebral extra/intra-cellular sodium ratio and amino acid metabolism. Furthermore, influence of ACTH and corticosteroids on acetylcholine metabolism (Torda and Wolf, 1952), on 5-hydroxytryptamine (Green and Curzon, 1968) and total DNA content of the brain (Howard, 1968) has also been reported.

However, an increasing number of data indicate that the brain stem and forebrain contains wide representations of somatic and endocrine functions; and also, that

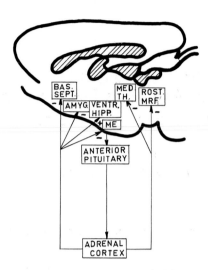

Fig. 1. Negative feedback effect of pituitary–adrenocortical hormones on fore- and midbrain structures regulating pituitary ACTH release.

these structures are sensitive to specific changes of the chemical environment. Thus,
antagonistic organization of the motivated behavioural reactions, as well as of the
pituitary–adrenal response on brain stem and diencephalic levels, has been suggested
by series of experiments in our laboratory (Lissák and Endröczi, 1964, 1967a, b;
Endröczi, 1969). The chemosensitivity, that is, the corticosteroid sensitivity of ascending facilitatory and descending inhibitory mechanisms has been shown by implantation
experiments. Thus, as seen in Fig. 1, a complex negative feedback relationship between
neural and hormonal control assures a dynamic regulation of adaptive pituitary–
adrenal responses. Corticosteroid feedback action manifests itself in inhibition of
facilitatory mechanism of ACTH release at mesencephalic and thalamic reticular,
amygdala or basal septal level, or else in modifying inhibitory actions at ventral
hippocampal level (Bohus et al., 1968b). An increasing number of electrophysiological
observations supports the idea of an antagonistic character of corticosteroid feedback
action on neural activity (Slusher et al., 1966; Endröczi et al., 1968; Steiner et al.,
1969). It is then deemed of interest whether the antagonistic character of corticosteroid feedback effect manifests itself in the control of behavioural reactions as well.
The object of this paper is to give a review of studies attempted to localize the site of
action and to clarify the mode of action of pituitary–adrenal hormones on extinction
of conditioned avoidance behaviour in the rats.

*Pituitary ACTH release and avoidance extinction of rats with cortisol implants in the
median eminence and mesencephalic reticular formation*

As mentioned in the introduction, pituitary ACTH and corticosteroids have an
opposite effect on the extinction of avoidance behaviour of rats. Thus, facilitation
of extinction of a conditioned avoidance response (CAR) was observed in rats treated

with corticosteroids, while ACTH treatment resulted in a delay of extinction (De Wied, 1967; Bohus *et al.*, 1968a; Bohus and Lissák, 1968). Since it has been shown that corticosteroids may suppress ACTH release in the median eminence or even at anterior pituitary level, it was of interest to study whether the influence of corticosteroids on ascending facilitatory or descending inhibitory mechanisms is of primary importance; or if facilitation of extinction is merely due to the suppression of ACTH release (Bohus, 1968).

Male albino rats of an inbred strain were conditioned to avoid the unconditioned stimulus of an electric shock by jumping onto a platform. As a conditional stimulus, a tone was presented 5 sec prior to the unconditioned stimulus. The rats were conditioned until the learning criterion — 24 or more CAR's out of 30 trials of three consecutive sessions — was achieved. Then crystalline cortisol (free-alcohol) was implanted in the anterior median eminence or the mesencephalic reticular formation. Reconditioning of the CAR was begun on the day following the implantation. After the learning criterion had been reached again, non-reinforced trials were presented for 7 days in order to study extinction of the CAR. Twenty-four hours after the last session of extinction, pituitary ACTH release of conditioned rats subjected to strange environment was assessed. The total corticosteroid production of adrenals *in vitro* as determined by the method of Van der Vies *et al.* (1960) served as an index of pituitary ACTH release.

Rapid extinction of the CAR took place in rats bearing cortisol implants in either the anterior median eminence or the rostral mesencephalic reticular formation (Fig. 2). It should be noted, however, that the extinction of CAR appeared faster in rats with cortisol implants in the reticular core. The total number of CAR's scored during extinction was significantly higher in rats bearing cortisol implants in the median eminence. Pituitary ACTH release in response to stress, on the other hand, was more suppressed in rats with cortisol implants in the median eminence (Table 1). When one correlates the total number of CAR's scored during extinction and the rate of ACTH release of each rat, a close correlation is found in rats bearing cortisol

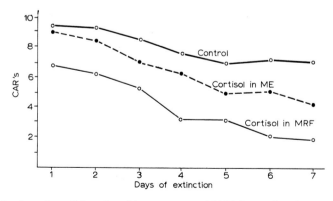

Fig. 2. Extinction of conditioned avoidance response (CAR) in rats bearing cortisol or cholesterol (control) implants in the anterior median eminence (ME) or in the rostral mesencephalic reticular formation (MRF).

TABLE 1

THE EFFECTS OF CORTISOL IMPLANTS IN THE MESENCEPHALIC RETICULAR FORMATION
OR IN THE MEDIAN EMINENCE ON EXTINCTION OF A CONDITIONED AVOIDANCE RESPONSE
AND ON STRESS-INDUCED ACTH RELEASE

Implantation	No. of rats	CAR's	p*	Corticosteroid production in µg/100 mg adrenal/h	p**
Cortisol in ME	11	44.9 ± 4.0***	< 0.005	11.9 ± 0.4	< 0.001
Cholesterol in ME	9	57.1 ± 3.8		24.1 ± 0.9	
Cortisol in MRF	12	29.0 ± 3.8	< 0.001	15.7 ± 0.8	< 0.001
Cholesterol in MRF	9	54.5 ± 2.7		22.2 ± 0.6	
Unoperated controls	10	56.2 ± 2.9		22.5 ± 0.7	

* Mann–Whitney U test (nonparametric).
** Student's t-distribution test.
*** Mean ± S.E.

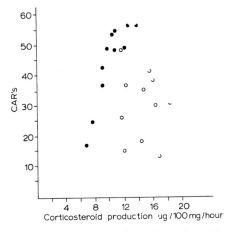

Fig. 3. Correlation between the total number of conditioned avoidance responses scored during
extinction and corticosteroid secretion in rats with mesencephalic (open circles) or hypothalamic
(solid circles) cortisol implants.

implants in the anterior median eminence. The stronger the suppression of the stress-
induced ACTH release, the faster was the avoidance extinction (Fig. 3). Such a
correlation could not be observed in rats with cortisol implants in the mesencephalic
reticular formation.

As a corollary to these observations, the direct neural influence of the corticosteroids on behavioural mechanisms is of primary importance. Evidence in favour
of a corticosteroid effect on CNS function, not mediated by the pituitary gland, has
also been reported by De Wied (1967). Moreover, the fact that suppression of ACTH
release may also facilitate the extinction suggests a supporting function of this mechanism on the primary direct neural action of corticosteroids.

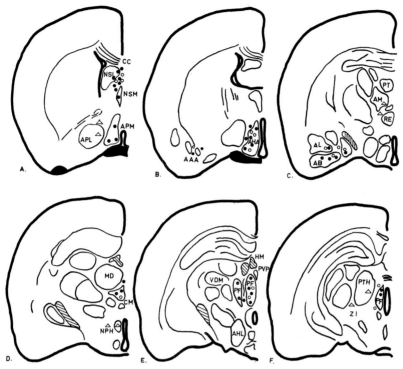

Fig. 4. Reconstruction of the sites of effective (solid circles) and ineffective (triangles) cortisol and of cholesterol (open circles) implants at septal-anterior hypothalamic (A), anterior hypothalamic-amygdala (B), amygdala (C), centro-median (D), parafascicular (E) and posterior (F) thalamic levels.

The effect of intracerebral implantation of cortisone acetate on retention and extinction of a pole-jumping avoidance response

As mentioned in the introduction, there has been abundant evidence supporting the hypothesis of the influence of corticosteroids implanted in the brain on the limbic–midbrain mechanisms controlling ACTH release, and on some electrophysiological parameters of the fore- and midbrain. It was considered to be of interest whether or not the implantation of corticosteroids affected the behavioural mechanisms at the limbic–diencephalic level.

Male albino rats were trained to avoid an electric shock by jumping onto a pole. As a conditional stimulus, the light of a 35-W bulb was presented 5 sec prior to the unconditioned stimulus of an electric shock of 0.5 mA. The acquisition period was run till the rats had reached the criterion of learning, that is, 24 or more avoidances during three consecutive sessions of 10 trials each. Then, crystalline cortisone acetate was implanted bilaterally in the brain according to De Groot's (1959) stereotaxic co-ordinates. On the day following the operation, reconditioning was begun. The rats were reconditioned until they reached the learning criterion again. Those rats that had achieved the criterion were subjected to the extinction procedure. Non-reinforced trials were presented for 7 days. At the end of the experiments, the brains

TABLE 2

EFFECT OF INTRACEREBRAL IMPLANTATION OF CORTISONE ACETATE ON RETENTION AND
EXTINCTION OF A POLE-JUMPING AVOIDANCE RESPONSE IN RATS

Site of implants	No. of rats	Retention		Extinction		p^*
		CAR's	RR's	Trials	CAR's	
Medial thalamus	12	$26.4 \pm 0.8^{**}$	5.2 ± 0.7	70	19.5 ± 3.1	< 0.01
Anterior hypothalamus	9	29.5 ± 1.2	5.5 ± 3.1	70	21.8 ± 3.6	< 0.01
Rostral septum	8	26.5 ± 0.9	3.5 ± 0.9	70	22.0 ± 3.6	< 0.01
Amygdala	7	26.7 ± 3.2	3.2 ± 0.5	70	37.5 ± 3.6	< 0.05
Lateral or anterior thalamus Posterior or lateral hypothalamus	6	27.0 ± 1.4	4.6 ± 0.8	70	57.5 ± 3.5	< 0.02
Control	14	27.3 ± 0.6	4.8 ± 0.7	70	47.6 ± 1.3	—

* Mann–Whitney U test.
** Mean $\pm$ S.E.

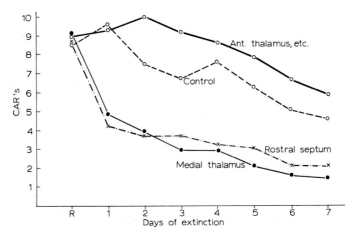

Fig. 5. Effect of cortisone acetate implantation on extinction of a pole-jumping avoidance response.

were fixed in Bouin solution, embedded in paraffin, and 10-μ-thick sections were stained with haematoxylin-eosin in order to localize the sites of implants. The sites of implants are shown in Fig. 4.

As can be seen in Table 2, the total number of CAR's scored during the reconditioning trials and that of the reinforced responses (RR's) were of the same order of magnitude in the rats bearing cortisone acetate implants in different forebrain and diencephalic structures as in those with cholesterol implants in the same regions. However, a rapid fall in avoidance performance was observed in rats bearing cortisone implants in the centro-median-parafascicular region of the medial thalamus or in the rostral septal area (Fig. 5). Avoidance extinction was also facilitated in the rats with cortisone implants in the anterior hypothalamus or in the amygdala (Fig. 6). If the implants were localized in the lateral or anterior thalamic nuclei, in the posterior or

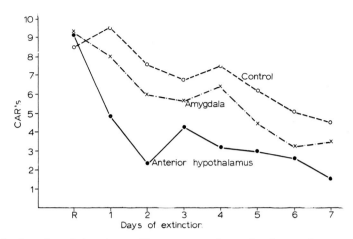

Fig. 6. Extinction of a pole-jumping avoidance response in rats bearing cortisone acetate implants in the anterior hypothalamus or in the amygdala.

lateral hypothalamus, avoidance extinction was similar to that in the controls bearing cholesterol implants (Fig. 5). The total number of CAR's scored during extinction was significantly less in the rats bearing cortisone implants in the medial thalamus, anterior hypothalamus, the rostral septum, or in the amygdala than that in the controls (Table 2). Inter-group analysis showed that the rats bearing cortisone implants in the amygdala scored more CAR's than either the rats with medial thalamic implants ($p < 0.01$) or those with rostral septal ($p < 0.05$) or anterior hypothalamic ($p < 0.05$) cortisone implants. It is worth mentioning that the rats with anterior or lateral thalamic and posterior or lateral hypothalamic implants scored more CAR's than the controls. This fact requires a more detailed investigation of the regions involved in the localization of implants.

Although the mode of action of cortisone on the function of these regions remains to be clarified, the results strongly suggest that the action of corticosteroids on avoidance behaviour of the rat is localized in several limbic–diencephalic or even mesencephalic regions. The importance of the parafascicular area in the action of dexamethasone and corticosterone on avoidance behaviour has also been stressed by Van Wimersma Greidanus and De Wied (1969).

It is generally acknowledged that extinction of a conditioned response is due to the action of internal inhibitory processes. Facilitation of extinction may mean that internal inhibitory processes are enhanced by corticosteroids. Evidence in favour of this hypothesis has been presented by this laboratory ever since the early 1960's (Endröczi and Lissák, 1962; Lissák and Endröczi, 1964; Bohus and Endröczi, 1965). Recent observations suggest that forebrain inhibitory mechanisms are involved also in behavioural inhibition, that is, forebrain inhibition may be connected with internal inhibitory processes (Lissák and Endröczi, 1965). The fact that implantation of cortisone in the rostral septal region and in the anterior hypothalamus resulted in facilitation of extinction of a conditioned avoidance response, suggests that corticosteroids affect the function of those structures which are involved in the organization of internal inhibitory processes.

The explanation that cortisone implanted in the medial thalamus might enhance inhibitory mechanisms is not acceptable. It seems also improbable that inhibition of a non-specific thalamic reticular function should result in a state in which forebrain inhibition may come into prominence. Nevertheless, the role of medial thalamic corticosteroid-sensitive mechanisms in the control of avoidance behaviour may be better explained in the light of the next experiments.

Effects of ACTH on extinction of a pole-jumping avoidance response in rats bearing intracerebral cortisone acetate implants

Adrenocorticotrophic hormone (ACTH) and corticosteroids have opposite effects on extinction of a conditioned avoidance response. It has been suggested that the physiological mechanisms underlying the extinction of an avoidance response could be under the well balanced influence of ACTH and corticosteroids in rats (Bohus and Korányi, 1969). The question may be raised as to whether the opposite effects of ACTH and corticosteroids are the result of an antagonistic action on the same mechanism, or of an influence exerted on different mechanisms. The forebrain structures involved in inhibitory mechanisms have been indicated as the sites of action of corticosteroids, although the thalamic and mesencephalic reticular system has also been demonstrated as the locus of action of corticosteroids. Observations of rats bearing lesions in the parafascicular area of the thalamus have indicated the involvement of a thalamic non-specific function in the effect of α-MSH — an ACTH-like peptide — on extinction of an avoidance response (Bohus and De Wied, 1967a). Thus, there is experimental evidence in favour of both hypotheses described above. Therefore, it was of interest to study the effect of ACTH on extinction of a pole-jumping avoidance response in rats bearing cortisone acetate implants in the brain.

The experimental protocol was the same as in the previous study. However, after being reconditioned, the rats bearing cortisone or cholesterol implants in different central nervous structures were randomly treated with either ACTH or a placebo. Immediately after the last training session, 10 μg of a long-acting zinc phosphate preparation of ACTH or, as placebo, zinc phosphate complex was administered subcutaneously. Treatment was given every other day during the extinction period.

ACTH delayed extinction of the avoidance response in rats bearing cortisone acetate implants in either the anterior hypothalamus or in the rostral septum and in the controls with cholesterol implants (Fig. 7). The total number of avoidance responses scored during extinction was significantly higher in the groups treated with ACTH than in the placebo-treated ones (Table 3). Latency of avoidance responses was significantly shorter in the controls treated with ACTH. However, the mean of the response latencies was of the same order of magnitude in the ACTH- and placebo-treated rats bearing cortisone implants in the anterior hypothalamus or in the rostral septum.

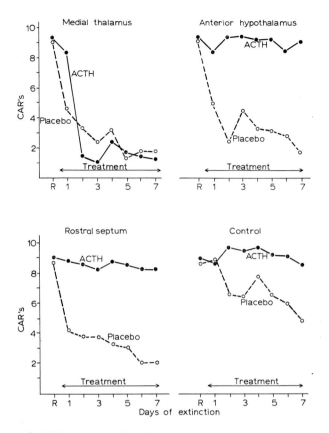

Fig. 7. Effects of ACTH on extinction of a pole-jumping avoidance response in rats with intra-cerebral cortisone implants.

TABLE 3

EFFECTS OF ADRENOCORTICOTROPHIC HORMONE ON EXTINCTION OF A POLE-JUMPING
AVOIDANCE RESPONSE IN RATS BEARING CORTISONE ACETATE IMPLANTS IN THE DIEN-
CEPHALON OR THE FOREBRAIN

Site of implants	Treatment	No. of rats	CAR's	p*	Mean response latency in sec	p*
Medial thalamus	ACTH	8	17.8 ± 1.8**	N.S.	3.87 ± 0.19	N.S.
	Placebo	8	17.6 ± 3.1		3.63 ± 0.33	
Anterior hypothalamus	ACTH	8	61.6 ± 1.0	< 0.01	3.51 ± 0.10	N.S.
	Placebo	9	21.8 ± 3.6		3.56 ± 0.38	
Rostral septum	ACTH	8	59.2 ± 2.9	< 0.01	3.35 ± 0.31	N.S.
	Placebo	8	22.0 ± 3.6		4.09 ± 0.45	
Control	ACTH	8	64.1 ± 0.7	< 0.01	2.91 ± 0.22	< 0.01
	Placebo	12	47.3 ± 1.3		3.57 ± 0.10	

* Mann–Whitney U test.
** Mean ± S.E.

References pp. 181–183

ACTH failed to delay extinction of the avoidance response in the rats with bilateral cortisone implants in the centro-median-parafascicular region of the thalamus. The total number of CAR's during the 7-day period of extinction, and the mean response latency, were of the same order in both groups treated with either ACTH or placebo.

The present experiments seem to indicate that the opposite effects of ACTH and corticosteroids on extinction of an avoidance response presuppose thalamic reticular mechanisms. It might be that both hormones act on the same area in the medial non-specific thalamic nuclei. If this were true, a competitive antagonism between the two hormones may be assumed. However, a competitive antagonism between the two hormones at the thalamic reticular level would mean that both hormones may pass the blood–brain barrier and reach the appropriate region. The present state of knowledge strongly suggests that corticosteroids enter the brain but there is no clear-cut evidence as to whether or not ACTH passes the blood–brain barrier.

As to the mode of action of corticosteroids in the medial thalamic nuclei, the experiments described in this chapter suggest an inhibition of reticular activation evoked by either hormonal and/or sensory stimuli. This idea is supported by numerous observations. Thus, rapid extinction of a shuttle-box avoidance response was observed in rats with bilateral lesions in the thalamic parafascicular region (Bohus and De Wied, 1967b). This rapid extinction could not be prevented by the administration of α-MSH (Bohus and De Wied, 1967a). Severe deficits in the retention of conditioned avoidance responses were demonstrated by Cardo and Valade (1965), Delacour and Libouban (1964) and Delacour and Santacana de Martinez (1967) in rats with lesions in the thalamic parafascicular area. There is also electrophysiological evidence in favour of an inhibitory action of corticosteroids on ascending reticular activation at the thalamic and mesencephalic levels. Thus, Slusher et al. (1966) reported that cortical potentials evoked by sciatic nerve stimulation were inhibited by local application of cortisol to the reticular core. Inhibition of potentials, recorded from the mesencephalic and pontine reticular formation and evoked by sciatic nerve stimulation, was achieved by the administration of corticosteroids (Endröczi et al., 1968).

It is of interest that ACTH delayed extinction of the conditioned avoidance response in rats bearing cortisone implants in the rostral septum or the anterior hypothalamus. In spite of the fact that the influence of ACTH upon forebrain inhibitory function became dominant, an analysis of response latency revealed that the rats with cortisone implants were still under a certain inhibitory influence.

GENERAL CONCLUSIONS

The results presented indicate that the CNS is the site of action of adrenocortical hormones in avoidance behaviour of rats. It has been revealed that the behavioural influence of corticosteroids presupposes at least two mechanisms, both of which are directly affected by these hormones. One of them consists of an enhancement of the descending forebrain influences upon the brain stem reticular core. The present results are direct evidence of corticosteroid action on internal inhibitory processes. The other mechanism is an inhibition of ascending reticular function. A medial thalamic locus of cortisone action provided evidence to the mode of the opposite effect of ACTH and corticosteroids on avoidance extinction. Furthermore, it is clear that the ascending reticular activating system is involved in the mediation of ACTH influence on avoidance behaviour. Nevertheless, the exact mode and site of action of ACTH and/or related peptides remain to be clarified.

As for the local effect of corticosteroids in the forebrain and brain stem structures, excitability changes may be the basic mechanism of action of corticosteroids. This assumption is supported by a number of studies indicating that the excitability of the brain (Woodbury, 1954), and in particular that of the above mentioned structures, (Endröczi, 1969) can be markedly affected by corticosteroids. ACTH may also influence brain excitability and it has been suggested that this effect is independent of the presence of the adrenal cortex (Feldman *et al.*, 1961; Wasserman *et al.*, 1965). Nevertheless, an inhibitory effect of corticosteroids at the thalamic and mesencephalic reticular levels might involve different mechanisms.

As mentioned in the introduction, antagonistic organization of the motivated behavioural reactions, as well as of the pituitary–adrenal response, exists at brain stem and diencephalic levels. In the light of this antagonistic organization, the complex negative feedback effect of pituitary–adrenocortical hormones influences the integrative neurohumoral function as follows. Environmental stimuli elicit activation of facilitatory and inhibitory mechanisms, which results in a certain somatic and viscero-endocrine response. The endocrine response involves the activation (or inhibition) of the pituitary–adrenocortical axis. The hormones then affect brain stem and forebrain facilitatory and inhibitory mechanisms, and the behavioural and the modified pituitary–adrenal responses appear. Since the pituitary–adrenocortical hormones *per se* do not evoke behavioural reactions, the character of their influence is highly dependent of the on-going nervous activity.

REFERENCES

BOHUS, B. (1968) Pituitary ACTH release and avoidance behaviour of rats with cortisol implants in mesencephalic reticular formation and median eminence. *Neuroendocrinology*, **3**, 355–365.

BOHUS, B. AND ENDRÖCZI, E. (1965) The influence of pituitary-adrenocortical function on the avoiding conditioned reflex activity in rats. *Acta Physiol. Acad. Sci. Hung.*, **26**, 183–189.

BOHUS, B. AND KORÁNYI, L. (1969) Hormonal conditioning of adaptive behavioural processes. In: *Results in Neurophysiology, Neuroendocrinology, Neuropharmacology and Behaviour, (Recent Developments of Neurobiology in Hungary*, Vol. II), K. LISSÁK (Ed.), Publishing House of the Hungarian Academy of Sciences, Budapest, pp. 50–76.

BOHUS, B. AND LISSÁK, K. (1968) Adrenocortical hormones and avoidance behaviour of rats. *Intern. J. Neuropharmacol.*, **7**, 301–306.

BOHUS, B. AND DE WIED, D. (1967a) Failure of α-MSH to delay extinction of conditioned avoidance behaviour in rats with lesions in the parafascicular nuclei of the thalamus. *Physiol. Behav.*, **2**, 221–223.

BOHUS, B. AND DE WIED, D. (1967b) Avoidance and escape behaviour following medial thalamic lesions in rats. *J. Comp. Physiol. Psychol.*, **64**, 26–30.

BOHUS, B., ENDRÖCZI, E. AND LISSÁK, K. (1963) Correlations between avoiding conditioned reflex activity and pituitary-adrenocortical function in the rat. *Acta Physiol. Acad. Sci. Hung.*, **24**, 79–83.

BOHUS, B., NYAKAS, CS. AND LISSÁK, K. (1968a) Involvement of suprahypothalamic structures in the hormonal feedback action of corticosteroids. *Acta Physiol. Acad. Sci. Hung.*, **34**, 1–8.

BOHUS, B., NYAKAS, CS. AND ENDRÖCZI, E. (1968b) Effects of adrenocorticotropic hormone on avoidance behaviour of intact and adrenalectomized rats. *Intern. J. Neuropharmacol.*, **7**, 307–314.

CARDO, B. AND VALADE, F. (1965) Rôle du noyau thalamique parafasciculaire dans la conservation d'un conditionnement d'évitement chez le rat. *C.R. Hébd. Séanc. Acad. Sci. (Paris)*, **261**, 1399–1402.

DE GROOT, J. (1959) The rat brain in stereotaxic co-ordinates. *Verh. Kon. Ned. Akad. Wet. Natuurkund.*, **52**, 1–40.

DE WIED, D. (1967) Opposite effects of ACTH and glucocorticosteroids on extinction of conditioned avoidance behavior. In: *Proc. 2nd Intern. Congress on Hormonal Steroids*, Excerpta Medica Intern. Congress Series, **132**, 945–951.

DE WIED, D., BOHUS, B. AND GREVEN, H. M. (1968) Influence of pituitary and adrenocortical hormones on conditioned avoidance behaviour in rats. In: *Endocrinology and Human Behaviour*, Oxford University Press, London, pp. 188–199.

DELACOUR, J. AND LIBOUBAN, S. (1964) Action différentielle de diverses lésions de noyaux relais thalamiques sur des conditionnements instrumentaux. *J. Physiol. (Paris)*, **56**, 555.

DELACOUR, J. AND SANTACANA DE MARTINEZ, M. P. (1967) Rôle du thalamus médian dans l'établissement et la rétention de conditionnements défensifs, classiques et instrumentaux. *Neuropsychologia*, **5**, 237–252.

ENDRÖCZI, E. (1969) Brain stem and hypothalamic substrate of motivated behaviour. In: *Results in Neurophysiology, Neuroendocrinology, Neuropharmacology and Behaviour, (Recent Developments of Neurobiology in Hungary*, Vol. II), K. LISSÁK (Ed.), Publishing House of the Hungarian Academy of Sciences, Budapest, pp. 27–49.

ENDRÖCZI, E. AND LISSÁK, K. (1962) Spontaneous goal-directed motor activity related to the alimentary conditioned reflex behaviour and its regulation by neural and humoral factors. *Acta Physiol. Acad. Sci. Hung.*, **21**, 265–283.

ENDRÖCZI, E., LISSÁK, K., KORÁNYI, L. AND NYAKAS, CS. (1968) Influence of corticosteroids on the hypothalamic control of sciatic-evoked potentials in the brain stem reticular formation and the hypothalamus. *Acta Physiol. Acad. Sci. Hung.*, **33**, 375–382.

ENDRÖCZI, E., TELEGDY, G. AND LISSÁK, K. (1957) Analysis of the individual variations of adaptation in the rat, on the basis of conditioned reflex and endocrine studies. *Acta Physiol. Acad. Sci. Hung.*, **11**, 393–398.

FELDMAN, S., TODT, J. C. AND PORTER, R. W. (1961) Effect of adrenocortical hormones on evoked potentials in the brain stem. *Neurology*, **11**, 109–115.

GREEN, A. R. AND CURZON, G. (1968) Decrease of 5-hydroxytryptamine in the brain provoked by hydrocortisone and its prevention by Allopurinol. *Nature*, **220**, 1095–1097.

HOWARD, E. (1968) Reduction in size and total DNA of cerebrum and cerebellum in adult mice after corticosterone treatment in infancy. *Exptl. Neurol.*, **22**, 191–208.

LEVINE, S. AND JONES, L. E. (1965) Adrenocorticotropic hormone (ACTH) and passive avoidance learning. *J. Comp. Physiol. Psychol.*, **59**, 357–360.

LISSÁK, K. AND ENDRÖCZI, E. (1964) Neuroendocrine interrelationships and behavioural processes. In: *Major Problems in Neuroendocrinology*, E. BAJUSZ AND G. JASMIN (Eds.), S. Karger, Basel/New York, pp. 1–16.

LISSÁK, K. AND ENDRÖCZI, E (1965) *The Neuroendocrine Control of Adaptation*, Pergamon Press, Oxford, pp. 180.

LISSÁK, K. AND ENDRÖCZI, E. (1967a) The role of the mesodiencephalic activating system in higher nervous activity: Its role in habituation, learning mechanisms and conditioned reflex processes. In: *Brain Reflexes, (Progress in Brain Research*, Vol. 22), E. A. ASRATYAN (Ed.), Elsevier Publishing Company, Amsterdam, pp. 297–311.

LISSÁK, K. AND ENDRÖCZI, E. (1967b) Involvement of limbic structures in conditioning, motivation, and recent memory. In: *Structure and Function of the Limbic System, (Progress in Brain Research*, Vol. 27), W. ROSS ADEY AND T. TOKIZANE (Eds.), Elsevier Publishing Company, Amsterdam, pp. 246–253.

MASON, J. W., BRADY, J. V. AND SIDMAN, M. (1957) Plasma 17-hydroxycorticosteroid levels and conditioned behaviour in the Rhesus monkey. *Endocrinology*, **60**, 741–752.

SLUSHER, M. A., HYDE, J. E. AND LAUFER, M. (1966) Effect of intracerebral hydrocortisone on unit activity of diencephalon and midbrain in cats. *J. Neurophysiol.*, **29**, 157–169.

STEINER, F. A., RUF, K. AND AKERT, K. (1969) Steroid-sensitive neurones in rat brain: Anatomical localization and responses to neurohumors and ACTH. *Brain Res.*, **12**, 74–85.

TORDA, C. AND WOLFF, H. G. (1952) Effect of adrenocorticotrophic hormone, cortisone acetate, and 17-hydroxycorticosterone-21-acetate on acetylcholine metabolism. *Amer. J. Physiol.*, **169**, 150–158.

VIES, J. VAN DER, BAKKER, R. F. M. AND DE WIED, D. (1960) Correlated studies on plasma free corticosterone and on adrenal steroid formation rate *in vitro*. *Acta Endocrinol.*, **34**, 513–523.

WASSERMAN, M. J., BELTON, N. R. AND MILLICHAP, J. G. (1965) Effect of corticotropin (ACTH) on experimental seizures. Adrenal independence and relation to intracellular brain sodium. *Neurology*, **15**, 1136–1141.

WERTHEIM, G. A., CONNER, R. L. AND LEVINE, S. (1969) Avoidance conditioning and adrenocortical functions in the rat. *Physiol. Behav.*, **4**, 41–44.

WIMERSMA GREIDANUS, TJ. B. VAN AND DE WIED, D. (1969) Effects of intracerebral implantation of corticosteroids on extinction of an avoidance response in rats. *Physiol. Behav.* **4**, 365–370.

WOODBURY, D. M. (1954) Effect of hormones on brain excitability and electrolytes. *Recent Progr. Hormone Res.*, **10**, 65–104.

WOODBURY, D. M., TIMIRAS, P. S. AND VERNADAKIS, A. (1957) Influence of adrenocortical steroids on brain function and metabolism. In: *Hormones, Brain Function and Behavior*, H. HOAGLAND (Ed.), Academic Press, New York, pp. 27–54.

DISCUSSION

DE WIED: I was very pleased with the results of the experiments with implantation of cortisol in the medial thalamus whereby the effect of ACTH on extinction of the CAR was inhibited. I would like to know whether you injected only one dose or also higher amounts of ACTH to determine the mode of the "antagonistic" action between cortisol and ACTH.

BOHUS: Only one dose of ACTH was used. However, observations on intact rats treated with ACTH suggest that when the dose of ACTH would be increased one might antagonize the facilitatory influence produced by medial thalamic cortisol implants.

MCEWEN: Did you also measure behavioral effects of hippocampal implants of cortisol?

BOHUS: I do not possess enough data to allow a conclusion on the effect of hippocampal corticosteroid implants.

MCEWEN: Did you also use corticosterone rather than cortisol, as the former steroid is the naturally occurring hormone in the rat and to my knowledge very little, if any, cortisol is present in the rat?

BOHUS: The effect of corticosterone implants will be the subject of another paper.

FELDMAN: How do you envisage the mechanism of the effects of steroids on extra-hypothalamic structures in relation to ACTH secretion?

BOHUS: My concept is that extra-hypothalamic corticosteroid feedback action is of physiological importance to change the properties of both facilitatory and inhibitory tracts of mesodiencephalic structures or in other terminology of the limbic system–midbrain circuit. Impulses from the circuit to the hypothalamus supply the information to CRF-producing neurones of the final common pathway.

DELACOUR: Is it possible to consider the medial thalamic structures simply as a pure activating system?

BOHUS: There are data which suggest that with some stimulus parameters one can evoke inhibitory responses as well in this area.

DELACOUR: The inhibitory processes postulated in the extinction of a CAR can be implicated in the extinction of food-motivated instrumental responses. What is the effect of steroid implants on the extinction of food-reinforced responses?

BOHUS: I have no data in this respect to comment on this point.

SACHAR: Could anything be learned from the shape of the extinction curves in the cortisone-implanted animals? The curves appear to be biphasic, with a sharp drop on the first day, then a slope very similar to that of the controls. Does this imply something about the nature of CNS inhibition produced by cortisone?

BOHUS: These "biphasic" curves obtained with rats bearing corticosteroid implants might be due to the conditioning procedure. Reconditioning which followed the acquisition period led to a relative resistance to extinction. In spite of the fact that the inhibition produced by corticosteroid implants is very marked, the resistance to extinction prevents complete extinction of the CAR.

WEIJNEN: The interpretation of the shapes of acquisition and extinction curves poses many problems· This is particularly the case if these curves only show the average performance of a group of animals·

The biphasic curve under discussion might be a fair approximation of the performance of the individual animals but might also be the result of averaging the extinction data of, say, 90% of the animals which show a very rapid extinction rate together with the data of 10% of the animals which show a very slow extinction rate.

BOHUS: I would fully agree with this comment. However, the shape of the biphasic extinction curve is the result of fairly uniform performance of the animals during extinction rather than an averaging artifact.

Effects of Steroids on Extinction of an Avoidance Response in Rats.
A Structure-Activity Relationship Study

TJ. B. VAN WIMERSMA GREIDANUS

Rudolf Magnus Institute for Pharmacology, Medical Faculty, University of Utrecht, Vondellaan 6, Utrecht (The Netherlands)

In recent years, attention has been focused upon the effect of ACTH and cortico-steroids on extinction of conditioned avoidance behavior. Subcutaneous injections of corticosterone, dexamethasone, or cortisone for 12 or 14 days during the extinction period leads to a dose-dependent facilitation of extinction of a conditioned avoidance response (CAR) (De Wied, 1967; Bohus and Lissák, 1968; De Wied, Bohus and Greven, 1968). The facilitating effect of adrenocortical steroids on extinction of the CAR might be the result of glucocorticoid activity rather than of mineralocorticoid activity, since the effect of aldosterone on extinction is small (De Wied, 1967). ACTH exhibits an opposite effect, *i.e.*, it delays extinction of the CAR. The facilitating effect of dexamethasone and corticosterone on extinction of the CAR, however, is not caused by inhibition of pituitary ACTH release since the steroids also facilitate extinction of the CAR in hypophysectomized animals (De Wied, 1967). Gyermek has shown that metabolites of progesterone are also effective in suppressing a conditioned avoidance performance of rats (Gyermek, Genther and Fleming, 1967). This suggests that the effect of steroids on extinction of the CAR is not specific for adrenocortical hormones. It was deemed of interest therefore to determine the relationship between structure and behavioral activity by using various chemically related steroids.

MATERIALS AND METHODS

Male albino rats of an inbred Wistar strain, weighing 110–120 grams at the start of the experiment, were conditioned in a pole-jumping box (De Wied, 1966; Van Wimersma Greidanus and De Wied, 1969). The box was equipped with a grid floor through which the unconditioned stimulus (US) of shock (0.2 mA) was delivered. The rats could avoid shock by jumping onto a pole which was placed vertically in the middle of the box. A light produced by a 40-W bulb placed on top of the box, was used as the conditioned stimulus (CS). It was presented for 5 sec prior to the US. The CS–US combination was terminated as soon as the animal jumped onto the pole. If the rat avoided shock within the 5 sec of CS pres-

References pp. 190–191

entation the light was switched off. Ten acquisition trials were given each day for 4 consecutive days with a variable intertrial-onset interval of 60 sec. On the fifth day extinction trials were run, the CS was terminated at the end of the 5-sec period; if no response had occurred, shock was not applied. Rats which made 8 or more positive responses in these ten extinction trials were randomly allocated to different treatment groups and used for experimentation.

The crystalline steroids were dissolved in heated 96% ethanol, diluted afterwards with 0.9% sodium chloride and administered subcutaneously, in two different dose levels, immediately after the first extinction session. The effect of the steroid was studied 4 h after injection in a second extinction session of ten trials.

The following steroids were used: dexamethasone (9α-fluoro-16α-methyl-pregna-1,4-diene-11β,17α,21-triol-3,20-dione), corticosterone (pregn-4-ene-11β,21-diol-3,20-dione), progesterone (pregn-4-ene-3,20-dione), pregnenolone (pregn-5-ene-3β-ol-20-one), 17β-ethyl-androst-4-ene-3-one, cholesterol (cholest-5-ene-3β-ol), testo-

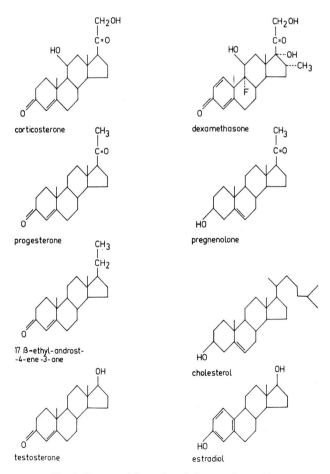

Fig. 1. Structural formulas of the tested steroids.

TABLE 1

EFFECT OF STEROIDS ON EXTINCTION OF A POLE-JUMPING AVOIDANCE RESPONSE

% CAR's 2nd extinction session	Number of animals	Treatment
80.7 ± 3.0 }$p < .01$	14	Placebo
62.0 ± 6.4	15	0.1 mg corticosterone
46.2 ± 6.6 }$p < .05$	16	0.5 mg corticosterone
87.8 ± 4.3 }$p < .005$	9	Placebo
60.0 ± 6.2	9	0.2 mg dexamethasone
36.0 ± 7.0 }$p < .05$	10	1.0 mg dexamethasone
80.0 ± 5.7 }$p < .005$	8	Placebo
55.0 ± 5.7	8	0.2 mg progesterone
32.2 ± 6.8 }$p < .05$	9	1.0 mg progesterone
89.2 ± 3.1 }$p < .005$	13	Placebo
67.9 ± 4.9	14	0.2 mg pregnenolone
50.7 ± 7.1 }$p < .05$	15	1.0 mg pregnenolone
76.4 ± 4.3 ⎫	11	Placebo
66.4 ± 7.0 ⎬ $p < .05$	11	0.2 mg 17β ethyl-adnrost-4-ene-3-one
58.2 ± 9.0 ⎭	11	1.0 mg 17β ethyl-adnrost-4-ene-3-one
61.0 ± 7.3	10	Placebo
66.2 ± 10.0	8	0.2 mg cholesterol
64.4 ± 7.8	9	1.0 mg cholesterol
80.0 ± 4.6	8	Placebo
82.2 ± 4.6	9	0.2 mg testosterone
81.2 ± 5.5	8	1.0 mg testosterone
64.5 ± 7.1	11	Placebo
67.3 ± 8.7	11	0.2 mg estradiol
69.1 ± 9.5	11	1.0 mg estradiol

sterone (androst-4-ene-17β-ol-3-one) and estradiol (estra-1,3,5(10)-triene-3,17β-diol) (see structural formulas, Fig. 1).

Statistical analysis was performed using Student's t test.

RESULTS

As seen from Table 1, the glucocorticosteroids, corticosterone — the major product of the rats' adrenal cortex — and dexamethasone, a synthetic product, both facilitated extinction of a pole-jumping avoidance response. The effect appeared to be dose dependent. The mean percentage CAR's in the second extinction session after placebo treatment was significantly higher than that after subcutaneous injection of 0.1 mg corticosterone ($p < 0.01$), which in turn was higher than the mean percentage CAR's after administration of 0.5 mg corticosterone ($p < 0.05$). Avoidance performance after injection of 0.2 mg dexamethasone was significantly lower than after pla-

References pp. 190–191

cebo treatment ($p < 0.005$) and significantly higher than after administration of 1.0 mg of this steroid ($p < 0.05$).

Progesterone and pregnenolone, from which all steroid hormones are derived, both facilitated extinction of the pole-jumping avoidance response. The effect appeared to be dose dependent. The significance of the differences between the treatment groups is shown in Table 1. 17β-Ethyl-androst-4-ene-3-one, which resembles progesterone except at the C_{20} position where progesterone possesses a keto group while this steroid is saturated with hydrogen, causes a significant facilitatory effect on extinction when administered in the amount of 1.0 mg. After injection of 0.2 mg, no significant facilitation of extinction of the CAR was observed compared with the placebo group. Cholesterol, which is converted to pregnenolone by cleavage of the side chain, showed no effect on extinction of the pole-jumping avoidance response at all. Testosterone and estradiol, the male and female sex hormone, were also inactive in facilitating the extinction of the CAR. So it appears that from the 8 tested steroids 5 were able to facilitate extinction of conditioned avoidance behavior. The effect of these 5 steroids on extinction is demonstrated in Fig. 2. Dexamethasone

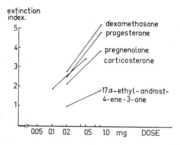

Fig. 2. The effect of steroids on extinction of a pole-jumping avoidance response. The extinction index represents the difference between the mean number conditioned avoidance responses after placebo treatment and after steroid administration.

corticosterone, progesterone and pregnenolone facilitate extinction in an equipotent manner, while 17β-ethyl-androst-4-ene-3-one appeared to have only a weak effect.

From these results it is clear that only pregnene type steroids, *i.e.* steroids containing 21 C atoms and a double bond, facilitate extinction of the CAR. The results with corticosterone, dexamethasone, progesterone and pregnenolone further suggest that the hydroxy group at C_{11} or at C_{21} is not important for the effect, since only corticosterone and dexamethasone possess these hydroxy groups; but all four steroids facilitate extinction in an equipotent manner. Thus, the common features of the active steroids are their double bond — two in the case of dexamethasone — in either ring A or B (pregnenolone), their keto or hydroxy (pregnenolone) group at C_3 and their keto group at C_{20}. The importance of the C_{20} keto group is clearly demonstrated by the results of the 17β-ethyl-androst-4-ene-3-one experiments. These results indicate that this keto group, although important, is not necessarily essential for the effect.

Accordingly, steroids of the pregnene type with the double bond in ring A or B, a keto group or hydroxy group at C_3, and with a keto group at C_{20} are able to facilitate extinction of a pole-jumping avoidance response. The effect is dose dependent. Substitution of the keto group at C_{20} by hydrogen appears to be detrimental to the effect.

Although extinction of the CAR is markedly affected by adrenocortical function (De Wied, 1967; Bohus and Lissák, 1968) the finding that progesterone, pregnenolone, dexamethasone and corticosterone affect extinction of conditioned avoidance behavior in an equipotent manner suggests that the facilitatory effect is not merely due to the glucocorticoid activity of the steroids.

DISCUSSION

Although there are discrepancies in the reported central activity of steroids, presumably due to the different methodology, it is suggested that steroids act on behavior by affecting the mesencephalic reticular activity or the diffuse thalamic projection system. Recent experiments support this hypothesis, since facilitation of extinction of the CAR is observed after implantation of cortisol in the mesencephalic reticular formation. Extinction is also enhanced in rats with cortisol implants in the median eminence but significantly less avoidances are made by rats bearing cortisol implants in the mesencephalic reticular formation (Bohus, 1968). Dexamethasone phosphate causes a rapid extinction of the CAR when implanted in the median or posterior thalamus or when implanted into the lateral ventricle, while corticosterone facilitates extinction of the CAR when implanted in the posterior part of the thalamus (Van Wimersma Greidanus and De Wied, 1969). Whether all the steroids used in the present experiments have the same site of action in the central nervous system (CNS) as the glucocorticosteroids remains to be elucidated.

In which way the steroids alter conditioned avoidance behavior is not clear. More than 25 years ago, Selye reported that certain hormonal steroids are capable of altering brain function and under certain conditions may exhibit an anesthetic effect. Those compounds which were oxygenated at the two extreme ends of the molecule exerted the highest anesthetic effect. Furthermore, it was found that if rings A or B contained one double bond their anesthetic effect was not critically affected. However, the presence of two or more of these double bonds inhibited the anesthetic effect (Selye, 1942). Although it has been reported that anesthesia is obtained if these steroids are administered intraperitoneally or intravenously, but not if they are injected subcutaneously, it is still worth noting that the steroids that cause facilitation of a pole-jumping avoidance response fulfill the above mentioned criteria for anesthetic activity.

Subsequent investigators have tried to explore the effect of steroids on the CNS. It has been shown that dexamethasone and hydrocortisone stimulate the rate of self-stimulation in rats with electrodes in the lateral hypothalamic–median forebrain bundle region. In contrast, decreased rates are found in rats with electrodes in the cerebral peduncle (Slusher, 1965). Progesterone, cortisone, and hydrocortisone cause a rise in the response rate of septal self-stimulation, while estradiol and testosterone are without effect (Campbell, 1968). These experiments indicate that the same structure-activity relationship exists in the effect of steroids on self-stimulation as on extinction of the CAR.

Other studies have indicated that brain excitability can be markedly affected by steroids. Administration of estradiol or testosterone to intact rats lowered electroshock seizure threshold (EST). Progesterone rapidly and significantly raised EST in female rats, but had no effect in males. Cholesterol, pregnenolone and corticosterone produced no effect on EST, but corticosterone normalized alterations in brain excitability or prevented an increase or a decrease in EST (Woodbury and Vernadakis, 1966, 1967).

Hydrocortisone and testosterone have been shown to affect the excitability of the mesencephalic reticular formation in male rats (Soulairac, Gottesmann and Thangaprégassam, 1963). Administration of adrenocortical steroids increased the excitability of "centrencephalic" structures of cats (Feldman, Todt and Porter, 1961). Metabolites of progesterone inhibit the electrocortical arousal elicited by stimulating the midbrain reticular formation in cats. This effect is induced by these metabolites in lower doses than by pregnenolone, which in turn has a lower minimal effective dose in suppressing the arousal from the reticular formation than progesterone (Gyermek, Genther and Fleming, 1967).

ACKNOWLEDGEMENT

The author is greatly indebted to the Organon Co., Oss, The Netherlands, for supplying the steroids.

REFERENCES

BOHUS, B. (1968) Pituitary ACTH release and avoidance behavior of rats with cortisol implants in mesencephalic reticular formation and median eminence. *Neuroendocrinology*, **3**, 355–365.

BOHUS, B. AND LISSÁK, K. (1968) Adrenocortical hormones and avoidance behaviour of rats. *Intern. J. Neuropharmacol.*, **7**, 301–306.

CAMPBELL, H. J. (1968) Acute effects of pregnene steroids on septal self-stimulation in the rabbit. *J. Physiol.*, **196**, 134P–135P.

DE WIED, D. (1966) Inhibitory effect of ACTH and related peptides on extinction of conditioned avoidance behavior in rats. *Proc. Soc. Exptl. Biol. Med.*, **122**, 28–32.

DE WIED, D. (1967) Opposite effect of ACTH and glucocorticosteroids on extinction of conditioned avoidance behavior. In: *Proc. Second Intern. Congr. Hormonal Steroids, Milan, May 1966, Excerpta Medica, Intern. Congr. Ser.* No. 132, L. MARTINI, F. FRASCHINI AND M. MOTTA (Eds.), Excerpta Medica Foundation, Amsterdam, pp. 945–951.

DE WIED, D., BOHUS, B. AND GREVEN, H. M. (1968) Influence of pituitary and adrenocortical hormones on conditioned avoidance behavior in rats. In: *Endocrinology and Human Behaviour*, R. P. MICHAEL (Ed.), Oxford University Press, London, pp. 188–199.

FELDMAN, S., TODT, J. C. AND PORTER, R. W. (1961) Effect of adrenocortical hormones on evoked potentials in the brain stem. *Neurology*, **11**, 109–115.

GYERMEK, L., GENTHER, G. AND FLEMING, N. (1967) Some effects of progesterone and related steroids on the central nervous system. *Intern. J. Neuropharmacol.*, **6**, 191–198.

SELYE, H. (1942) Correlations between the chemical structure and the pharmacological actions of the steroids. *Endocrinology*, **30**, 437–458.

SLUSHER, M. A. (1965) Influence of adrenal steroids on self-stimulation rates in rats. *Proc. Soc. Exptl. Biol. Med.*, **120**, 617–620.

SOULAIRAC, A., GOTTESMANN, CL. AND THANGAPRÉGASSAM, M.-J. (1963) Variations de l'excitabilité nerveuse centrale chez le rat sous l'influence de diverses hormones stéroïdes. *J. Physiol. (Paris)*, **55**, 340–341.

VAN WIMERSMA GREIDANUS, TJ. B. AND DE WIED, D. (1969) Effects of intracerebral implantation of corticosteroids on extinction of an avoidance response in rats. *Physiol. Behav.*, **4**, 365–370.

WOODBURY, D. M. AND VERNADAKIS, A. (1966) Effects of steroids on the central nervous system. In: *Steroidal Activity in Experimental Animals and Man, Methods in Hormone Research*, Vol. V, R. I. DORFMAN (Ed.), Academic Press, New York, pp. 1–58.

WOODBURY, D. M. AND VERNADAKIS, A. (1967) Influence of hormones on brain activity. In: *Neuroendocrinology*, Vol. II, L. MARTINI AND W. F. GANONG (Eds.), Academic Press, New York, pp. 335–376.

DISCUSSION

MONEY: This paper really fascinates me tremendously. Extrapolation from animal to man may be dangerous, but your data remind me of a recently observed clinical phenomenon in the use of anti-androgens for the control of really bad sex behavior in sex offenders. I first learned about this in 1966, in Hamburg, where they were using cyproterone (6-chlor-$\triangle$6-1,2α-methylene-17α-hydroxy-progesterone), which, I believe, has since been used more widely in Germany and Switzerland with good effects on sex offenders. Dr. Claude Migeon and I have used anti-androgen in Baltimore for a small group of sex offenders. We have not had cyproterone available to us. So we have used Depo-Provera (6α-methyl-17α-hydroxyprogesterone acetate). The effect on patients, when it is effective, is sudden and dramatic. It has the effect of abolishing the sexual response, including potency and the ejaculate, as well as sexual desire. Whether this effect is integrated into the total psychic economy depends on the general attitude of the patient and the nature of his symptoms and perhaps the amount of counselling and psychotherapy that is given. For example, one very compulsive exhibitionist I saw, required very little counselling because he was so extremely pleased to be relieved of what he called his nervousness. He didn't have to exhibit himself, which had been as often as ten times a day. In addition to its use with regard to the sex offenders, Provera has a further psychiatric application. Dr. D. Blumer who has been working with me, and who is in the neurosurgery department, decided to try the drug with temporal lobe epileptics who had attacks of rage or violence, so that they became dangerous and impossible to live with, in the family. These people happen to have hyposexual functioning associated with their temporal lobe epilepsy. They experienced sudden and dramatic relief from their attacks of violence, and were able to go back to school if they were young, or back to work if they were older.

BOHUS: What is the minimal dose of steroids of the pregnene type that can facilitate the extinction of avoidance behavior?

VAN WIMERSMA GREIDANUS: To answer your question I should have tested a wide range of doses of pregnene-type steroids. However, I only have investigated the effects of 2 doses per steroid. In general I can say that dexamethasone-21-sodium phosphate is much more potent than the free alcohol of dexamethasone.

The Relation between Pretraining Plasma Corticosterone Levels and the Acquistion of an Avoidance Response in the Rat

A. M. L. VAN DELFT

Rudolf Magnus Institute for Pharmacology, Medical Faculty, University of Utrecht, Vondellaan 6, Utrecht (The Netherlands)

Data regarding the role of the hormones of the pituitary–adrenal system on extinction of a conditioned avoidance procedure indicate that ACTH has an inhibitory effect on extinction, while corticosteroids facilitate extinction (Bohus and De Wied, 1966; De Wied, 1967; Van Wimersma Greidanus, this volume, page 155; Van Wimersma Greidanus and De Wied, 1969). The influence of the pituitary–adrenal system on acquisition of conditioned avoidance behaviour is less well established, although interesting interrelationships have been noted between individual differences in learning capacity and pituitary–adrenal activity. Endröczi, Telegdy and Lissák (1957) using rats in a conditioned food reward situation, interrupted by electric shock, showed that those animals which resumed pre-shock behaviour first, had the lowest ACTH secretion in response to a noxious stimulus after the training period. In dogs exposed to the same situation, fastest recovery to pre-shock behaviour was also observed in animals with a low secretion rate of corticosteroids, in particular, hydrocortisone (Lissák, Endröczi and Meggyesy, 1957). In monkeys, Mason, Brady and Tolliver (1968) showed that in a Sidman avoidance situation, animals with low pre-avoidance lever-pressing and high avoidance lever-pressing had lowest 17-OH corticosteroid secretion. Contradictory results were reported by Bohus, Endröczi and Lissák (1963) who found a high corticosterone secretion rate in animals with the greatest number of avoidance responses. Wertheim, Conner and Levine (1969) found that animals with higher pre-training stress responses attained greater avoidance performance proficiency in a Sidman avoidance situation.

Although the pituitary–adrenal system is activated during acquisition of conditioned responses (Mason, Brady and Sidman, 1957; Mason *et al.*, 1968; Takeda, Kawa, Ogawa, Inamori, Okamoto and Kanehisa, 1957) neither ACTH nor corticosteroids seem to be essential for the acquisition of an avoidance response (De Wied, 1964; De Wied, 1967; Miller and Ogawa, 1962; Bohus and Endröczi, 1965; Bohus and Lissák, 1968; Van Delft, unpublished).

The results of the aforementioned studies indicate that the exact influences of the pituitary–adrenal system on avoidance acquisition are still obscure. It was deemed of interest therefore to study the activity of this system in rats before and during a

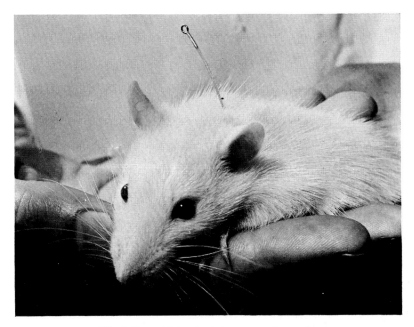

Fig. 1. Rat with implanted permanent cannula.

conditioned avoidance procedure using a technique by which repeated measurements of plasma corticosterone were possible. For this reason, animals were implanted with a permanent cannula for blood sampling and subsequently subjected to a conditioned avoidance procedure.

EXPERIMENTAL

Male rats of an inbred Wistar strain, weighing 120–140 g, were used. They were housed in separate cages under laboratory-controlled light–dark 12-h conditions.

Cannulation was performed under ether anesthesia. A polyethylene cannula was inserted into the left carotid artery and guided under the skin, in the back of the animal, right behind the head. The cannula was filled with a heparin solution in saline (1.0 mg/ml) and closed with a metal pin. For blood sampling the pin was removed, a needle connected with a syringe was pushed into the cannula and 0.3 ml blood was withdrawn. Anesthesia was never applied during blood sampling. The cannula was filled again with the heparin/saline solution and closed. Blood was immediately centrifuged and corticosterone was determined in 0.1 ml of plasma after methylene-chloride extraction by measuring the fluorescence in alcoholic sulphuric acid (Glick, Von Redlich and Levine, 1964). All animals were allowed 5 days of recovery after cannulation before the experiments were begun.

Avoidance learning was conducted in a pole-jumping conditioning box. The box had a grid floor through which the unconditioned stimulus (US) of shock (540 V, 0.22 mA) was delivered. The conditioned stimulus (CS) was a light emitted by a

40-W bulb on top of the box. The CS was presented for 5 sec prior to the US, and both were terminated when the rat jumped onto a pole (placed in the middle of the box) or when the rat made no response 25 sec after the onset of US. A conditioned avoidance response (CAR) meant that the rat had jumped onto the pole within 5 sec after presentation of the CS. Inter-trial responses (ITR) were scored each time the rat jumped onto the pole when the CS was not presented. Ten conditioning trials (with a variable inter-trial onset interval) were administered in a 10 min-session during each of 3 consecutive days.

Adrenal sensitivity to ACTH was determined *in vitro* by measuring the rate of corticosteroid production (Van der Vies, Bakker and De Wied, 1960). Both adrenals were removed, quartered and separately incubated for 1 h at 37°C in a Krebs–Ringer buffer. After 1 h, adrenals were incubated again in fresh medium. To one of each pair of flasks, 20 mU ACTH (A_1 peptide) was added. The amount of corticosteroids produced during this second hour was used as an index of ACTH activity.

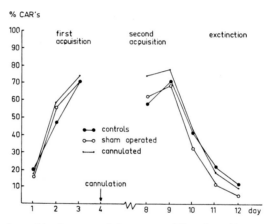

Fig. 2. Effect of carotid artery cannulation on conditioned avoidance acquisition.

Preliminary experiments were performed to investigate the effect of cannulation on avoidance behaviour of the animals and on adrenal sensitivity to ACTH. Forty-five rats were trained during 3 days for pole-jumping. After training, they were divided into 3 groups, matched for avoidance and inter-trial responses. One group was cannulated, the second sham-operated, and the third remained undisturbed. Four days after operation, reconditioning was started for 2 days after which extinction was studied during 3 consecutive days. In the extinction period, the CS was presented for 5 sec and never followed by the US of shock. After operation, no differences were found in avoidance behaviour between the 3 groups of animals (Fig. 2).

TABLE 1

EFFECT OF CANNULATION OF 8-DAYS DURATION ON ADRENAL WEIGHT

Controls	29.0 ± 0.95 mg
Sham-operated	28.5 ± 0.98 mg
Cannulated	29.8 ± 0.89 mg

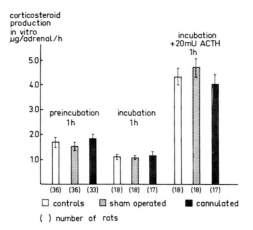

Fig. 3. Effect of carotid artery cannulation on adrenal responsiveness to ACTH.

At the end of the experiment, animals were weighed and decapitated. Adrenals were removed and weighed and adrenal sensitivity to ACTH was determined.

RESULTS

No effect of cannulation on adrenal weight was found (Table 1). Although a temporary decrease in body weight had occurred, there was no significant difference in body weight between the 3 groups of animals at the end of the experiment. As shown in Fig. 3, the sensitivity of the adrenal glands to ACTH in rats bearing a cannula did not differ from that of control animals. From these experiments, it can be concluded that no drastic changes, either in avoidance behaviour nor in pituitary–adrenal function, were introduced by the cannulation procedure.

In a second series of experiments, basal levels of corticosterone concentration in plasma were determined on the first day of the acquisition period. Between 8 a.m. and 9 a.m., when lowest concentrations of corticosterone during the circadian rhythm are expected, blood was collected. In the course of this day and the two following days, rats were trained in the pole-jumping box. The total number of positive responses of 30 trials for each individual was plotted against the basal level of plasma corticosterone (Fig. 4). A significant (Spearman rank correlation test $p = 0.025$) negative correlation between the two parameters was found. If the total number of inter-trial responses of each individual was plotted against the initial level of plasma corticosterone, a similar negative correlation was found ($p < 0.01$; Fig. 5).

In another group of animals, the rise in plasma corticosterone level was investigated 10 min after an ether stress of 1-min duration, in order to test the possibility that differences in performance could be attributed to a concomitant difference in corticosterone secretion. Fig. 6 depicts initial and stress levels of corticosterone of 13 animals. There is a remarkably constant rise in corticosterone 1 min after ether stress. The magnitude of the increase in all animals is the same irrespective of the initial basal level of corticosterone.

References p. 198

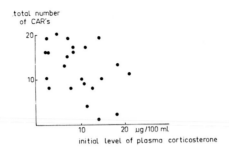

Fig. 4. Correlation between pre-training level of plasma corticosterone and total number of conditioned avoidance responses in 3 days of avoidance acquisition.

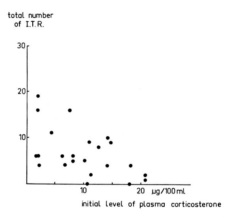

Fig. 5. Correlation between pre-training level of plasma corticosterone and the total number of intertrial responses in 3 days of avoidance acquisition.

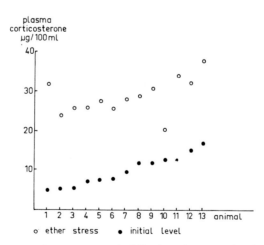

Fig. 6. Rise in circulating corticosterone 10 min following ether stress in relation to initial level of plasma corticosterone. Animals are arranged according to magnitude of initial level.

DISCUSSION

The present experiments indicate that pre-training levels of pituitary–adrenocortical activity, as well as the rise in corticosterone secretion following ether stress, are associated with learning ability of rats in a conditioned avoidance situation. The higher the pre-conditioning level of corticosterone, the lower the ability of the rat to acquire the avoidance response. It has been suggested by Smelik (1963) that the rise in plasma corticosterone due to stress is rather independent of pre-existing levels of circulating corticosterone. In fact, the present experiments indicate that the rise in plasma corticosterone is very constant in the various individual animals, and that the final concentration of corticosterone depends on the initial level.

The present findings are in contrast with those of Bohus et al. (1963) who demonstrated that the performance of a conditioned avoidance reflex in individual rats is more intensive in animals showing higher resting corticosterone secretion; also with those of Wertheim et al. (1969) who found that animals which exhibited higher pre-training adrenal responses to stress attained a greater avoidance performance proficiency. They are in agreement with findings of Mason et al. (1968), Endröczi et al. (1957), Lissák et al. (1957) according to which low pituitary–adrenal activity was correlated with superior avoidance learning. They are also in agreement with the experiments of Levine and Soliday (1960) with median eminence-lesioned rats. These animals, which had a measurable diabetes insipidus and in which stress-induced ACTH release was blocked, were found to be markedly superior to the rate of avoidance acquisition.

The pre-training plasma corticosterone level reflects the stress situation of an animal. Apparently, this level is negatively correlated with learning ability in an avoidance situation. Thus, the more severe the stress situation, the lower is the learning ability of the animal. It may be that the circulating hormones of the pituitary–adrenal system affect avoidance learning by a direct effect on the central nervous system. However, adrenalectomy (Miller and Ogawa, 1962; Bohus et al., 1963; Bohus and Endröczi, 1965; De Wied, 1967; Van Delft, unpublished) does not interfere with learning behaviour in rats. The pre-training corticosterone level is a reflection of an activity of central nervous system structures controlling pituitary function. It is possible that alterations are induced as well in those structures in the central nervous system which participate in the acquisition of conditioned avoidance behaviour.

It is interesting to note that the number of inter-trial responses is also negatively correlated with pre-training corticosterone levels; that is, the higher the corticosterone level, the lower the number of inter-trial responses. Since ACTH markedly suppresses inter-trial response activity in an avoidance situation (Bohus and Endröczi, 1965), it is quite probable that inter-trial response activity is controlled by the circulating hormones of the pituitary–adrenal system, presumably by an action on the central nervous system.

The extent to which individual differences may be basically hereditary or experiential, cannot be determined at present. The extent of stress experience in the animal's past history might be of relevance as well (Mason *et al.*, 1968). In this respect, it is noteworthy that pre-training levels of corticosterone are rather high in some of the cannulated animals, and it is possible that experimentally produced higher basal levels of a chronic nature, as introduced by the cannulation procedure, might have important effects on the central nervous system and consequently on avoidance behaviour.

REFERENCES

BOHUS, B. AND DE WIED, D. (1966) Inhibitory and facilitatory effect of two related peptides on extinction of avoidance behavior. *Science*, **153**, 318–320.

BOHUS, B. AND ENDRÖCZI, E. (1965) The influence of pituitary-adrenocortical function on the avoiding conditioned reflex activity in rats. *Acta Physiol. Acad. Sci. Hung.*, **26**, 183–189.

BOHUS, B., ENDRÖCZI, E. AND LISSÁK, K. (1963) Correlations between avoiding conditioned reflex activity and pituitary-adrenocortical function in the rat. *Acta Physiol. Acad. Sci. Hung.*, **24**, 79–83.

BOHUS, B. AND LISSÁK, K. (1968) Adrenocortical hormones and avoidance behaviour of rats. *Intern. J. Neuropharm.*, **7**, 301–306.

DE WIED, D. (1964) Influence of anterior pituitary on avoidance learning and escape behavior. *Amer. J. Physiol.*, **207**, 255–259.

DE WIED, D. (1967) Opposite effects of ACTH and glucocorticoids on extinction of conditioned avoidance behavior. *2nd Intern. Congr. on Hormonal Steroids, Milan 1966, Excerpta Medica Intern. Congress Series*, **132**, 945–951.

ENDRÖCZI, E., TELEGDY, G. AND LISSÁK, K. (1957) Analysis of the individual variations of adaptation in the rat, on the basis of conditioned reflex and endocrine studies. *Acta Physiol. Acad. Sci. Hung.*, **11**, 393–398.

GLICK, D., REDLICH, D. VON AND LEVINE, S. (1964) Fluorimetric determination of corticosterone and cortisol in 0.02–0.05 milliliters of plasma or submilligram samples of adrenal tissue. *Endocrinology*, **74**, 653–655.

LEVINE, S. AND SOLIDAY, S. (1960) The effects of hypothalamic lesions on conditioned avoidance learning. *J. Comp. Physiol. Psychol.*, **53**, 497–501.

LISSÁK, K., ENDRÖCZI, E. AND MEGGYESY, P. (1957) Somatisches Verhalten und Nebennierenrindentätigkeit. *Pflügers Arch. Ges. Physiol.*, **265**, 117–124.

MASON, J. W., BRADY, J. V. AND SIDMAN, M. (1957) Plasma 17-hydroxycorticosteroid levels and conditioned behavior in the Rhesus monkey. *Endocrinology*, **60**, 741–752.

MASON, J. W., BRADY, J. V. AND TOLLIVER, G. A. (1968) Plasma and urinary 17-hydroxycorticosteroid responses to 72-h avoidance sessions in the monkey. *Psychosomatic Med.*, **30**, 608–630.

MILLER, R. E. AND OGAWA, N. (1962) The effect of adrenocorticotrophic hormone (ACTH) on avoidance conditioning in the adrenalectomized rat. *J. Comp. Physiol. Psychol.*, **55**, 211–213.

SMELIK, P. G. (1963) Failure to inhibit corticotrophin secretion by experimentally induced increase in corticoid levels. *Acta Endocrinol.*, **44**, 36–46.

TAKEDA, S., KAWA, A., OGAWA, T., INAMORI, Y., OKAMOTO, O. AND KANEHISA, T. (1967) The levels of adrenal corticosterone in conditioned avoidance response and conditioned emotional response in the rat. *Acta Med. Univ. Kagoshima*, **9**, 161–164.

VAN DER VIES, J., BAKKER, R. F. M. AND DE WIED, D. (1960) Correlated studies on plasma free corticosterone and on adrenal steroid formation in vitro. *Acta Endrocrinol.*, **34**, 513–523.

VAN WIMERSMA GREIDANUS, TJ. B. AND DE WIED, D. (1969) Effect of intracerebral implantation of corticosteroids on extinction of an avoidance response in rats. *Physiol. Behav.*, **4**, 365–370.

WERTHEIM, G. A., CONNER, R. L. AND LEVINE, S. (1969) Avoidance conditioning and adrenocortical function in the rat. *Physiol. Behav.*, **4**, 41–44.

DISCUSSION

LEVINE: It is important to discriminate between various types of avoidance behavior. The effects of hormones may be very different depending on the task. In one situation, the animal is learning a timing response as he learns in Sidman-avoidance. In another situation, he is learning the relationship between a conditioned and a non-conditioned stimulus. And in yet another situation, he is learning not to go as opposed to going. These are not the same behaviors. Comparisons between experiments must take into account the nature of the task.

DELACOUR: It is indeed necessary to distinguish between different types of avoidance behavior. For instance, the same lesion, such as a lesion in the centrum medianum parafascicularis nuclei, can impair a two-way shuttle box response but fails to influence a one-way shuttle box response or passive avoidance behavior.

There exists a significant correlation between locomotory activity in an open field and some kinds of avoidance behavior. I wonder whether you have investigated a possible relationship between the basal level of plasma corticosteroids and open field activity?

VAN DELFT: No, I have not. I started these experiments by trying to measure corticosterone secretion during extinction of conditioned avoidance behavior. By chance, I observed the correlation with the performance in the acquisition period.

RINGOLD: On simple question. It is possible that animals with high plasma corticosterone levels have a reduced pain threshold? This might complicate the interpretation of shock-motivated conditioned behavior.

VAN DELFT: It is possible, but relatively high doses of both corticosterone or dexamethasone injected either chronically or acutely in adrenalectomized rats, have no effect on acquisition in the pole-jumping situation as compared to non-injected control rats.

HENKIN: Dr. Ringold's point is quite relevant, because animals or humans with Cushing's syndrome have markedly elevated thresholds for a number of sensory stimuli. Adrenalectomized rats have markedly depressed thresholds for these stimuli. So one would expect some stimuli to be less effective in producing a CAR in rats with an elevated plasma steroid level than with a lowered level.

McEWEN: As far as sensitivity to shock is concerned: in our study on passive avoidance, we found no difference in conditioning in the unaltered apparatus between normal, ADX and hypophysectomized rats. We did observe tremendous differences when we altered the training box and reduced the number of specific cues which indicate punishment. This effect we attribute to the predominance of hormonal factors when specific fear cues are weak and it is consistent with hormonal effects on extinction of various types of avoidance behavior.

LEVINE: Everybody working in this area is concerned about the pain problem. It is very hard to measure pain. However crude these studies may be, we attempted to look at thresholds of adrenalectomized rats. We found no differences between adrenalectomized rats and controls in the amount of shock necessary to drive animals across the barrier to the safe side. We have done a few other things attempting to get a pain threshold. We have never found any difference between adrenalectomized and non-adrenalectomized rats.

MARKS: Where are the ACTH receptors in the studies described? Have we ruled out peripheral receptor mechanisms?

VAN DELFT: It is not implicated in this study that ACTH has either a central or a peripheral effect or both. We believe that the negative correlations found only say something about possible connections in the central nervous system between the regulatory mechanisms of avoidance behavior and pituitary–adrenal activity. Van Wimersma Greidanus (unpublished) observed that implantation of ACTH-(1-10) in the posterior thalamic area has marked effects on extinction, similar as found after subcutaneous injections of the same peptide or of the intact ACTH hormone. In addition, Gispen, van Wimersma Greidanus and DE WIED (*Physiol. Behav.*, 1969, in press) found no effect of injected ACTH-(1-10) on shock responsivity in both normal and hypophysectomized rats.

The Uptake and Action of Corticosterone: Regional and Subcellular Studies on Rat Brain

BRUCE S. McEWEN AND JAY M. WEISS

Rockefeller University, New York, N.Y. (U.S.A.)

INTRODUCTION

Because we are interested in the action of adrenal steroids on brain biochemistry and on neural processes and behavior, we have begun a program of investigation in which we have attempted to determine the availability of corticosterone, the principal adrenal steroid in the rat (Bush, 1953), to the rat brain. In the course of our studies we have obtained evidence which relates to three important questions concerning the interaction of corticosterone with the brain: (1) Does corticosterone circulating in the blood enter the brain, and are changes in the blood level reflected in changes in brain level of this steroid? (2) Can one obtain evidence as to the neuroanatomical and intracellular site of action of steroids, such as corticosterone, by means of uptake studies with radioactive hormone? (3) What are the biochemical effects that corticosterone has on the brain? Because of a fundamental interest in genetic regulation in the brain, we have placed particular emphasis on action in the cell nucleus and on the control by corticosterone of enzyme levels in the brain. In this paper we also plan to discuss a general conceptual framework within which behavioral effects of corticosterone can be recognized and studied. Much of the work referred to in this paper has been published or submitted for publication elsewhere (McEwen, Weiss and Schwartz, 1968, 1969, 1970; Weiss, McEwen, Silva and Kalkut, 1969, 1970); the experimental procedures will be found in these papers.

Increased blood levels are reflected in increased brain levels of corticosterone

The primary requirement for the brain to act as a sensing device for the regulation of ACTH secretion and as a target organ for corticosterone to influence neural activity and behavior is that the hormone be able to enter the brain in increasing amounts as the blood level increases, as it does in stress. We have determined the amount of [1,2-^{3}H]corticosterone entering the cortex, hypothalamus, septum, and hippocampus as a result of the administration of a physiological range of doses (0.7 to 50 μg) to adrenalectomized rats. The results, presented in Fig. 1, show that the amount entering the cortex, hypothalamus, and septum is proportional to the dose administered. In contrast, the capacity of the hippocampus shows a pronounced tendency to be satur-

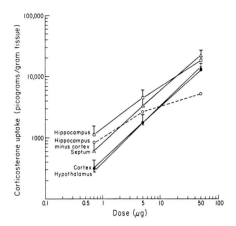

Fig. 1. The concentration of corticosterone (picograms per gram tissue) as a function of dose given intraperitoneally in four regions of brain from adrenalectomized rats. Animals were sacrificed two hours after hormone injection and brain tissue was extracted for radioactivity determinations as described elsewhere (McEwen *et al.*, 1969a).

ated by the hormone as the dose increases. The dotted line in Fig. 1 is the difference in concentration of radioactive corticosterone between the hippocampus and the cortex. This shows the saturability of the hippocampal retention mechanism even more clearly. It will be seen below that radioactive corticosterone uptake by the septum can be saturated by very high doses (3000 μg) of corticosterone even though it is not saturated by the corticosterone found in the blood of a normal, stressed rat.

Retention of corticosterone by hippocampus and septum, as indicated by the time course of disappearance of [1,2-³H]corticosterone

An important characteristic of a limited-capacity retention mechanism in a hormone target tissue is that it retains the hormone at higher concentrations and for a longer time than other tissues. The time course of disappearance of intraperitoneally administered [1,2-³H]corticosterone from blood and various brain regions of normal and adrenalectomized rats is shown in Fig. 2. The brain and blood level of the hormone at all times after injection is higher in the adrenalectomized animals than in the normal, and this difference may be due to a reduction in the capacity of the liver to inactivate the hormone as a result of adrenalectomy. The time course of disappearance of hormone is very similar in the blood and in brain structures such as cortex and hypothalamus, and this indicates a free and rapid exchange of hormone between brain and blood. On the other hand, the septum of the normal rats and the septum and hippocampus of the adrenalectomized animals show a pronounced tendency to retain the hormone at higher concentrations and for longer times than the other brain structures. As indicated in the previous section, the absence of hormone retention in the hippocampus of normal rats is due to the saturation of the limited-capacity uptake mechanism by the circulating levels of corticosterone in the normal animal subjected to the stress of handling and hormone injection. Bilateral adrenalectomy

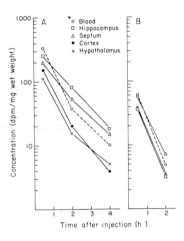

Fig. 2. Time course of disappearance of labelled corticosterone from blood and four brain regions of adrenalectomized (A) and normal (B) rats. Tissue samples were extracted and radioactivity determined as described elsewhere (McEwen *et al.*, 1969).

produces within two hours a two-fold increase in the amount of labelled corticosterone taken up by the hippocampus (McEwen *et al.*, 1969).

We have checked by thin-layer chromatography the identity of the steroid extracted from the hippocampus of adrenalectomized rats (McEwen *et al.*, 1969), and found that most of it could be recovered in a spot moving with the R_F of corticosterone. We obtained the following results according to the time interval between hormone injection and sacrifice: 30 min, more than 90% as corticosterone; 1 h, 80%; 2 h, approximately 70%; 4 h, 85%; 6 h, 40%. In general, the percentage of radioactivity recovered as corticosterone was only slightly greater in the hippocampus than in the rest of the brain, but all brain areas had a higher percentage of the hormone than did the blood. We have not identified all of the metabolites to which [1,2-³H]corticosterone is converted, but we have determined that only 10% or less has the R_F of 11-dehydrocorticosterone, a metabolite of corticosterone which can be formed by the brain (Grosser, 1966).

Studies of intracellular distribution of corticosterone: the phenomenon of binding to hippocampal cell nuclei

In a number of hormone target tissues, the retention of a particular steroid hormone by that tissue is correlated with the presence of high concentrations of that hormone tightly bound within cell nuclei (King and Gordon, 1967; Bruchovsky and Wilson, 1968; Jensen, Suzuki, Numata, Smith and DeSombre, 1969; Shyamala and Gorski, 1969). Current thinking on the mode of action of these bound hormones favors the idea that the nuclear binding factor is a regulator of genetic activity and that the hormone helps to inactivate the repressor-like activity of the binding factor and thereby produces a burst of genetic activity leading to the production of ribonucleic acid and protein molecules by the cell (Hamilton, 1968; Jensen *et al.*, 1969).

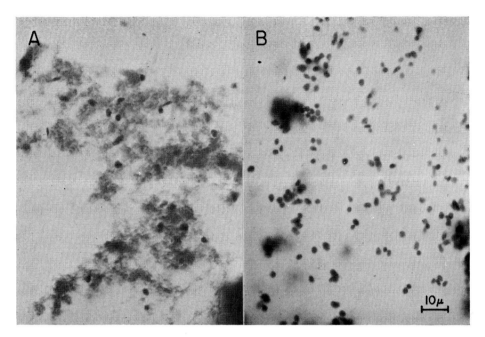

Fig. 3 A. Photomicrograph of whole homogenate of rat hippocampus. B. Purified cell nuclei obtained from hippocampus by method of Løvtrup-Rein and McEwen (1966). Magnification × 200. Bar indicates 10 μ. Dark spots in B are clumps of isolated nuclei which are not in focus; they do not indicate contamination.

In order to see if a similar parallel exists between tissue and nuclear retention of [1,2-³H]corticosterone in the hippocampus of adrenalectomized rats, we carried out a series of cell fractionation and nuclear isolation experiments on brain regions removed from rats injected one hour before sacrifice with 100 μC of the hormone. Nuclei were isolated by the method of Løvtrup-Rein and McEwen (1966), which uses a detergent, Triton-X-100, to remove cytoplasmic debris; it can be seen in Fig. 3B that the resulting nuclei are free of visible cytoplasmic debris. For comparison, Fig. 3A presents a photomicrograph of a whole homogenate of hippocampus, showing the large amount of cytoplasmic material which is removed during the isolation procedure.

In the initial experiments, the brain sample was fractionated into particulate and soluble cytoplasmic fractions and cell nuclei. The hippocampal nuclei had the highest concentration of any fraction. In seven experiments, the hippocampal nuclei had a mean of 12.1 ± 2.5 % of the radioactivity of the whole homogenate, and a concentration of 7.34 ± 1.95 times that of hippocampal tissue. If we correct for the nuclear yield of 33 % (based on recovery of DNA), then 36 % of the corticosterone in hippocampus is associated with cell nuclei. In order to eliminate several possible sources of artifact, we carried out several types of control experiments. First, nuclear binding did not occur after the tissue was disrupted, since after mixing [1,2-³H]corticosterone with the whole hippocampal homogenate from an adrenalectomized rat and isolating nuclei, we found no nuclear-bound radioactivity. Second, the uptake is not a property of the general steroid molecular shape, since [1,2-³H]cholesterol administered to an adrenalectomized rat was not found in hippocampal cell nuclei. More than 90% of the nuclear-bound radioactivity has the R_F of corticosterone (McEwen *et al.*, 1970).

Similar nuclear isolation experiments were performed on other regions of the brains of adrenalectomized rats which had been given [1,2-³H]corticosterone. No other brain region showed the same high degree of nuclear binding of the hormone, although all regions of the brain, particularly amygdala and cerebral cortex, show some degree of nuclear retention. This retention can be reduced to almost nothing by a saturating dose (see below) of unlabelled corticosterone (McEwen *et al.*, 1970). Our present interpretation of these results is that cells whose nuclei retain corticosterone are concentrated in the hippocampus and, to a lesser extent, in other parts of the brain. We would expect to find that each nucleus, irrespective of its location in the brain, binds the same amount of radioactive corticosterone, and we are conducting autoradiographic studies to verify this prediction.

The time course of retention of corticosterone in hippocampal nuclei is shown in Fig. 4, compared with the time course of disappearance of the hormone from the whole homogenate from which the nuclei were isolated. It can be seen that the nuclei retain the hormone over the first two hours and then lose it rapidly in the third and fourth hours. This tendency is emphasized in Fig. 4 by the dotted line, which represents the percentage of the total radioactivity recovered in the nuclear pellet. The process by which the nuclear binding is terminated after several hours is not easily explained, but may be due to the destruction of the binding factors themselves or to a competing reaction which removes the hormone from the nucleus. We believe that this timed retention has physiological significance, since the cessation of binding would signal the end of the cellular events over which the hormone has control and enable the rat to return to its original state in preparation for another stressful event (McEwen *et al.*, 1970).

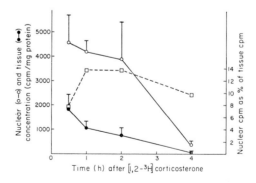

Fig. 4. Time course of retention of labelled corticosterone by cell nuclei from hippocampus compared with disappearance of the hormone from the whole homogenate. Dotted line indicates ratio of nuclear to whole homogenate hormone concentration. For procedural details, see McEwen *et al.* (1970).

Competition for corticosterone uptake by other steroids

In order to establish the specificity of the uptake mechanism for corticosterone, we conducted several competition experiments in brain tissue and isolated nuclei. In the first of these, which is presented in Fig. 5, adrenalectomized rats were given 3 mg of unlabelled steroid 30 min prior to the injection of radioactive corticosterone, and the brain was analyzed according to the radioactive concentration in seven brain regions and the pituitary. The hormone concentration was normalized for each animal by dividing the concentration in each brain region by the concentration in cerebral cortex. Only two regions showed any significant effect of the competition: in hippocampus and septum, tissue concentrations were reduced by prior injection of corticosterone, dexamethasone, and cortisol, but not by cholesterol. As noted above, endogenous levels of corticosterone in normal rats saturated the hippocampal mechanism but not that in the septum.

Competition experiments with a lower dose of steroid (0.5 mg) revealed a high degree of specificity for corticosterone in hippocampus, particularly at the nuclear level. These results are presented in Table 1. Tissue uptake was reduced by 0.5 mg of corticosterone to 40% of control, to a lesser extent by dexamethasone, desoxycorticosterone, and aldosterone, and not at all by cortisol and cholesterol. Nuclear uptake

TABLE I

COMPETITION FOR NUCLEAR AND TISSUE UPTAKE IN HIPPOCAMPUS BY 0.5 mg OF UNLABELLED STEROID

Steroid	Nuclear uptake		Tissue uptake	
	$[^3H]$ Cortico-sterone in nucleus % $\pm$ SEM	Per cent control	H/C $\pm$ SEM	Per cent control
Vehicle (n = 4)	6.34 $\pm$ 0.35	100	3.04 $\pm$ 0.39	100
Cholesterol (n = 2)	9.12, 6.22	143, 98	3.98, 3.71	131, 122
Hydrocortisone (n = 2)	8.98, 8.38	142, 132	3.05, 2.96	100, 97
Dexamethasone (n = 4)	8.35 $\pm$ 2.02	132	2.02 $\pm$ 0.39	66
Corticosterone (n = 4)	1.34 $\pm$ 0.41	21	1.29 $\pm$ 0.16	42
Desoxycorticosterone (n = 4)	6.35 $\pm$ 2.36	99	1.93 $\pm$ 0.35	63
Aldosterone (n = 2)	4.76, 5.37	75, 85	2.19, 2.20	72, 72

Nuclear uptake is presented as the percentage of labelled corticosterone recovered in the nuclear pellet; tissue uptake as the ratio of the concentration of labelled hormone in hippocampus to that in cortex (McEwen *et al.*, 1969a). Unlabelled steroid was injected 30 min before the labelled corticosterone, and animals were sacrificed 1 h after radioactive hormone administration.

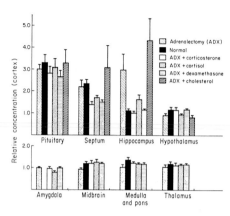

Fig. 5. Competition for uptake and retention of labelled corticosterone in pituitary and seven rat-brain regions. Three mg of each competing steroid was injected 30 min prior to the labelled cortico-sterone, and animals were sacrificed 2 h after injection of radioactive hormone. ADX = adrenalectomy.

was reduced to 20 % of control by corticosterone, to a very slight extent by aldosterone, and not at all by dexamethasone, desoxycorticosterone, cortisol, and cholesterol. The enhanced nuclear retention observed with cholesterol, cortisol, and dexamethasone may reflect a displacement of radioactive corticosterone from cytoplasmic into nuclear binding sites, since the nuclear uptake process is apparently much more specific than the tissue (*i.e.*, cytoplasmic) uptake process.

Comparison of uptake of radioactive corticosterone and estradiol

Reports from a number of laboratories have indicated that estradiol tends to localize in the preoptic region and hypothalamus (Eisenfeld and Axelrod, 1965; Kato and Villee, 1967; Pfaff, 1968, Stumpf, 1968; McEwen and Pfaff, unpublished), where it is believed to act in regulating gonadotrophic hormone release and in promoting sexual behavior (Lisk, 1967). The different regions of the brain involved in the retention and action of estradiol, on the one hand, and of corticosterone on the other, would seem to indicate that the brain is differentiated with respect to sites of steroid hormone sensitivity. Mr. Richard Zigmond, in the authors' laboratory, has examined nuclear retention of estradiol and has found very pronounced retention by cell nuclei, amount-ing to over 40 % of the tissue radioactivity, in the hypothalamus and preoptic area. (Zigmond and McEwen, 1970) A lesser degree of nuclear retention was observed in the amygdala, and very little was found in nuclei from hippocampus and cerebral cortex. We are therefore in the position of having observed nuclear binding of estradiol in the brain region which shows highest tissue retention of that hormone, and nuclear binding of corticosterone in the brain region which shows the highest tissue con-centration of that hormone.

Dependence of the levels of certain brain enzymes on corticosterone

Binding of a hormone by the cell nucleus appears to involve the action of the hormone on the transcription of genetic information leading to an altered synthesis of protein molecules within the affected cells. We have therefore attempted to see if there are any enzymes in the brain, the levels of which are controlled by corticosteroids. One such enzyme is glycerolphosphate dehydrogenase, as reported by DeVellis and Inglish (1968). Another such enzyme is tryptophan hydroxylase, a key step in serotonin biosynthesis, according to work now being carried out by Mr. Efrain Azmitia in the authors' laboratory (Azmitia and McEwen, 1969). Mr. Azmitia has found that adrenalectomy results in reduced levels of this enzyme, and that corticosteroid administration to adrenalectomized rats returns the level of tryptophan hydroxylase toward normal in as little as four hours. The effects of corticosterone can be prevented by intracranial administration of a protein synthesis inhibitor, cycloheximide. This finding not only shows the type of effect which corticosterone has in some brain cells but raises intriguing possibilities with respect to the interaction between adrenal steroids and biogenic amines such as serotonin, norepinephrine, and dopamine.

Some indications of the physiological and behavioral role of corticosterone action in the brain

We are particularly interested in determining the physiological and behavioral consequences of corticosterone action on the hippocampus and other regions of the brain. There is a growing body of evidence which indicates that adrenal steroids act directly on the brain to regulate release of ACTH from the pituitary (Mangili, Motta and Martini, 1966) and to moderate neural activity underlying behavioral responses (Woodbury and Vernadakis, 1966). Lesion and electrical stimulation studies of the limbic system (Mangili *et al.*, 1966) indicate that the hippocampus, as part of a delicately counterbalanced system of excitation and inhibition converging on the median eminence, has an inhibitory influence on ACTH release. One way that corticosterone could influence this system is by altering the activity of the hippocampus and thereby leading to an altered threshold for the release of ACTH. A corticosteroid-produced refractory period for ACTH release elicited by certain mild stressors has been described (Brodish and Long, 1958; Smelik, 1963; Hodges and Jones, 1964). This period does not appear until an hour or more after corticosterone blood levels have reached their peak and it lasts for eight hours or more thereafter. The time course for retention of corticosterone by hippocampal nuclei described above, and certain biosynthetic reactions resulting from corticosterone action on the nucleus, would seem able to provide a basis for the time course of this refractory period (McEwen *et al.*, 1970).

The hippocampus may also act as an important source of internal inhibition affecting behavior (Kimble, 1968). The behavioral effects of corticosterone in the rat have received very little attention; and because of our interest in this hormone and its effects on the hippocampus, we have begun to determine if corticosterone also influences behavior. In view of the ability of fear and pain-producing events to elicit corticosterone secretion, we first examined the role of corticosterone in fear-motivated behavior. It is evident that we must also understand the function of ACTH in such behavior if we wish to understand the role of corticosterone secretion.

Corticosterone secretion reaches a peak 15 or more minutes after the onset of stress and is relatively insensitive to stress intensity, but rather is "all-or-none" in nature. Therefore it seemed to us that in fear situations this hormone would be a poor mediator of defensive responses but might have a restorative function. On the other hand, ACTH is secreted rapidly after stress. This, together with the pioneering studies of Miller and Ogawa (1962) and of De Wied and colleagues (De Wied, 1966; Bohus and De Wied, 1966; De Wied, 1967) on behavioral effects of ACTH, suggested that ACTH might have the opposite role of potentiating the behavioral excitation evoked by the stressful event. Therefore we designed a series of experiments to test the notion that ACTH and corticosterone operate antagonistically in an elegant feedback circuit to regulate fear-motivated responding.

According to this hypothesis, ACTH has general excitatory effects which potentiate fear-motivated responding. However, ACTH also initiates the "shut-off" of this excitatory influence by stimulating secretion of corticosterone, which restores excitability to a normal level. This "normalizing" function of corticosterone is consistent with the physiological role proposed for this hormone in the central nervous system (Woodbury and Vernadakis, 1966). Corticosterone, according to these authors, may be unique among corticosteroids in having this type of effect. It is important to point out that we believe corticosterone to counteract excitatory effects of ACTH and not necessarily to have a suppressive action of its own in the absence of ACTH.

In a series of studies, some of which have been published (Weiss et al., 1969, 1970), we have found results consistent with the above hypothesis: Hypophysectomized rats, which lack ACTH, were found to be deficient in both active and passive avoidance responding when compared with normal rats; and given ACTH, these hypophysectomized animals improved their avoidance behavior toward normal. Adrenalectomized rats, which lack corticosterone and release excessive amounts of ACTH, showed more pronounced avoidance behavior than normals; given corticosterone, their avoidance responding diminished toward normal.

We have found certain conditions under which these hormones are maximally effective, which suggest to us that ACTH and corticosterone are not primarily responsible for reactions to clearly-signalled, imminent dangers but are more important in affecting the responses of the animal to what might be called a general level of anxiety. For example, when we measured suppression to foot shock of bar-pressing for food and water (the "Conditioned emotional response" or CER), we found that suppression to a tone presented several seconds before a strong shock did not differentiate the groups. But the suppression we observed to the training box alone during extinction produced clear differences between normal, hypophysectomized, and adrenalectomized rats. An even clearer demonstration that ACTH and corticosterone have their principal influence under conditions of mild, generalized fear can be seen in one of the passive avoidance experiments (Weiss et al., 1969). In this experiment, animals stepped from a small compartment into a larger one, and there received a foot shock. When placed back in the small compartment, hypophysectomized rats showed slightly more willingness to re-enter the larger compartment (i.e., less avoidance) than did normal or adrenalectomized rats. We then altered the entire apparatus, making the previously clear plexiglass walls opaque white and changing the grid-bar floor to a solid, white one. This procedure reduces the rat's fear by eliminating various conditioned fear stimuli and decreasing the number of specific danger signals in the larger compartment. Under these conditions, enormous behavioral differences were observed: hypophysectomized rats entered the larger compartment almost as fast as they had before they were shocked, and much faster than normals; adrenalectomized rats continued to show pronounced avoidance behavior and re-entered the larger compartment much more slowly than normal animals. This observation, that the hormonal state is more effective in influencing behavior when fear is weak and generalized than when fear is strong and clearly signalled, is consistent with previous findings of behavioral differences during extinction (Miller and Ogawa, 1962; De Wied, 1966). It also seems logical to us that a hormonal system, which is relatively slow-acting, would influence the general level of excitability and that other systems, probably neural, would be largely responsible for immediate reactions to clear dangers.

If ACTH and corticosterone indeed alter the general level of excitability or emotionality, a wide range of responses might well be affected by their secretion, depending upon the stimulus characteristics of the situation. We recently tested adrenalectomized, hypophysectomized, and normal rats, and animals treated with ACTH or corticosterone, in a discrimination task with food reinforcement to determine if hormone effects would be evident. High ACTH levels produced accelerated rates of responding just before the onset of reinforcement periods, whereas the presence of corticosterone reduced this effect. Thus, the excitatory influence of ACTH and the counter-excitatory influence of corticosterone can also pertain to appetitive behavior. The role of the hippocampus in this kind of appetitive situation is indicated by recent studies of Haddad and Rabe (1969).

ACKNOWLEDGEMENTS

This research was supported by USPHS grants NB 07080 to Dr. McEwen and MH13189 to Dr. N. E. Miller. We are grateful to Mrs. Leslie S. Schwartz for excellent technical assistance in these studies.

REFERENCES

AZMITIA, E., JR. AND MCEWEN, B. S. (1969) Effect of adrenalectomy and corticosterone-replacement therapy on tryptophan hydroxylase levels in midbrain of rat. *Science*, in press.
BOHUS, B. AND DE WIED, D. (1966) Inhibitory and facilitatory effect of two related peptides on extinction of avoidance behavior. *Science*, **153**, 318–320.
BRODISH, A. AND LONG, C. N. H. (1958) Changes in blood ACTH under various experimental conditions studied by means of a cross-circulation technique. *Endocrinology*, **59**, 666–676.
BRUCHOVSKY, N. AND WILSON, J. D. (1968) The intranuclear binding of testosterone and 5α-androstane-17β-ol-3-one by rat prostate. *J. Biol. Chem.*, **243**, 5953–5960.
BUSH, I. E. (1953) Species differences in adrenocortical secretion. *J. Endocrinol.*, **9**, 95–100.
DEVELLIS, J. AND INGLISH, D. (1968) Hormonal control of glycerol phosphate dehydrogenase in the rat brain. *J. Neurochem.*, **15**, 1061–1070.

DE WIED, D. (1966) Inhibitory effect of ACTH and related peptides on extinction of conditioned avoidance behavior in rats. *Proc. Soc. Exptl. Biol. Med.*, **122**, 28–32.

DE WIED, D. (1967) Opposite effects of ACTH and glucocorticoids on extinction of conditioned avoidance behavior. In: *Proc. 2nd Intern. Congr. on Hormonal Steroids, Milan, 1966*, L. MARTINI, F. FRASCHINI AND MOTTA (Eds.), Excerpta Medica Foundation, Amsterdam, pp. 945–951.

EISENFELD, A. J. AND AXELROD, J. (1965) Selectivity of estrogen distribution in tissues. *J. Pharmacol. Exptl. Therap.*, **150**, 469–475.

GROSSER, B. I. (1966) 11β-Hydroxysteroid metabolism by mouse brain and glioma 261. *J. Neurochem.*, **13**, 475–478.

HADDAD, R. K. AND RABE, A. (1969) Modified temporal behavior in rats after large hippocampal lesions. *Experimental Neurol.*, **24**, 310–317.

HAMILTON, T. H., (1969) Control by estrogen of genetic transcription and translation. *Science*, **161**, 649–661.

HODGES, J. R. AND JONES, M. T. (1964) Changes in pituitary corticotrophic function in the adrenalectomized rat. *J. Physiol.*, **173**, 190–200.

JENSEN, E. V., SUZUKI, T., NUMATA, M., SMITH, S., AND DESOMBRE, E. R. (1969) Estrogen-binding substances of target tissues. *Steroids*, **13**, 417–427.

KATO, J. AND VILLEE, C. A. (1967) Preferential uptake of estradiol by the anterior hypothalamus in the rat. *Endocrinology*, **80**, 567–575.

KIMBLE, D. P. (1968) Hippocampus and internal inhibition. *Psychol. Bull.*, **70**, 285–295.

KING, R. J. B. AND GORDON, J. (1967) The association of [6,7-³H]oestradiol with a nuclear protein. *J. Endocrinol.*, **39**, 533–542.

LISK, R. D. (1967) Sexual behavior: hormonal control. In: *Neuroendocrinology*, Vol. 2, L. MARTINI AND W. GANONG (Eds.), Academic Press, New York, pp. 197–240.

LØVTRUP-REIN, H. AND MCEWEN, B. S. (1966) Isolation and fractionation of rat brain nuclei. *J. Cell Biol.*, **30**, 405–416.

MANGILI, G., MOTTA, M. AND MARTINI, L. (1966) Control of adrenocorticotrophic hormone secretion. In: *Neuroendocrinology*, Vol. 1, L. MARTINI AND W. GANONG (Eds.), Academic Press, New York, pp. 297–370.

MCEWEN, B. S., WEISS, J. M. AND SCHWARTZ, L. S. (1968) Selective retention of corticosterone by limbic structures in rat brain. *Nature*, **220**, 911–912.

MCEWEN, B., WEISS, J. M. AND SCHWARTZ, L. (1969) Uptake of corticosterone by rat brain and its concentration by certain limbic structures. *Brain Research*, **16**, 227–241.

MCEWEN, B. S., WEISS, J. M., AND SCHWARTZ, L. S. (1970) Retention of corticosterone by cell nuclei from brain regions of adrenalectomized rats. *Brain Research*, in press.

MILLER, R. AND OGAWA, N. (1962) The effect of adrenocorticotrophic hormone (ACTH) on avoidance conditioning in the adrenalectomized rat. *J. Comp. Physiol. Psychol.*, **55**, 211–213.

PFAFF, D. W. (1968) Autoradiographic localization of radioactivity in rat brain after injection of tritiated sex hormones. *Science*, **161**, 1355–1356.

SHYAMALA, G. AND GORSKI, J. (1969) Estrogen receptors in the rat uterus: Studies on the interaction of cytosal and nuclear binding sites. *J. Biol. Chem.*, **244**, 1097–1103.

SMELIK, P. G. (1963) Relation between blood level of corticoids and their inhibiting effects on the hypophyseal stress response. *Proc. Soc. Exptl. Biol. Med.*, **113**, 616–619.

STUMPF, W. E. (1968) Estradiol-concentrating neurons: Topography in the hypothalamus by dry-mount autoradiography. *Science*, **162**, 1001–1003.

WEISS, J. M., MCEWEN, B. S., SILVA, M. T., AND KALKUT, M. S. (1969) Pituitary-adrenal influences on fear responding. *Science*, **163**, 197–199.

WEISS, J. M., MCEWEN, B. S., SILVA, M. T., AND KALKUT, M. S. (1970) Pituitary-adrenal alterations and fear-responding. *Amer. J. Physiol.*, in press.

WOODBURY, D. M. AND VERNADAKIS, A. (1966) Effects of steroids in the cerebral nervous system. In: *Methods in Hormone Research*, Vol. 5, R. I. DORFMAN (Ed.), Academic Press, New York, pp. 1–57.

ZIGMOND, R. AND MCEWEN, B. S., (1970) Selective retention of estradiol by cell nuclei in specific brain regions of the ovariectomized rat, *J. Neurochem.*, in press.

DISCUSSION

GLASSMAN: Do nuclei from liver, which is also affected by cortisone, show a similar behavior as hippocampal nuclei?

McEwen: Liver nuclei do show a slight tendency to retain corticosterone by a mechanism which can be saturated by the unlabelled hormone.

Glassman: Since liver and hippocampus differ, is it not possible that the binding by hippocampal nuclei is an artifact not related to normal corticosterone action?

McEwen: It should be remembered that most enzyme induction experiments on liver have been done with cortisol or cortisone. We have found that cortisol does not compete for nuclear binding of corticosterone at physiological doses. Hence cortisol and corticosterone, by virtue of their different structures, are apparently completely different in action on the hippocampal nucleus and may be different in their effect on the liver. Furthermore, the literature on enzyme induction in liver is by no means clear regarding a direct nuclear effect of corticosteroids. Finally, the high degree of specificity of nuclear binding in hippocampus precludes any kind of "artifact", as the term is generally used.

McNeil: Did you notice any difference in distribution of uptake between adrenalectomized and non-adrenalectomized rats?

McEwen: Yes, we did. The hippocampus does not retain corticosterone in the normal rat but does so in the adrenalectomized animal.

McNeil: How long after adrenalectomy did you inject the labelled compounds? Is there a difference in distribution if you wait, say several days, instead of giving immediately injections?

McEwen: Two hours after adrenalectomy we can detect nuclear binding and tissue retention in the hippocampus. We usually use rats adrenalectomized 3–7 days previously.

McNeil: What would be the function of the hormone in the brain itself, especially in the hippocampus?

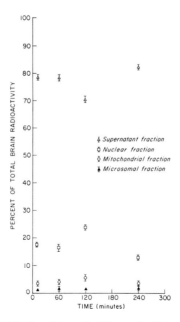

Fig. 1. Per cent of total radioactivity found in each of four subcellular fractions of brain 10 min to 4 h after intravenous injection of [1,2-^{3}H]-F in eviscerated cats.

McEwen: I wish I knew the answer at the physiological or behavioral level. We postulate that at the cellular level, certain enzymes are under direct genetic regulation.

Henkin: We have recently published data demonstrating the time course of the localization of radioactive cortisol (^{3}HF) in brain nuclei of eviscerated cats (Fig. 1). After a single i.v. injection of ^{3}HF, brain cell nuclei rapidly take up the hormone to achieve a highest concentration at 2 h after injection; at 4 h the concentration is lower again. There is a concomitant decrease in ^{3}HF in the supernatant fraction 2 h after injection and a concomitant increase at 4 h. There were no significant changes in ^{3}HF concentration in brain cell mitochondria or microsomes.

Harris: Some years ago, Drs. Taurog, Tong, Chaikoff and myself found that the uptake of labelled thyroxine and tri-iodothyronine by the posterior pituitary gland of the normal rabbit occurred against a concentration gradient, and that a similar high uptake occurred (weight for weight) if the posterior pituitary was inactive and atrophied to one-third of its weight by pituitary stalk section. One possible explanation is that the connective tissue was primarily responsible for the phenomenon. I wonder if, in this connection, you have any evidence that the hippocampal nuclei involved in your observations are really the nuclei of nerve cells and not the nuclei of neuroglial cells.

McEwen: Autoradiographs by Pfaff and by Stumpf have shown very clearly neuronal localization for [^{3}H]estradiol and [^{3}H]testosterone. Glial cells do not concentrate the hormone. We do not yet have autoradiographs for [^{3}H] corticosterone but do have preliminary evidence from density gradients that the hormone is bound to the large neuronal nuclei.

Marks: Is the difference between the brain regions due to a difference in the nuclei or to a difference in nerve cell transport?

McEwen: We believe that there exists in the cytoplasm of nerve cells where there is nuclear binding of corticosterone a binding protein which may be involved in subsequent nuclear binding. This may be one reason why we cannot obtain binding on isolated nuclei *in vitro*. This situation is analogous to that in uterus for estradiol uptake and binding as described by Jensen's group and by Gorski and colleagues. We also believe that only some nuclei have a binding protein for corticosterone (and that they exist in cells with the cytoplasmic uptake mechanism). The cytoplasmic uptake process is less specific towards corticosterone while the nuclear mechanism as we have shown, is highly selective.

Hodges: The lack of correlation between plasma corticosterone concentration and hippocampal nuclei corticosterone concentration reminds me of the similar dissociation between plasma steroid levels and inhibition of ACTH release. Do you consider that your work supports the concept of a negative feedback mechanism controlling ACTH release and that the site of the corticoid-sensitive controller is in the hippocampus?

McEwen: I would like to say "yes", and in fact we recently have written some speculations, which say just what you are saying. But the results of corticosterone implants in hippocampus, showing a positive feedback in ACTH release (Bohus — this meeting) are contradictory to this idea and are very puzzling. They prevent me from giving an unqualified "Yes".

Weijnen: You have pointed out that you believe corticosterone to counteract excitatory effects of ACTH and not necessarily to have a suppressing action of its own in the absence of ACTH. This implicates that no effect of corticosterone on, for instance, extinction of conditioned avoidance behavior would be predicted in hypophysectomized animals. However, De Wied (1967) demonstrated that extinction of shuttle box avoidance behavior was facilitated both by corticosterone and dexamethasone in hypophysectomized rats which were treated with a substitution therapy consisting of cortisone acetate, testosterone proprionate and *l*-thyroxine. (For reference to De Wied, see bibliography above.)

McEwen: We have made such a statement *only* because it has been the most cautious interpretation of the evidence at hand. However, De Wied's findings which you refer to provide the first direct evidence for an ACTH-independent action of corticosterone, although the general applicability of his findings to other behavioral situations remains to be established. We would like to see such an independent action of corticosterone because of our biochemical experiments indicating binding of corticosterone in hippocampus and other areas of the brain.

Anterior Pituitary Peptides and Avoidance Acquisition of Hypophysectomized Rats

D. DE WIED AND A. WITTER

Rudolf Magnus Institute for Pharmacology, Medical Faculty, University of Utrecht, Vondellaan 6, Utrecht (The Netherlands)

AND S. LANDE

Section of Dermatology, Department of Medicine, Yale University, School of Medicine, New Haven, Conn. (U.S.A.)

It is well established that the pituitary–adrenal system plays an essential role in the defense mechanism of the organism in response to noxious stimuli. These stimuli, which may be of neurogenic or emotional and of somatic or systemic character, invariably cause the discharge of ACTH from the adenohypophysis and the subsequent secretion of adrenocortical hormones. A number of studies have attempted to relate the activity of the pituitary–adrenal axis to behavior; in recent years, evidence has accumulated that this system may affect conditioned avoidance behavior (see for review De Wied, 1969). It has been shown that removal of the whole pituitary gland or the adenohypophysis alone, causes a severe deficit in the ability to acquire a conditioned avoidance response (Applezweig and Baudry, 1955; Applezweig and Moeller, 1959; De Wied, 1964). The administration of adrenal maintenance doses of adrenocorticotrophic hormone (ACTH) improves the rate of avoidance acquisition of hypophysectomized (Applezweig and Baudry, 1955) or adenohypophysectomized rats (De Wied, 1964). The effect of ACTH on avoidance acquisition, however, seemed not to be mediated by the adrenal cortex since adrenalectomized rats are similar to sham-operated animals in their ability to acquire the avoidance response (Moyer, 1958; Miller and Ogawa, 1962; De Wied, 1967). This suggests that ACTH might play a role in avoidance acquisition in some manner other than its trophic effect on the adrenal cortex. In fact, the administration of ACTH analogues materially devoid of corticotrophic activities like α-MSH, the decapeptide ACTH 1-10, or the heptapeptide ACTH 4-10, stimulates the rate of acquisition of the avoidance response of hypophysectomized rats in a way similar to that of synthetic or natural ACTH (De Wied, 1969).

Further studies with the heptapeptide ACTH 4-10 in hypophysectomized rats revealed that it had no effect on adrenal weight, plasma corticosterone, or thymus weight, indicating the absence of corticotrophic activities. Nor does the peptide affect the gonads, since atrophy of the testes in the hypophysectomized rat is not influenced by chronic treatment with ACTH 4-10. Body weight loss, which occurs as a result of hypophysectomy, also is not affected by treatment with this heptapeptide. The peptide affects neither plasma glucose of hypophysectomized rats, nor plasma insulin levels which are significantly decreased in the hypophysectomized rat. Accordingly, ACTH 4-10 does not affect endocrine functions. Lack of demonstrable systemic effects in the hypophysectomized rat indicates that this polypeptide exhibits a specific effect on behavior. Behavioral deficiency of the hypophysectomized rat certainly is linked in some extent to metabolic derangements and physical weakness, which occur as a result of hypophysectomy. In fact, a replacement therapy consisting of cortisone, testosterone, and thyroxin favourably affects the rate of acquisition of the avoidance response and also improves the motor and/or sensory capacities of the hypophysectomized animal (De Wied, 1964). Nevertheless, the heptapeptide ACTH 4-10, which neither affects the metabolic derangement nor the physical condition of the hypophysectomized rat, does restore the rate of acquisition of the avoidance response towards nearly normal levels. Interestingly, the effect of peptide hormones generally disappears if the size of the peptide chain is reduced. However, the studies reviewed above demonstrated that a small entity of the ACTH molecule still carries full behavioral activity. This prompted us to postulate that the pituitary gland might contain peptides which normally operate in the formation of conditioned and other adaptive responses. These neurogenic peptides may be represented by ACTH, α- or β-MSH, or by peptides related to these hormones. In order to test this hypothesis, a study was undertaken with the aim of isolating relatively small peptides related to the afore-mentioned hormones, from the pituitary.

In all experiments, hypophysectomized male rats, weighing between 130–160 g, were used. Hypophysectomy was performed via the trans-auricular route under ether

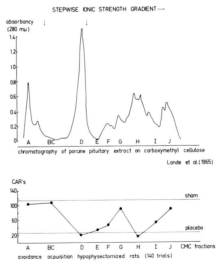

Fig. 1. Effect of CMC sub-fractions (Lande *et al.*, 1965) on the rate of acquisition of a shuttle-box avoidance response of hypophysectomized male rats. Fractions were administered as long-acting zinc phosphate preparations in a dose of 20 μg injected subcutaneously every other day for 14 days.

anesthesia. Animals were allowed to recover from the operation for 1 week. Avoidance training in a shuttle box was started 1 week after the operation. The conditioned stimulus (CS) was a buzzer presented for 5 sec prior to the unconditioned stimulus (US) of shock. Ten trials were given each day for 10 or 14 days with a mean inter-trial onset interval of 60 sec presented in a random sequence. All peptide fractions were administered as long-acting zinc phosphate preparations (De Wied, 1966). Treatment was started the day before avoidance training was begun. Peptide fractions were injected subcutaneously every other day during avoidance training. The total number of positive avoidances (CAR) was used as a measure of avoidance acquisition.

The starting material was a fraction with high MSH activity from hog pituitaries. Preparation of the starting material has been described by Schally, Lipscomb and Guillemin (1962). This fraction was separated by ion exchange chromatography on CMC into 10 fractions, numbered A–J (Lande, Lerner and Upton, 1965). It is clear from Fig. 1 that 4 fractions were highly active in stimulating the rate of avoidance acquisition in hypophysectomized rats. None of these fractions affected body weight loss, or adrenal- and testes atrophy of the hypophysectomized animals, indicating the absence of ACTH and gonadotrophic hormones. It is remarkable that fraction D, which contains β-MSH, and fraction H, which consists mainly of α-MSH, were inactive. Synthetic α-MSH and purified β-MSH both were found to be highly active in previous experiments. No explanation for the discrepancy in the results with these peptides and the fractions D and H can be given at present.

Fraction BC exhibited the strongest effect. This fraction had a rather low MSH activity, although the presence of β-MSH was demonstrated by paper electro-phoresis (Lande et al., 1965). The absorbancy at 280 mμ of this fraction was relatively low, and from its behavior on CMC it could be concluded that it consisted of weakly

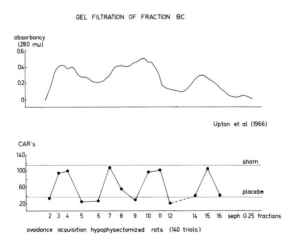

Fig. 2. Effect of Sephadex G-25 sub-fractions of BC (Upton et al., 1966) on the rate of acquisition of a shuttle-box avoidance response of hypophysectomized male rats. Fractions were administered as long-acting zinc phosphate preparations in a dose of 20 μg injected subcutaneously every other day for 14 days.

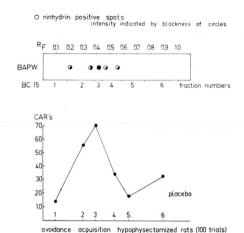

Fig. 3. Effect of sub-fractions of BC 15 separated by paper chromatography on the rate of acquisition of a shuttle-box avoidance response of hypophysectomized male rats. Fractions were administered as long-acting zinc phosphate preparations injected subcutaneously every other day for 10 days.

acidic peptides. For these reasons, fraction BC was used for further purification studies. Gel filtration of fraction BC on Sephadex G-25 yielded 17 sub-fractions numbered 1–17 as based on the absorbancy at 280 mμ and the Folin reaction (Upton, Lerner and Lande, 1966). Evaluation of the behavioral activity of these sub-fractions is depicted in Fig. 2. Activity was found in 6 sub-fractions. Because of the rather high activity of fraction BC 15 and its presumed low molecular weight, further paper-chromatographic purification was attempted with this fraction.

Paper chromatography on Whatman 3 MM paper, pre-washed with the solvent system, in BAPW (*n*-butanol–acetic acid–pyridine–water, 15 : 3 : 10 : 12 (by vol.)) was carried out with 400 μg BC 15/spot. Detection of peptide material was carried out with 0.4 % ninhydrin in 96 % ethanol–collidine, 20 : 1 (v/v).

As seen from Fig. 3, the behavioral activity was found in sub-fractions BC 15-2 and 3. The latter had the highest activity. This coincided with the strongest ninhydrin-positive spot in the BAPW paper chromatogram. The sub-fraction BC 15-3 was therefore rechromatographed after elution in BAW = 4 : 1 : 5 (upper phase of *n*-butanol–acetic acid–water = 4 : 1 : 5 (by vol.)). Again, the Whatman 3 MM paper was pre-washed with the solvent. The main spot BC 15-3^d, R_F = 0.42 in BAW 4 : 1 : 5, was the only active component in the acquisition test (Table 1). Only minor fractions were present besides the main spot.

Amino acid analysis of fraction BC 15-3^d could not be adequately performed due to lack of enough purified material, and experiments are in progress to purify the material for amino acid- and structure analysis.

The isolated peptide is materially devoid of ACTH, MSH, and vasopressor activities. This suggests that it is not ACTH, MSH, or vasopressin. Since neither histidine, nor tryptophane, nor arginine could be detected by specific colour reactions on the chromatogram, it seems highly improbable that the peptide is structurally related to

TABLE 1

EFFECT OF SUB-FRACTIONS BC 15-3 ON THE RATE OF AVOIDANCE LEARNING, NUMBER OF INTERTRIALS (IT'S), BODY WEIGHT, ADRENAL, TESTES AND THYMUS WEIGHT OF HYPOPHYSECTOMIZED MALE RATS TREATED FOR 10 DAYS (BAW)

Sub-fractions long-acting preparations	CAR's*	IT's	Body weight difference between initial and final weight g	Adrenal weight mg	Testes weight mg	Thymus weight mg	Number of animals
BC 15-3a+b+c	30 ± 1**	20 ± 2	−35 ± 2	9.5 ± 0.7	707 ± 48	218 ± 33	6
BC 15-3d	72 ± 2	17 ± 1	−35 ± 2	9.8 ± 1.0	630 ± 54	204 ± 19	7
Placebo	20 ± 2	13 ± 1	−35 ± 5	10.6 ± 0.6	604 ± 98	237 ± 38	6

* Number of positive avoidances of 100 trials during 10 days.
** Mean ± Standard Error of the Mean.

References p. 218

ACTH 4–10, which represents the common core of ACTH, α- and β-MSH. Although the elution volume of the Sephadex separation indicates a mean molecular weight for BC 15 in the range of a heptapeptide, the behavior on CMC demonstrates a significant more acidic character for the BC 15 material than for the ACTH 4-10 peptide. However that may be, a factor of pituitary origin has been isolated which is capable of stimulating the rate of acquisition of the avoidance response of the hypophysectomized rat. The potency of this factor appeared to be higher than that of the heptapeptide ACTH 4-10 and related ACTH analogues. It seems, therefore, that a new hitherto unknown factor has been isolated. Definite proof however has to await structure analysis of the isolated peptide. If this proves to be different from the known anterior pituitary hormones then it may indicate that the pituitary indeed contains a specific peptide which stimulates the acquisition of an avoidance response. Such a neurogenic peptide presumably acts on central nervous structures involved in motivational, learning, and memory processes. Whether this pituitary neurogenic peptide is involved in conditioned avoidance behavior can be demonstrated only by determining a relationship between release of such a factor from the anterior pituitary and the acquisition of conditioned avoidance behavior.

REFERENCES

APPLEZWEIG, M. H. AND BAUDRY, F. D. (1955) The pituitary-adrenocortical system in avoidance learning. *Psychol. Rep.*, **1**, 417–420.
APPLEZWEIG, M. H. AND MOELLER, G. (1959) The pituitary-adrenocortical system and anxiety in avoidance learning. *Acta Psychol.*, **15**, 602–603.
DE WIED, D. (1964) Influence of anterior pituitary on avoidance learning and escape behavior. *Amer. J. Physiol.*, **207**, 255–259.
DE WIED, D. (1966) Inhibitory effect of ACTH and related peptides on extinction of conditioned behavior in rats. *Proc. Soc. Exptl. Biol. Med.*, **122**, 28–32.
DE WIED, D. (1967) Opposite effects of ACTH and glucocorticosteroids on extinction of conditioned avoidance behavior. *Proc. Second Intern. Congr. on Hormonal Steroids, Milan, May, 1966*, Exc. Med. Intern. Congress Series, No. **132**, 945–951.
DE WIED, D. (1969) Effects of peptide hormones on behavior. In: *Frontiers in Neuroendocrinology*, W. F. GANONG AND L. MARTINI (Eds.), Oxford University Press, New York, pp. 97–140.
LANDE, S., LERNER, A. B. AND UPTON, G. V. (1965) Isolation of new peptides related to β-melanocyte-stimulating hormone. *J. Bio!. Chem.*, **240**, 4259–4263.
MILLER, R. E. AND OGAWA, N. (1962) The effect of adrenocorticotrophic hormone (ACTH) on avoidance conditioning in the adrenalectomized rat. *J. Comp. Physiol. Psychol.*, **55**, 211–213.
MOYER, K. E. (1958) Effect of adrenalectomy on anxiety motivated behavior. *J. Genet. Psychol.*, **92**, 11–16.
SCHALLY, A. V., LIPSCOMB, H. S. AND GUILLEMIN, R. (1962) Isolation and amino acid sequence of α_2-corticotrophin-releasing factor (α_2-CRF) from hog pituitary glands. *Endocrinolkogy*, **71**, 164–173.
UPTON, G. V., LERNER, A. B. AND LANDE, S. (1966) Pituitary peptides. Resolution by gel filtration. *J. Biol. Chem.*, **241**, 5585–5589.

DISCUSSION

KRIVOY: I wonder if you might say something about the mechanism of action of these peptides and how they normalize the impaired learning of hypophysectomized rats.

DE WIED: To speculate about the mode of action of the peptide is rather difficult. The inability to acquire the avoidance response might be due to a general debilitation of the hypophysectomized organism and to central nervous system defects. Since the peptide did not visibly affect the general health and condition of the hypophysectomized rat, an effect on the function of the nervous system is plausible. Actually, the work presented by Gispen and Schotman (this conference) suggests an effect on macromolecular metabolism in the brain of hypophysectomized rats under the influence of the peptide during avoidance learning. The exact mode of action of the peptide in this respect is not known.

KRIVOY: I wonder also about the nomenclature. You called the peptide a "neurogenic" peptide. We have been calling them "neurotropic" peptides because they tend to act on the nervous system. I would be willing to use either term if we can reach agreement.

DE WIED: The choice of the right term has been troubling me. Thank you for your comment, let us reconsider the issue together.

LEVINE: Do you conceive that these peptides are released individually, independently of other peptides? Or would they be contained in the mass release of pituitary peptides under the appropriate conditions?

DE WIED: An individual release of the peptide, independently of other peptides is not likely. At the end of my paper I said that in order to relate avoidance acquisition with release of neurogenic peptides, a demonstration between the release of such a factor during avoidance conditioning should be demonstrated.

LARON: You mentioned that the peptide does not resemble ACTH-(4-10), but you did not say whether it resembles ACTH-(1-10). Have you considered the possibility that the peptide is part of one or of several pituitary hormones? We know, for example, that digestion of human growth hormone up to 90% still leaves or even increases, its lipolytic acitivity (Kowadlo-Silbergeld and Laron (1966) *Israel J. Med. Sci.*, **2**, 22). This shows that this property is related to a small part of the big molecule.

WITTER: The available knowledge on the amino acid composition of the isolated peptide indicates that it does not resemble ACTH-(1-10) either. The definite answer to your question regarding the possibility that the isolated peptide is part of a larger pituitary hormone must, of course, await the amino acid sequence analysis. We certainly do not want to exclude this possibility. The behavioral results obtained with ACTH fragments, like the 4-10 peptide, keep us alert for such a possibility. We also cannot exclude the possibility that the peptide is an isolation artifact, but this is not likely.

DE WIED: If it would be an artifact then it is a very interesting one, because the isolated peptide is more active than the ACTH-(4-10) molecule.

GLASSMAN: There is no question that you have isolated a compound of immense potential importance. However, it is possible that like many compounds that have such properties, the effect is to stimulate performance rather than to augment learning and memory processes. Have you any data that would distinguish between these possibilities?

DE WIED: I am not sure if hypophysectomized rats would perform better with stimulating compounds during avoidance training. I do not think this has been demonstrated. It is, of course, important that the nature of the performance modification should be investigated when more of the peptide becomes available. It should be mentioned, however, that we did not notice any effects on behavior during the experiments.

CLEGHORN: The perspectives opened up by this work have great implications for the psychologist and the psychiatrist. What the meaning may be regarding the influence of such peptides on avoidance learning remains to be seen. What avoidance learning means in other central nervous system terms is open to the most exciting speculation.

MARKS: Do peptides of this type occur in the brain itself?

WITTER: The investigation was carried out with hog pituitaries, nothing can be said therefore about other parts of the brain or about other species. For many years we have attempted to isolate peptides from the brain. It would be interesting to test peptide fractions of the brain on avoidance acquisition. However, isolation of peptides from the brain is even more difficult than isolation from the pituitary; this is not only caused by the complexity of the composition of the peptides in the CNS, but also to a great extent by the very low concentrations of the active peptides.

LEVINE: ACTH and MSH are naturally occurring peptides which can affect conditioned avoidance behavior. Now one more peptide with neurogenic properties has been isolated. It seems that there may be a variety of peptides which are active in a similar way.

DE WIED: That might be true, and it would be interesting to isolate more of these peptides. But it is a little difficult and the problem is that we do not have enough starting material.

The point I want to stress is that this peptide is more active than the peptides we used up to now. It will be very interesting to see what substance we have been using and whether or not it resembles ACTH-(1-10) or ACTH-(4-10).

MIRSKY: In the posterior pituitary there are 90 peptides, if not more. The fact that more than one has a specific function is really of very little importance until each is identified. Then one can determine their specificity. Many of these compounds which exert extra-adrenal activity (but are regarded as adrenocorticotropic) act by an interesting mechanism in that they stimulate adenylcyclase and induce an increase in cyclic AMP, as Dr McEwen started to mention, acting as the so called "second messenger" within the brain, as within other tissues. It is interesting to note that some of these peptides, or related peptides, did exert a metabolic activity *in vitro*. Some of them act like insulin on hypothalamic tissue. So the whole question is wide open until we can really identify all these peptides and test them.

Effects of ACTH-Analogues on Extinction of Conditioned Behavior

J. A. W. M. WEIJNEN AND J. L. SLANGEN

Rudolf Magnus Institute for Pharmacology, University of Utrecht, Medical Faculty, Vondellaan 6, Utrecht (The Netherlands)

In many studies on the effects of ACTH on behavior it is not quite clear whether the obtained effects are due to the direct action of ACTH on the nervous system or rather to corticosteroids which have been secreted following stimulation of the adrenals by ACTH. This is particularly confusing as ACTH and corticosteroids are reported to exhibit an opposite effect on extinction of conditioned behavior in studies which were designed to elucidate the roles of the separate hormones: ACTH can inhibit extinction of conditioned avoidance behavior, whilst glucocorticosteroids — and some other steroids as well — can facilitate the rate of extinction (Miller and Ogawa, 1962; De Wied, 1967; Weiss, McEwen, Silva and Kalkut, 1969; Van Wimersma Greidanus, this volume, page 185). Interference by adrenocortical steroid action in some ACTH studies could be minimized or excluded by administering low doses of ACTH in a long-acting preparation or by using adrenalectomized rats. The action of corticosteroids in absence of endogenous ACTH was studied in hypophysectomized rats.

The study of the effects of ACTH on the behavior of intact animals received a new impetus after the discovery that fragments of this hormone containing the first 10 amino acids — or even smaller peptides like ACTH-(4-10) — could still exhibit a similar behavioral effect as ACTH. These peptides lack the well-known biological activities of the intact hormone such as stimulation of the adrenals. The behavioral effect of ACTH could now be studied in intact animals independently of concomitant steroid action (De Wied, 1966; Greven and De Wied, 1967).

Labelling these peptides as "ACTH-analogues" is more a matter of habit than of precise description since also α- and β-MSH, which exert a similar inhibiting effect on extinction of conditioned avoidance behavior as ACTH, share the amino acid sequence that we conveniently call ACTH-(4-10).

Interesting data were reported by Bohus and De Wied (1966) in a study where ACTH-(1-10) and [D-phe⁷]-ACTH-(1-10) were used. In the latter peptide the phenylalanine in the 7th position is replaced by the D form. Effects of the two peptides — 10 μg/48 h of a long-acting zinc phosphate preparation — on extinction of shuttlebox avoidance behavior were studied in daily 10-trial sessions. During the extinction sessions foot-shock is not applied any more and the conditioned stimulus (CS), the sound of a buzzer, is response-terminated or ended after 5 sec by the experimenter in case the rat fails to make the conditioned response. The results are shown in Fig. 1.

References p. 233

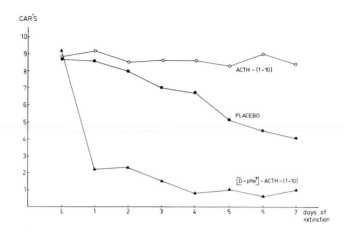

Fig. 1. Effects of ACTH-(1–10), [D-phe⁷]-ACTH-(1–10), and placebo on the extinction of a shuttle-box avoidance response. (From Bohus, B. and De Wied, D., *Science* vol. 153, pp. 318–320, 15 July 1966. Copyright 1966 by the American Association for the Advancement of Science.)

ACTH-(1-10) inhibited extinction again, but the D-peptide facilitated extinction. This effect could not be explained by a direct antagonism between the D-peptide and structurally related L form peptides of pituitary origin.

The study and replications of the experiment, also by other investigators, in the shuttle-box and pole-jumping situations stimulated our research into the nature of the behavioral modifications obtained after administration of ACTH-analogues (Greven and De Wied, 1967; De Wied and Pirie, 1968; De Wied, 1969).

The possibility of a peptide effect on the general activity level of the rat or of a peptide-induced development of a behavior pattern that might interfere with conditioned avoidance behavior deserved our attention. It is obvious for instance that administration of a drug that incapacitates an animal to move will result in a dramatic reduction of avoidance behavior. Bohus and De Wied (1966) had shown already that

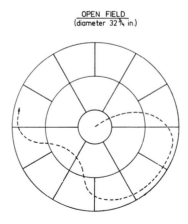

Fig. 2. Scoring ambulation in the open field. A rat path, as indicated by the dashed line would be scored as 10 (floor units entered).

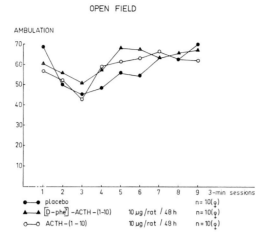

Fig. 3. Mean ambulation scores for 3 treatment groups over 9 sessions in the open field.

in a single 3-min session during which the activity of the rat was observed in a simple open-field no effects of ACTH-(1-10) and of the D-peptide could be detected on ambulation, rearing, grooming and defecation.

This study was extended to observation during repeated sessions. An open-field (for dimensions see Broadhurst, 1960) was used, illuminated by a 75-watt bulb suspended 20 inch above the field centre. Ambulation was measured by counting the number of floor units entered by the rat during the daily 3-min session (Fig. 2). Three groups of 10 female white rats each of our inbred Wistar strain took part in the experiment; mean body weight 126 g at the beginning of the experiment. ACTH-(1–10) and the D-peptide were administered as long-acting Zn phosphate preparations (De Wied, 1966). The treatment started the day before the first session. Subcutaneous injections of 10 μg/48 h of the peptides in a suspension of 0.5 ml were given. Zinc phosphate complex without peptide served as a placebo, like in all other experiments we performed. As a rule "double"-blind conditions were observed in our experiments.

TABLE I

THE EFFECT OF β-MSH ON AMBULATION AND DEFECATION OF RATS IN THE OPEN FIELD

Mean total scores, summed over 5 sessions, are given.

Treatment/24 h		n	Sessions	Ambulation		Boli	
β-MSH	5 μg	10 ♀	5 × 3 min	232.7	n.s.*	28.4	n.s.*
Placebo		10 ♀	5 × 3 min	220.6		24.3	
β-MSH	5 μg	10 ♀	5 × 5 min	245.0	n.s.*	27.9	n.s.*
Placebo		10 ♀	5 × 5 min	253.8		24.2	
β-MSH	10 μg	10 ♀	5 × 5 min	234.0	n.s.*	34.0	n.s.*
Placebo		10 ♀	5 × 5 min	232.6		33.0	

* Not significant at 5% level (Mann-Whitney U test, two tailed).

References p. 233

Y-MAZE

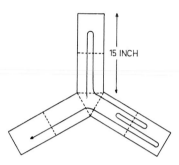

Fig. 4. Scoring ambulation in the Y-maze. A rat path as indicated by the line in the diagram would be scored as 10 (half-arm units).

Results are shown in Fig. 3. The activity scores of the rats, summed over 9 sessions, did not differ from each other at the 5% level. (Mann-Whitney U test, two tailed.) We repeated this experiment several times with β-MSH at two dose levels, with 3- and 5-min sessions (Table 1). No significant results were obtained.

In these open-field experiments we used dose levels comparable to those that are effective in modifying the extinction rate in avoidance conditioning. However, no change in activity level, expressed in floor units entered by the rat, could be detected. The hypothesis that an action of ACTH analogues on the general activity level of the rats might account for the reported effects is not supported by our data.

In the open-field experiments rats were not subjected to foot-shock. In another series of experiments therefore, we investigated whether differences in activity might show up in rats which had experienced foot-shock in the test situation.

A symmetrical Y-shaped maze (Steinberg, Rushton and Tinson, 1961) equipped with a grid floor was used. Ambulation is measured by counting the number of times a rat entered a half-arm unit with all four feet (Fig. 4). In this test situation a short period of inescapable foot-shock results in a low ambulation level of the rats. This suppression of ambulation is frequently named: Conditioned Emotional Response (CER). With subsequent sessions ambulation scores can increase again to the level of nonshocked control rats, if no shock is applied any more. Marked drug effects can be demonstrated in this situation (Weijnen, 1969).

If we suppose that a low ambulation level in the Y-maze after foot-shock is a consequence of fear conditioning, and if we would interpret the effect of ACTH-analogues on avoidance extinction in terms of an influence on fear motivation, then we should predict a low ambulation level in the Y-maze for ACTH-(1-10)-treated rats and a high level for rats treated with the D-peptide during sessions following foot-shock.

Note that the previously mentioned working hypothesis that effects of ACTH-analogues might be due to a nonspecific general activity effect, would have predicted opposite results.

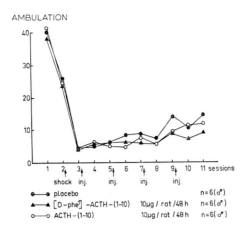

Fig. 5. Mean ambulation scores for 3 groups of male rats. Foot-shock was applied at the end of session 2. Session-3 scores were used to divide the animals into matched treatment groups; peptide and placebo administration (10 μg/rat) followed, and was repeated every 48 h.

Three experiments will be reported. Ambulation was measured during daily 3-min sessions; scrambled foot-shock was applied at the end of the second session (300 V a.c. with a 600 000-ohm series resistor). Following session 3, rats were allocated to treatment groups matched for ambulation, using session-3 scores as a criterion. ACTH-(1-10) and the D-peptide were administered. Fig. 5 shows the results obtained with male rats; mean body weight 160 g at day 1. These rats received foot-shock for 15 sec in three bursts of 5 sec. Ten μg of the peptides/rat/48 h were administered. Statistical analysis did not reveal any differences between the treatment groups. Since ambulation levels after foot-shock stayed quite low, shock duration was diminished in the next two experiments: 5 sec only, again with a short circuit value of 0.5 mA. Moreover, female rats rather than males took part in these experiments. Female rats overcome the ambulation-suppressing effects of foot-shock sooner than male rats. Fig. 6 shows the results of an experiment with animals weighing approx. 150 g, at day 1 and receiving 10 μg peptide/48h. Fig. 7 presents the data of a comparable experiment with a dose level twice as high.

No meaningful differences in ambulation scores during the treatment periods could be detected. Rearing, grooming and defecation had also been scored. No consistent differences were found.

We have investigated ACTH-analogue effects in another test situation in which a suppression of on-going behavior was measured. In a conventional Skinner box female rats were trained to press a lever for a water reward on a 30-sec variable interval schedule with a $2\frac{1}{2}$-sec limited hold. This schedule ensured a fairly high and constant rate of lever pressing during the entire 40-min session.

Two conditioning trials per session were superimposed on the lever-pressing performance. The CS consisted of auditory and visual stimuli. A 5-min presentation of the CS was terminated contiguously with an inescapable 1-sec scrambled foot-shock of 0.5 mA (short circuit value). The general procedure of superimposing a

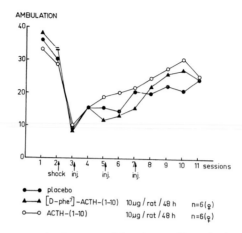

Fig. 6. Mean ambulation scores for 3 groups of female rats. Foot-shock was applied at the end of session 2. Session-3 scores were used to divide the animals into matched treatment groups; peptide and placebo administration (10 μg/rat) followed, and was repeated after 48 and 96 h.

stimulus terminating with a noxious stimulus on a base line of on-going behavior is called the Estes–Skinner procedure. In a well trained animal the CER appears as a decrease of the animal's lever-pressing behavior during presentation of the CS. However, both before and after the CS period a constant rate of lever pressing is maintained. Having obtained an almost complete suppression of on-going behavior during the CS we started an extinction procedure by omitting the shock in subsequent sessions.

The effect of ACTH-(4-10) was studied on this extinction of the suppression of lever pressing for water. Neither in the first experiment of this type we performed, nor in the replication of the study did we observe any differences between the group of rats

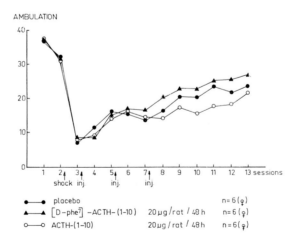

Fig. 7. Mean ambulation scores for 3 groups of female rats. Foot-shock was applied at the end of session 2. Session-3 scores were used to divide the animals into matched treatment groups; peptide and placebo administration followed, and was repeated after 48 and 96 h. In this experiment 20, instead of 10 μg/rat of the long-acting zinc phosphate preparation was injected.

ELEVATED RUNWAY

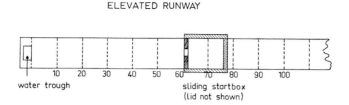

Fig. 8. Elevated runway with sliding startbox at the 60-cm position (top view).

treated with ACTH-(4-10) and the group treated with the placebo.

The two sets of experiments in which extinction of suppression of on-going behavior was studied did not bring evidence in support of the hypothesis that ACTH-analogues might modify conditioned behavior through an influence on a hypothetical "fear motivation" level.

There exists a fundamental difference between extinction sessions in the described suppression of on-going behavior studies and extinction sessions in active avoidance experiments, with the shuttle-box for instance. If in the latter situation the animal responds in time during extinction sessions, the situation does not differ from the training period. Only an animal that fails to respond in time can experience that no shock is presented any more. On the other hand in the studies concerning the suppression of behavior, shock appearance did not depend on the behavior of the rat. Therefore extinction sessions differ distinctly from training sessions. The relevance of this distinction for the interpretation of ACTH-analogue effects on extinction of conditioned behavior is tested in current experiments.

Besides studying extinction of negatively reinforced behavior, we also investigated whether we could modify the extinction of positively reinforced behavior. Modification of behavior resulting from this type of study might mean that noxious stimulation by foot-shock is not essential in obtaining ACTH-analogue effects.

Rats were trained to run for water on an elevated runway (Fig. 8). Starting at a distance of 0 cm — sliding startbox against water trough — animals were trained to run eventually 100 cm for 1.25 ml of water per trial. There were five trials per day, approx. 30–45 min apart. No water had been available to the rats in the living cage since 48 h before the start of the experiment. Access to food was normal, also during the intertrial interval.

A rat that is gently dropped in the startbox soon learns to run straight to the trough and it is interesting to note that most animals ran back to the startbox immediately after they had drunk the water. During extinction sessions water was available at the first trial of the day only. At the end of each day another 5 ml was presented to each rat in a drinking cage equipped with a trough.

After 7 training days animals were allocated to treatment groups, matched for performance during the training period; this was followed by administration of ACTH -(1-10) and D-peptide: 20 μg/rat/48 h. We performed 2 experiments with female rats; mean body weight 120 g at the day the water regime began. The water intake restrictions during the experiment kept the body weight of the rats at a fairly constant level

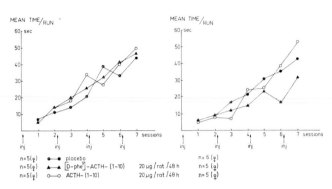

Fig. 9. Extinction of running for water on an elevated runway. The mean time per non-rewarded run is shown for the 3 treatment groups over 7 sessions.

of approx. 95 g. Fig. 9 shows the results of both experiments. The mean time it took the animals of each treatment group to reach the water trough during the non-reinforced runs of the extinction sessions are presented. Animals which did not reach the trough within 60 sec were taken from the runway, or startbox, and put back in the living cage until the next extinction trial. (An animal that exceeded the 60-sec limit during training was put at the trough.)

Neither an analysis of the results per session, nor an analysis of the results per trial produced evidence in favour of ACTH-analogue effects on extinction of this type of positively reinforced behavior.

It would be interesting to perform similar experiments with food as the reinforcing stimulus since the very effects of partial dehydration of rats, with a concomitant release of endogenous Anti-Diuretic Hormone (ADH), on extinction of conditioned behavior have not been thoroughly studied. This is not just an academic problem as administration of ADH or, more precisely, of a long-acting preparation of purified lysine vasopressin or of pitressin tannate in oil can markedly modify extinction of avoidance behavior in the shuttle-box situation (De Wied, 1965; De Wied and Bohus, 1966).

In interpreting results obtained in experiments on the effects of drugs and hormones on behavior, a possible interaction between the drug and the primary reinforcer should be taken in consideration. For example, a substance that reduces the water intake of animals might therefore reduce performance during water-reinforced behavior experiments, in training and in extinction sessions. In our avoidance behavior studies we escaped the problem of a possible interaction between the peptides and the US — foot-shock — by administering ACTH-analogues during extinction sessions only, foot-shock being not applied any more. With the study of extinction of water-reinforced behavior the situation is different. In these extinction studies the animal is still on a restricted water intake schedule.

The rather negative results of the described set of experiments made it preferable to further study the nature of the extinction modification of avoidance behavior itself, instead of investigating situations which are chosen to test various hypotheses. Shuttle-box experiments are quite complicated and time-consuming; the pole-jumping situation is not too attractive either as a research tool. Complications in this latter type of experiments arise from the fact that the experimenter has to intervene often, since rats do not always quit the pole spontaneously after an escape or avoidance reaction. Moreover it was thought necessary to create a situation that could easily be automated so that standard conditions are easily maintained and it is not left to the experimenter to decide in ambiguous cases whether the response of the animal is in time or not.

A box fitted with a retractable jump-on ledge was chosen as the instrument for further investigation (Fig. 10). The apparatus is a slightly modified version of the test situation described by Baum (1965), and is entirely automatically operated. Interrupting the light beam following jumping onto the ledge constitutes the response.

Four experiments will be described. The procedure in the first 3 experiments was as follows.

At the beginning of each daily session the rat is put on the ledge which is retracted after 10 sec. The animal drops on the grid floor $6\frac{1}{2}$ inch below. One minute later the ledge comes in and the CS is switched on. The CS consists of the noise of a running-time counter that is attached to the apparatus. Five seconds after CS onset scrambled foot-shock is applied via the grid floor (300 V a.c. with a 1-megohm series resistor). Both CS and US are response terminated, or ended 20 sec after CS onset in case the animal fails to escape. Ten seconds after the response the ledge is retracted again. A variable intertrial interval of 60 sec is used and there are 10 trials per session. During extinction sessions, no shock is applied and maximum CS duration is 5 sec.

This procedure was chosen in an attempt to mimic pole-jumping conditions. Training sessions were continued until a mean avoidance level of approx. 75 % was reached. Only animals with a markedly inferior performance level during training were

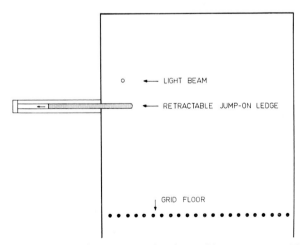

Fig. 10. Schematic representation of the automated active avoidance apparatus. The rat can escape or avoid foot-shock by jumping onto the ledge. Breaking the light beam constitutes the response.

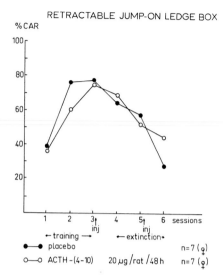

Fig. 11. Performance as a function of sessions during training and extinction of an active avoidance response (retractable jump-on ledge box). The peptide and the placebo were administered during the extinction period only.

discarded at the end of the training period (respectively 1, 0, 6, and 4 animals of the 4 reported experiments). A definite conditioning criterion has not yet been determined for this type of experiments. (A conditioning criterion is frequently used, but mostly arbitrarily set.)

At the end of the last training session rats were allocated to treatment groups, matched for performance during training sessions. The result of the first experiment can be seen in Fig. 11. No effect of 20 μg ACTH-(4-10)/rat/48 h was observed on the

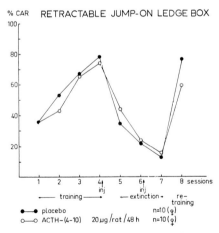

Fig. 12. Performance as a function of sessions during training, extinction and re-training of an active avoidance response (retractable jump-on ledge box). The peptide and the placebo were administered during the extinction and re-training period.

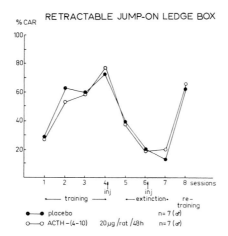

Fig. 13. Performance as a function of sessions during training, extinction and re-training of an active avoidance response (retractable jump-on ledge box). The peptide and the placebo were administered during the extinction and re-training period.

extinction of the conditioned avoidance response in the group of 7 female rats. The same holds for the next experiment with 10 female rats per treatment group (Fig. 12). Also re-training scores did not differ at a satisfactory level of statistical significance.

The third experiment (Fig. 13) was performed with groups of 7 male rats. Again no difference between the ACTH-(4-10) group and the placebo group could be detected on extinction and re-training scores. The procedure in the last experiment differed on some points. The first trial started at the moment the ledge was retracted. There was no other CS than the retracting of the ledge that was immediately returned into the box. Following the escape or avoidance response the rat could stay on the ledge until the next trial.

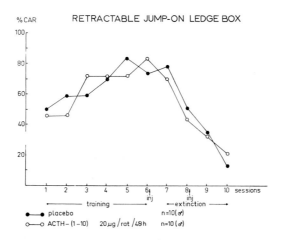

Fig. 14. Performance as a function of sessions during training and extinction of an active avoidance response (retractable jump-on ledge box). The peptide and the placebo were administered during the extinction period only.

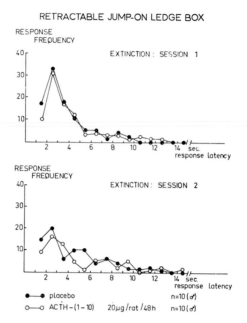

Fig. 15. Response–latency distributions obtained during the first two extinction sessions.

The experiment was performed with two groups of 10 male rats, and 20 μg ACTH-(1-10)/rat/48 h was administered, during extinction only as usual. Neither the difference between the number of avoidance responses (jump onto the ledge within 5 sec) nor the difference between the response–latency distributions did warrant a positive statement concerning the effects of ACTH-analogues on extinction of conditioned avoidance behavior in this situation (Figs. 14 and 15).

The absence of any modifying effect of ACTH-analogues on behavior in the reported experiments, particularly in the last 4, had not been expected. It was decided that it would now first of all be necessary to directly replicate the well demonstrated ACTH-analogue effects in the original pole-jumping or shuttle-box situations.

In conclusion: The results reported so far could not yet contribute to a further elucidation of the behavioral effects of ACTH-analogues.

ACKNOWLEDGMENTS

The ACTH-analogues were generously supplied by N.V. Organon, Oss, The Netherlands and the purified β-MSH by Dr. Roger Guillemin. We also acknowledge the assistance of Miss M. A. van Aardenne and of Messrs. P. Akkerboom, P. R. Beneder, J. van Ree and M. E. A. Reith with some of the experiments.

REFERENCES

BAUM, M. (1965) An automated apparatus for the avoidance training of rats. *Psychol. Rept.*, **16**, 1205–1211.

BOHUS, B. AND DE WIED, D. (1966) Inhibitory and facilitatory effect of two related peptides on extinction of avoidance behavior. *Science*, **153**, 318–320.

BROADHURST, P. L. (1960) Experiments in psychogenetics: Applications of biometrical genetics to the inheritance of behaviour. In: *Experiments in Personality*: Vol. 1, *Psychogenetics and Psychopharmacology*, H. J. EYSENCK (Ed.), Routledge & Kegan Paul, London, p. 30.

DE WIED, D. (1965) The influence of the posterior and intermediate lobe of the pituitary and pituitary peptides on the maintenance of a conditioned avoidance response in rats. *Intern. J. Neuropharmacol.*, **4**, 157–167.

DE WIED, D. (1966) Inhibitory effect of ACTH and related peptides on extinction of conditioned avoidance behavior in rats. *Proc. Soc. Exptl. Biol. Med.*, **122**, 28–32.

DE WIED, D. (1967) Opposite effects of ACTH and glucocorticosteroids on extinction of conditioned avoidance behavior. In: *Proc. Second Intern. Congr. on Hormonal Steroids*, Milan 1966, Excerpta Medica Intern. Congr. Ser., Vol. 132, pp. 945–951.

DE WIED, D. (1969) Effects of peptide hormones on behavior. In: *Frontiers in Neuroendocrinology*, W. F. GANONG AND L. MARTINI (Eds.), Oxford University Press, New York, pp. 97–140.

DE WIED, D. AND BOHUS, B. (1966) Long term and short term effects on retention of a conditioned avoidance response in rats by treatment with long acting Pitressin and α-MSH. *Nature*, **212**, 1484–1486.

DE WIED, D. AND PIRIE, G. (1968) The inhibitory effect of ACTH 1-10 on extinction of a conditioned avoidance response: its independence of thyroid function. *Physiol. Behav.*, **3**, 355–358.

GREVEN, H. M. AND DE WIED, D. (1967) The active sequence in the ACTH molecule responsible for inhibition of the extinction of conditioned avoidance behaviour in rats. *Europ. J. Pharmacol.*, **2**, 14–16.

MILLER, R. E. AND OGAWA, N. (1962) The effect of adrenocorticotrophic hormone (ACTH) on avoidance conditioning in the adrenalectomized rat. *J. Comp. Physiol. Psychol.*, **55**, 211–213.

STEINBERG, H., RUSHTON, R. AND TINSON, C. (1961) Modification of the effects of an amphetamine-barbiturate mixture by the past experience of rats. *Nature*, **192**, 533–535.

WEIJNEN, J. A. W. M. (1969) Effects of amphetamine–amylobarbitone mixtures on ambulation of rats in the Y-maze. *Europ. J. Pharmacol.*, **5**, 180–184.

WEISS, J. M., McEWEN, B. S., SILVA, M. T. A. AND KALKUT, M. F. (1969) Pituitary–adrenal influences on fear responding. *Science*, **163**, 197–199.

DISCUSSION

LEY: Have you checked the time course of open-field or *in-situ* activity during your daily observations of ambulation?

WEIJNEN: Ambulation was scored over successive 1-min periods during each session. No effect of the treatment could be observed.

LEY: Have you tested the daily open field activity of animals in active-avoidance training and extinction?

WEIJNEN: No, but I have been looking at the ambulation of animals during intertrial intervals. The rats were trained to make a light–dark discriminated avoidance response in a Y-maze. Neither treatment with α-MSH, nor with β-MSH resulted in data that warranted any conclusion about treatment effects during training.

LEY: As a comment on your H_2O-appetitive studies: In my research I have failed to replicate the effects of ACTH on active avoidance that you mention in your introduction, but I have recently generated a tentative suggestion of a strong effect of ACTH on H_2O-appetitive behavior.

McEWEN: I should like to make a brief comment, more or less as a representative for my colleague Jay Weiss, who has been responsible for most of our behavioral studies. There is an important factor which must be considered in looking for effects of ACTH and steroids on behavior. That is the question whether the behavioral response is clearly signalled, or weakly and ambiguously signalled. In the former situation hormonal factors are not seen, while in the latter strong hormonal effects on behavior are observed. (See McEwen and Weiss, this book.)

WEIJNEN: Your data have, of course, attracted my attention. However, I wonder whether these results can be easily generalized. You used the hypophysectomized and the adrenalectomized animal as a model to investigate effects of ACTH and steroids on behavior, and these animals were already subjected to surgery before training started. We only used intact animals, and peptides were only administered after training had been completed. Secondly, I wonder how your hypothesis could explain the reported effects of ACTH and steroids on extinction of conditioned behavior in the shuttle-box and pole-jumping situation. The signals used in these experiments are quite clear and unambiguous.

It is obvious that we should consider your data carefully in designing new experiments.

LEVINE: There are many discrepancies between laboratories, We have obtained positive results in many situations in which you obtain negative results. Some of these studies were performed with mice, and mice may react very different from rats.

WEIJNEN: The study of these discrepancies you refer to should not be neglected. Quite a few test situations and differences in procedure can be indicated. They make a direct comparison of your studies and our own experiments rather difficult.

DELACOUR: Your avoidance test, with the retractable ledge, seems to be less difficult for rats than the two-way shuttle-box situation. Your test seems more similar to the one-way shuttle box: the CS is, at least partly, the retractable ledge. This is a spatial and well located cue. In the two-way shuttle box the CS is sporadic and rather diffuse. Do you think that these differences could explain the lack of effect of ACTH analogues?

WEIJNEN: If I would not be aware of the effects shown in experiments with the pole-jumping test I might have answered your question with a speculative "could be".

HENKIN: It is very important and appropriate to restate in a slightly different form what Dr. McEwen has said previously about the nature of the sensory stimulus and the "learning experience" surrounding it. I think that this point has not been emphasized and I think the word learning as applied to the integration of sensory signals has been incorrectly applied. Thus, it might be well to recognize the limitations of the meaning of these words and concepts. Dr. Glassman also pointed out this difficulty when he tried to ascertain what it was in his experimental situation that was being "learned". What I mean is that there are classes of sensory signals, some of which are well controlled by hormones and others which are not. In general, those stimuli which are hormonally controlled appear to be what McEwen termed "weak" stimuli. I think that one can redefine this in different terms and call these stimuli "isolated" or relatively simple stimuli. In general, the sensory milieu to which we are exposed in our everyday life is complex and the sensory information content present in this normal environment is greatly overdetermined. When I speak, the meaning is not conveyed alone by the words which I am saying but also by the inflection in my voice, the emotion behind it, my facial expression and body movement and everything in my personality that strives to convey the meaning that I wish you to understand. This is an overdetermined set of sensory signals dependant upon visual, auditory and cognitive stimuli. In general, these complex stimuli are not hormonally controlled mainly because there are so many signals going into so many sensory systems that it is impossible to isolate the effect of one hormone on one sensory stimulus. However, if it were possible to isolate one aspect of these multiple stimuli, one taste quality, one olfactory signal, one sinusoidal frequency at one intensity, then the sensory signal could be evaluated and hormonal effects on this signal could be measured. This operational concept in which learning is in part made up of the integration of numerous sensory signals allows for an experimental approach to the concept of the effects of hormones on sensory signals which result in the acquiring of information.

VAN RIEZEN: Many experimenters have explored the effects of ACTH on behavior. The modification of avoidance behavior during extinction sessions seems to be well demonstrated. Effects on habituation to repeated stimuli have also been reported. The study of the behavior of hypophysectomized rats might suggest a function of ACTH in the acquisition of conditioned behavior, but not much experimental evidence obtained with intact animals has been published. A failure to demonstrate ACTH effects on acquisition might be due to the methods employed.

We decided to study the effects of the peptide consisting of the first 10 amino acids of ACTH, on the homing response of pigeons. This peptide has the behavioral effects of ACTH, but it lacks the corticotropic activity of this hormone (De Wied, 1966).

In the first experiment we trained unexperienced pigeons to home from 8 different directions. They were released individually from their home cage. We then measured their performance after treatment with 0.2 ml of 0.2 mg/ml of the peptide in a zinc phosphate suspension or with 0.2 ml of the placebo solution. The substances were administered every other day. The pigeons were individually released at twice the training distance, again from 8 different directions, at 5-minute intervals. Statistical evaluation of the results revealed no effect of the peptide on the homing response. The transport to the starting point might have stressed the animals and the subsequently released ACTH might have confounded the effect. The animals might also have been overtrained. So another experiment was designed.

Unexperienced pigeons were trained, once at 5, once at 15, and once at 30 km. They were divided in pairs of equal performance and one animal out of each pair was treated with the peptide the day before a 60-km flight. The pigeons were transported to the starting point one day before this flight in order to eliminate a behavioral effect of stress-induced ACTH release. Twenty-five pairs of animals were used and the results were analysed with the help of a sequential test. No peptide effect at all could be detected on the performance of the animals in two flights.

We were still not inclined to accept these results as sufficient evidence for our final conclusion. And we remembered that the same peptide with a D-form instead of an L-form amino acid at the 7th position of ACTH-(1-10) had a behavioral effect opposite to the effect of the all L-peptide (Bohus and De Wied, 1966). Therefore we repeated the second experiment with this 7-D-peptide. However, also this experiment did not show any effect of the treatment on the performance of the animals.

As we studied only one dose and the peptides were only injected once, these results are no absolute evidence to deny a role of ACTH on performance or aquisition in this type of experiment. Although it is hazardous to compare entirely different experimental situations it should be mentioned that the lack of success in finding effects on the homing performance of pigeons agrees with the absence of an effect of the same peptides on runway performance of rats which are motivated by unavoidable shock, as shown by Bohus and De Wied (1966). (For references see p. 233).

Effect of Hypophysectomy and Conditioned Avoidance Behavior on Macromolecule Metabolism in the Brain Stem of the Rat

W. H. GISPEN

Rudolf Magnus Institute for Pharmacology, Medical Faculty, University of Utrecht, Vondellaan 24a 6, Utrecht

AND

P. SCHOTMAN

Laboratory for Physiological Chemistry, Medical Faculty, University of Utrecht, Vondellaan, Utrecht (The Netherlands)

In recent years several studies have related biochemical processes in the brain to acquisition and extinction of learned behavior. A close association between RNA synthesis (Hydén, 1967; Shashoua, 1968; Gaito, 1966; Machlus *et al.*, 1968; Zemp *et al.*, 1966, 1967; Adair *et al.*, 1968a, b; Dellweg *et al.*, 1968; Bowman *et al.*, 1969) and/or protein synthesis (Flexner *et al.*, 1967; Hydén, 1968) in the brain and learning processes of animals has been demonstrated.

The pituitary–adrenal system also seems to play an essential part in conditioned avoidance behavior (see for review: De Wied, 1969). It has been shown that hypophysectomy impairs the acquisition of a shuttle-box conditioned avoidance response, while ACTH analogues can restore the response performance of the hypophysectomized rat without detectable endocrine, metabolic or systemic effects (De Wied, 1969).

Biochemically it has been demonstrated that the synthesis of macromolecules is decreased in peripheral organs, such as the liver, following hypophysectomy (Staehelin, 1965; Tata, 1967a; Korner, 1965). Although the effect of hypophysectomy on macromolecular metabolism in nervous tissue has not been intensively studied, some studies indicate an altered metabolism since amino acid incorporation is decreased in brain cell-free systems after hypophysectomy (Dunn *et al.*, 1966) and that the RNA/DNA ratio in the brain stem is reduced (De Vellis *et al.*, 1968).

In view of these findings it was deemed of interest to investigate the effect of hypophysectomy on macromolecule metabolism in the brain of rats. In addition, it was felt desirable to determine whether the defective learning behavior of the hypophysectomized rat would be reflected in macromolecule metabolism of the brain and finally, if this were the case, to study the influence of pituitary fractions known to stimulate avoidance learning in hypophysectomized rats.

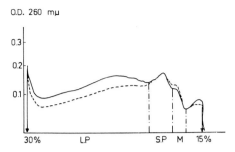

Fig. 1. Polysome pattern of three pooled brain stems. The polysomes are layered over a continuous sucrose gradient (15–30%) and centrifuged 2 h at 63000 g_{av} in Spinco Rotor S.W. 25. The UV extinction at $\lambda = 260$ mμ is measured in a Vanguard photospectrometer. ——— control, ---- hypophysectomized. M = monomers; S.P = small polysomes; L.P = large polysomes

I. THE EFFECT OF HYPOPHYSECTOMY ON BRAIN STEM POLYSOMES IN THE RAT

Male Wistar rats weighing approximately 110–120 g were used. Hypophysectomy was performed via the transauricular route under ether anesthesia. Operated rats were used three weeks after operation. Control rats were of the same weight. Loss of body weight and adrenal atrophy and macroscopic inspection of the sella turcica were indications that hypophysectomy had been correctly performed.

After decapitation of the rats, dissected brain stems of 3 animals similarly treated were pooled, immersed in the homogenization buffer and weighed. The polysome isolation procedure was performed at 0–4° C. The procedure was a slightly modified technique as described by Adair *et al.* (1968a). The isolated polysomes were suspended and layered over a 25-ml linear (15–30%) sucrose gradient (Sucrose: Merck P. A.). They were then centrifuged for 2 h in a Spinco L2 Rotor SW-25.1 at 63000 g_{av}. After centrifugation the gradients were extracted using a density displacement method with a 50% sucrose solution and measured continuously in a Vanguard spectrophotometer at 260 mμ against water and fractions of 0.5 ml were collected (Fig. 1).

The material was further identified as polysomal aggregates by electron microscopy

TABLE 1

EXTINCTION RATIOS AND TOTAL RNA CONTENT OF THE CENTRIFUGED POLYSOME FRACTION

	SP/M	*LP/M*	*mg RNA/100 g fresh tissue*
Controls	1.55 ± 0.05**	1.25 ± 0.06	10.1 ± 0.3 (9)
Hypox	1.58 ± 0.04	1.02 ± 0.05*	8.2 ± 0.6* (9)

( ) Number of groups of 3 rats.
* $P \leqslant 0.05$ (U-test).
** Mean ± Standard Error of the Mean.
M = monomers. SP = small polysomes. LP = large polysomes. Extinction ratios are calculated from the polysome pattern. Total RNA content was determined by pooling the fractions of the gradient and by measuring the E_{260} in a Zeiss spectrophotometer. $E_{260} = 20\,000$ in 0.1% RNA solution.

and by its sensitivity to ribonuclease digestion. These procedures are criteria used by several other workers (Appel *et al.*, 1967; Adair *et al.*, 1968a; Campagnoni and Mahler 1967).

After hypophysectomy a decrease in the content of large polysomes in the brain stem (Fig. 1, Table 1) and also a decrease in total RNA content of the gradient (Table 1) was found.

It has been shown that hypophysectomy reduces the content of polysomes in the rat liver (Korner, 1965; Staehelin, 1965). The isolated polysomes are also less active in amino acid incorporation systems *in vitro* (Korner, 1965; Staehelin, 1965; Tata *et al.*, 1967b).

Anterior pituitary growth hormone (STH) restores the reduced incorporation activity of the isolated polysomes (Korner, 1965; Tata *et al.*, 1967b). STH also raises the total RNA synthesis *in vivo* in the liver of hypophysectomized rats (Korner, 1965; Gupta *et al.*, 1968).

The reduced amount of large polysomes (Table 1), the less active amino acid incorporation *in vitro* (Dunn *et al.*, 1966) and the lower RNA/DNA ratio (De Vellis, 1968) all are evidence for a lower rate of macromolecular metabolism in the brain after hypophysectomy. The effect of hypophysectomy on the metabolism in the brain stem is therefore comparable to that found in the liver.

II. THE EFFECT OF HYPOPHYSECTOMY ON INCORPORATION OF RADIO-URIDINE INTO RAPIDLY LABELED RNA

A double labeling method as described by Zemp *et al.* (1966) was used to eliminate differences introduced by the isolation procedure. Hypophysectomized and control rats received alternatively [5-^{3}H] or the [2-^{14}C]uridine, as a specific precursor of RNA-synthesis. After 70 min in one experiment and 3 h in the others, rats were decapitated. RNA was subsequently isolated in various cell fractions of the brain stem and the radioactivity, incorporated into rapidly labeled RNA, was measured. The proportional change in the isotope ratio of various RNA-containing cell fractions, in comparison to the isotope ratio of the precursor nucleotides, was calculated, to determine the effect of hypophysectomy. To relate the effect of hypophysectomy on conditioned avoidance acquisition to molecular events in the brain, the effect of hypophysectomy on the synthesis of messenger-RNA was studied first. For this purpose, polysomes which contain *m*-RNA involved in protein synthesis were isolated from the cytoplasmic fraction, and the isotope ratio in the incorporated uridine was determined after sucrose gradient sedimentation analysis.

Rats were used as described in part I. Injections were carried out intradiencephally by the method of Valzelli (1964). Cell fractionation was performed slightly modified according to Zemp *et al.* (1966). The incorporation of labeled uridine into three RNA fractions is shown in Table 2. A negative proportional change reflects a lower incorporation of uridine by the ^{3}H-injected animal; a positive proportional change reflects a lower incorporation of uridine by the ^{14}C-injected animal. A significant

TABLE 2

PROPORTIONAL CHANGES IN THE ISOTOPE RATIO OF THE RNA FRACTIONS COMPARED TO
THAT OF THE PRECURSOR POOL AFTER 70 AND 180 min OF URIDINE INCORPORATION

No. of group	A	B	C	D	E	F	G
Time (min)	70	70	70	180	180	180	180
[³H]uridine	control	hypox	hypox	control	control	hypox	control
[¹⁴C]uridine	control	control	control	control	hypox	control	hypox
Total RNA	−5%	−35%	−31%	−5%	+61%	−18%	+40%
Nuclear RNA	−7	−37	−43	−6	+76	−24	+48
Cytoplasmic RNA	−2	−36	−29	−6	+56	−17	+39

Hypox = hypophysectomized. Hypophysectomized and control rats were injected intradiencephally with [5-³H] or [2-¹⁴C]uridine and sacrificed after 70 or 180 min. Brainstems of a hypophysectomized and a control rat, or those of two control rats, were pooled and total, nuclear and cytoplasmic RNA were isolated. The isotope ratios of the RNA fractions were compared to the ratio in the precursor pool, purified by charcoal treatment.

decrease in incorporation of radioactive uridine into rapidly labeled RNA in the rat brain stem was found after hypophysectomy (Table 2).

Table 3 shows the incorporation of labeled uridine into RNA of the polysomes. As a result of hypophysectomy there is a decreased incorporation of uridine into RNA after both periods of incorporation.

The optical density pattern at 260 mμ shows some slowly sedimenting material in the first 10 fractions (Fig. 2A and B), followed by the 80 S monomers, localized around fraction 12. The labeling pattern of the polyribosomes is different after 70 and 180 min of incorporation. After 70 min of labeling, the radioactivity is wholly concentrated in the first 16 fractions with the fraction of maximum radioactivity sedimenting more slowly than 80 S (Fig. 2A). As seen from Fig. 2B, radioactivity is spread out over

TABLE 3

PROPORTIONAL CHANGES IN THE ISOTOPE RATIO OF THE POLYSOMAL RNA COMPARED TO
THAT OF THE PRECURSOR POOL AFTER 70 AND 180 min OF URIDINE INCORPORATION

No. of group	A	B	C	D	E
Time (min)	70	70	70	180	180
[³H]uridine	control	hypox	control	control	control
[¹⁴C]uridine	control	control	hypox	hypox	hypox
Polysomes	+12%	−66%	+61%	+69%	+93%

* Hypox = hypophysectomized.
Hypophysectomized and control rats were injected intradiencephally with [5-³H]- or [2-¹⁴C]uridine and sacrificed after 70 and 180 min. Brainstems of a hypophysectomized and a control rat, or those of two control rats, were pooled and polysomes were isolated. The mean isotope ratio of the gradient fractions was compared to the ratio in the precursor pool, purified by thin-layer chromatography.

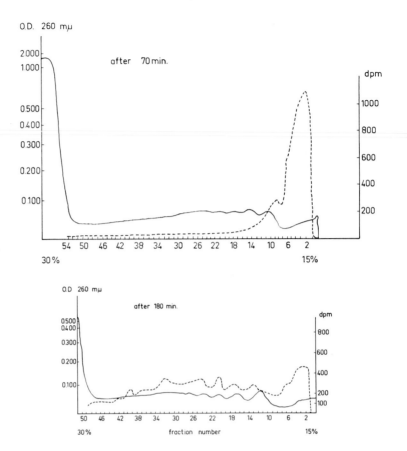

Fig. 2A, 2B. Labeling pattern of the polysome fractions after two periods of uridine incorporation. Polyribosomes were suspended and layered over a 25-ml linear (15–30%) sucrose. Centrifugation was performed for 2 h in a Spinco L2 Rotor SW-25 at 63000 g_{av}. Gradients were measured continuously in a Vanguard spectrophotometer at 260 mμ against water. Fractions of 0.5 ml were collected and assayed for radioactivity via a Mark I Nuclear Chicago scintillation spectrometer. ——— = O.D. 260 mμ. ----- = radioactivity in dpm.

the total gradient with two broad peaks, one in the same region as shown in Fig. 2A, another corresponding with the large polysomes. The slowly sedimenting fractions 1–16 (exclusively labeled after 70 min) resemble nucleoprotein particles, as is suggested from preliminary experiments. This fraction is first labeled in the cytoplasm. It is partly washed out by a purification step with 2 M sucrose, and also by treatment with 1% sodium deoxycholate.

From the total ribosome fraction and from the labeled fractions after centrifugation RNA was isolated and identified as heterogenous RNA which sediments between 5 and 20 S with a maximum near 12 S. This indicates that these are ribonucleoprotein particles (Samec *et al.*, 1967, 1968).

III. RELATION OF CONDITIONED AVOIDANCE ACQUISITION TRAINING OF HYPOPHYSECTOMIZED RATS TO POLYSOME CONTENT IN THE BRAIN STEM

Recently, evidence has been presented which suggests an increase in the number of large polysomes in the rat brain as a result of animal training (Dellweg et al., 1968). It was deemed of interest to investigate if conditioned avoidance acquisition training might have an effect on the fraction of large polysomes in the brain stem.

As mentioned above, hypophysectomy impairs the response performance of the rat in the acquisition training in the shuttle-box. ACTH analogues can restore the response performance to almost normal levels. It was therefore of interest to study the behavior of the fraction of large polysomes in the brain stem during conditioned avoidance learning of hypophysectomized rats. In addition, the effect of peptides known to restore the response performance of the hypophysectomized animal was investigated. The peptide used in the present experiments was the one isolated from a peptide fraction (BC-15) obtained from hog anterior pituitaries by Lande et al. (1965) (De Wied et al., p. 213). The peptide had the same behavioral activity as ACTH or its analogues. Like the ACTH-analogues, this peptide had no detectable corticotrophic activities. Avoidance training was begun one week after operation and treatment was started one day before the first session (see, for details, De Wied et al., p. 213).

The active peptide or placebo was injected subcutaneously as a long-acting Zn phosphate preparation, every other day for 10 days during the acquisition period. On the 11th day the brain stems of 3 rats, which had been subjected to the same treatment were pooled and the polysome fractions were isolated as described above. The density gradient centrifugation was carried out in a I.E.C. ultracentrifuge Rotor SB 110 2.5 h 63000 g_{av}.

The results demonstrate an increase in the fraction of large polysomes in those rats, who showed the restored acquisition rate as a result of the treatment with the active

TABLE 4

RELATION BETWEEN POLYSOME PATTERN, ISOLATED FROM THE BRAIN STEM, AND THE RATE OF ACQUISITION OF A SHUTTLE-BOX AVOIDANCE RESPONSE IN HYPOPHYSECTOMIZED RATS

	SP/M	LP/M	Total number of conditioned avoidance responses (100 trials)
Placebo	1.34 ± 0.07*	1.18 ± 0.08	21 ± 2 (4)
Active fraction from anterior pituitary	1.41 ± 0.04	1.55 ± 0.08**	64 ± 2** (4)

* Mean ± Standard Error of the Mean.
** $P \leqslant 0.05$ (U-test).
( ) Number of groups of 3 rats.
M = monomers; SP = small polysomes; LP = large polysomes. Extinction ratios are calculated from the polysome pattern.

References pp. 242–243

peptide (Table 4). RNA content of the gradient of the homogenate was not significantly changed. Because of lack of enough purified material a control experiment was carried out with ACTH 1–10.

This experiment was performed with ACTH 1–10 zinc phosphate (20 μg/0.5 ml s.c. every 2 days for 10 days) and placebo treatment in hypophysectomized rats without the training procedure, to investigate if peptide treatment had any effect by itself. The ACTH 1-10 treatment had no detectable influence on the biochemical parameters (Table 5).

TABLE 5

EFFECT OF ACTH 1-10 TREATMENT ON THE POLYSOME PATTERN IN THE BRAIN STEM

	SP/M	LP/M
Placebo	1.32 ± 0.07*	1.65 ± 0.11 (5)
ACTH 1–10	1.32 ± 0.05	1.60 ± 0.11 (5)

* Mean ± Standard Error of the Mean.
( ) Number of groups of 3 rats.
M = monomers; SP = small polysomes; LP = large polysomes. Extinction ratios are calculated from the polysome pattern.

One might conclude, therefore, that the peptide treatment itself has no influence on the metabolism of large polysomes. The effect on the large polysomes, as found in the present experiments, might therefore be a result of the combination of peptide treatment and shuttle-box training, or a result of the shuttle-box training by itself.

Pilot experiments were done to determine whether the effect of training is specific for the brain or not, whereby liver was used as a control tissue.

Both after treatment with the active peptide in combination with training in the shuttle-box, and after treatment with ACTH 1-10 alone, no differences were found in the fraction of large polysomes of the liver as compared to that of the placebo group. Accordingly, the increase in the fraction of large polysomes in the brain stem of rats as a result of conditioned avoidance training provoked by peptide treatment seems to be specific for the brain. Further work is in progress to corroborate this observation.

REFERENCES

ADAIR, L. B., WILSON, J. E. AND GLASSMAN, E. (1968a) Brain function and macromolecules. III. Uridine incorporation into polysomes of mouse brain during short-term avoidance conditioning. *Proc. Natl. Acad. Sci. U.S.*, **60**, 606–613.
ADAIR, L. B., WILSON, J. E. AND GLASSMAN, E. (1968b) Brain function and macromolecules. IV. Uridine incorporation into polysomes of mouse brain during different behavioral experiences. *Proc. Natl. Acad. Sci. U.S.*, **60**, 917–922.
APPEL, S. H., DAVIS, W. AND SCOTT, S. (1967) Brain polysomes: Response to environmental stimulation. *Science*, **157**, 836–838.
BOWMAN, R. E., AND STROBEL, D. A. (1969) Brain RNA metabolism in the rat during learning. *J. Comp. Physiol. Psychol.*, **67**, 448–456.

CAMPAGNONI, A. T. AND MAHLER, H. R. (1967) Isolation and properties of polyribosomes from cerebral cortex. *Biochemistry*, **6**, 956–967.

DELLWEG, H., GERNER, R. AND WACKER, A. (1968) Quantitative and qualitative changes in ribonucleic acids of rat brain dependent on age and training experiments. *J. Neurochem.*, **15**, 1109–1119.

DE VELLIS, J. AND INGLISH, D. (1968) Hormonal control of glycerol phosphate dehydrogenase in the rat brain. *J. Neurochem.*, **15**, 1061–1071.

DE WIED, D. (1969) Effects of peptide hormones on behavior. In: *Frontiers in Neuroendocrinology*, W. F. GANONG AND L. MARTINI, (Eds.), Oxford University Press, New York, pp. 97–140.

DUNN, A. J. AND KORNER, A. (1966) Hypophysectomy and amino acid incorporation in a rat brain cell free system. *Biochem. J.*, **100**, 76 P.

FLEXNER, L. B., FLEXNER, J. B. AND ROBERTS, R. B. (1967) Memory in mice analyzed with antibiotics. *Science*, **155**, 1377–1383.

GAITO, J. (1966) *Macromolecules and Behavior*, Meredith Publ. Co., New York.

GUPTA, S. L. AND TALWAR, G. P. (1968) Effect of growth hormone on RNA metabolism. *Biochem. J.*, **110**, 401–406.

HYDÉN, H. (1967) Behavior, neural functions and RNA. *Progr. Nucleic Acid Res. Mol. Biol.*, **6**, 187–217.

HYDÉN, H. AND LANGE, P. W. (1968) Protein synthesis in the hippocampal pyramidal cells of rats during a behavioral test. *Science*, **159**, 1370–1373.

KORNER, A. (1965) Growth hormone control of biosynthesis of protein and ribonucleic acid. In: *Recent Progress in Hormone Research*, Vol. XXI, G. PINCUS (Ed.), Academic Press, New York and London, pp. 205–240.

LANDE, S., LERNER, A. B. AND UPTON, G. V. (1965) Isolation of new peptides related to β-melanocyte-stimulating hormone. *J. Biol. Chem.*, **240**, 4259–4263.

MACHLUS, B. AND GAITO, J. (1968) Unique RNA species developed during a shock avoidance task. *Psychon. Sci.*, **12**, 111–112.

SAMEC, J., MANDEL, P. AND JACOB, M. (1967) Occurrence of light ribonucleoprotein (RNP) particles in the microsomal fraction of adult rat brain. *J. Neurochem.*, **14**, 887–892.

SAMEC, J., JACOB, M. AND MANDEL, P. (1968) Occurrence of light particles carrying DNA-like RNA in the microsomal fraction of adult rat brain. *Biochim. Biophys. Acta*, **161**, 377–385.

SHASHOUA, V. E. (1968) RNA changes in goldfish brain during learning. *Nature*, **217**, 238–240.

STAEHELIN, M. (1965) Effect of hypophysectomy on rat liver polyribosomes. *Biochem. Z.*, **342**, 459–468.

TATA, J. R. (1967a) The formation and distribution of ribosomes during hormone-induced growth and development. *Biochem. J.*, **104**, 1–15.

TATA, J. R. AND WILLIAMS-ASHMAN, H. G. (1967b) Effects of growth hormone and tri-iodothyronine on amino acid incorporation by microsomal subfractions from rat liver. *Europ. J. Biochem.*, **2**, 366–374.

TATA, J. R. (1968) Hormonal regulation of growth and protein synthesis. *Nature*, **219**, 331–337.

VALZELLI, L. (1964) A simple method to inject drugs intracerebrally. *Med. Exptl.*, **11**, 23–26.

ZEMP, J. W., WILSON, J. E., SCHLESINGER, K., BOGGAN, W. O. AND GLASSMAN, E. (1966) Brain function and macromolecules. I. Incorporation of uridine into RNA of mouse brain during short-term training experience. *Proc. Natl. Acad. Sci. U.S.*, **55**, 1423–1431.

ZEMP, J. W., WILSON, J. E. AND GLASSMAN, E. (1967) Brain function and macromolecules. II. Site of increased labeling of RNA in brains of mice during a short-term training. experience. *Proc. Natl. Acad. Sci. U.S.*, **58**, 1120–1125.

DISCUSSION

GLASSMAN: Could I just ask you, did you train any hypophysectomized rats without peptide administration?

GISPEN: Yes, but these rats did not acquire the shuttle-box response well enough and no increase in the fraction of large polysomes was found.

LEVINE: Hypophysectomized rats will not learn a conditioned avoidance response. This does not mean, of course, that the animal is not learning something.

GLASSMAN: I have raised this point because in my paper I am going to present data obtained with hypophysectomized rats that did learn the task. These rats showed an increase in the labelling of the polysomes.

GISPEN: Indeed, the one does not exclude the other; in your experiment hypophysectomy did not interfere with learning as it did in our experiments.

VAN RIEZEN: I would like to know if you had any special reason for analysing brain stems instead of taking the whole brain.

GISPEN: Yes, there is some evidence that, following injection of uridine into the brain, most of the label is found in the diencephalic area after a short incorporation time (Zemp *et al.*, 1967). This is one of the reasons for concentrating our efforts on the brain stem. I would also like to mention that De Vellis (1968) showed in hypophysectomized rats that, whereas the RNA/DNA ratio did not change in the cerebrum, it was altered in the brain stem.

LEY: Did you control the effect of a possible interaction of foot-shock *per se* with the peptide treatment, by shocking some subjects in the absence of a learning opportunity?

GISPEN: In this experiment we did not control this possibility.

The Effect of Short Term Experiences on the Incorporation of Uridine into RNA and Polysomes of Mouse Brain

EDWARD GLASSMAN AND JOHN E. WILSON

Department of Biochemistry and the Neurobiology Curriculum, University of North Carolina, Chapel Hill, North Carolina (U.S.A.)

There is a considerable amount of literature indicating that training experiences can have marked effects on the macromolecules of the nervous system. Unfortunately, a number of difficulties mar unequivocal interpretation of these studies. First, the behavioral task is often too long or is too complicated to allow clear-cut conclusions concerning the critical behavioral components responsible for the chemical response. Second, there is often no comparable examination of chemical changes in tissues other than the nervous system to be sure the response is specific to it. Third, often either the entire brain is homogenized or only a very small part is examined, and an extensive inventory of all the major portions of the brain and even of the cells involved in the response is not available. A lack of consideration of these problems has led many investigators to conclude that their findings are relevant to memory research when, in fact, there is often a lack of critical data to establish such relevance. These considerations have made it difficult, if not impossible, to draw any conclusions concerning the possible cause-and-effect relationships between the experience or the behavior and the chemical change. Nor are there any data to indicate the role that the chemicals are playing in the responding cells.

This work is an attempt to approach this problem. The mouse was chosen because it has been used extensively in behavioral, biochemical, and genetical studies. To minimize genetic variation, only 6 to 8 week old males of strain C57B1/6J, supplied by the Jackson Laboratories, were used.

Conditioned avoidance training was carried out in the jump box described previously (Zemp *et al.*, 1966; Schlesinger and Wimer, 1967). It consists of a box divided into two sections with a common electric grid floor. One mouse is placed in each section. A light and a buzzer are attached to the outside of the box so that each mouse receives equal stimulation. The sections are identical except that one side has a shelf onto which the mouse in that section can jump. The light and buzzer are presented for 3 sec before the electric shock is applied. Initially, both mice jump in response to the shock and the animal that has the shelf uses it as a haven. The shock is terminated as soon as it does so. The mouse is then removed from the shelf and placed on the grid floor, and another trial then commences. The training lasts for 15 min, and between 30 and 35 trials are carried out during this period. The mouse that has the shelf will usually start to avoid the shock in response to light and buzzer by the fifth trial

References p. 249

and is performing to a criterion of 9 out of 10 by 5 min. It should be noted that when the trained mouse avoids the shock, the animal on the other side also does not receive one. The untrained mouse also receives equivalent handling at random during the training. Thus with respect to lights, buzzers, shocks, handling, and injections, the untrained mouse is *yoked* to the *trained* mouse.

The biochemical analysis utilizes a double isotope-labeling method. One mouse of a pair was injected intracranially with [^{14}C]uridine, the other with [^{3}H]uridine. Thirty minutes later, one of the mice was trained for 15 min in the jump box while the other served as the yoke animal. After the training period, the brains of both mice were homogenized simultaneously in the same homogenizer, after which the homogenate was fractionated into nuclei, ribosomes, and a supernatant fraction (Zemp *et al.*, 1966). UMP was isolated from the supernatant fraction and RNA was extracted from each of the subcellular components: the amount of ^{14}C and ^{3}H in each was determined (Zemp *et al.*, 1966). The purpose of using two labels in this way is to avoid the problem of differential losses of RNA that occur during the complicated manipulations we had to employ to isolate the RNA. The ratio of ^{3}H to ^{14}C in the UMP is a useful indication of the relative efficiency of the injection and of the relative amount of uridine that entered brain cells, and is used to correct the observed ratio of ^{3}H to ^{14}C in the RNA.

In 25 of such blind double-labeling experiments, all trained mice incorporated more radioactivity into RNA than did the untrained mice (Zemp *et al.*, 1966). The average increase in RNA isolated from nuclei was 38% and the range was 6.5 to 119%. The average increase in RNA isolated from the ribosomal pellet was 64% and the range was 7 to 180%. This difference between the incorporation into brain RNA of the trained and untrained mice cannot be unequivocally ascribed to *increased synthesis* of RNA in the trained animal. It could, for example, be due to *decreased destruction* of RNA, to *increases in permeability* of the cells or their nuclei to uridine, to a decrease in the synthesis of endogenous uridine, or to any one of a number of other alternatives. Thus we refer only to the *change in incorporation* and do not specify a mechanism.

By injecting radioactive uridine intraperitoneally as well as intracranially, it was possible to show that there were no differences between trained and untrained animals in the incorporation of radioactive uridine into liver and kidney RNA or polysomes, even though these same animals showed pronounced differences in the brain (Zemp *et al.*, 1966; Adair *et al.*, 1968a). It was concluded, therefore, that although tissues other than the liver and kidney might be responding, the effect may be specific to brain.

The effect also seems to be limited to specific areas in the brain. Gross dissection revealed that the increased incorporation of uridine into RNA took place entirely in the diencephalon and associated structures (Zemp *et al.*, 1967); there was a small but significant decrease in the cortex. Autoradiography confirmed this (Kahan *et al.*, 1970). Although there was similar labeling in comparable neurons in all mice, the trained mouse showed more incorporation into many neurons in the limbic system, whereas the untrained yoke mouse incorporated more [^{3}H]uridine into some neurons in the neocortex. These results indicate how important it is to know the full extent of the involvement of the brain in chemical responses to behavioral stimuli in order to gain proper perspective on the phenomenon being observed.

Yoked and quiet mice had similar amounts of incorporation of radioactive uridine into brain RNA and polysomes (Zemp *et al.*, 1966; Adair *et al.*, 1968b). It was concluded that non-specific stimuli, such as the lights, buzzers, shocks, and handling that the yoke mouse received are not sufficient to have any effect by themselves. To test this idea further, the incorporation of radioactive uridine into RNA taken from the brains of *quiet* mice was compared with that in mice subjected to 30 electric shocks given at random over the 15-min period. The data clearly show that the radioactivity in the RNA and polysomes was similar in both mice, thus giving further credence to the idea that mere stimuli and activity were not responsible for the effect we observed (Zemp *et al.*, 1966; Adair *et al.*, 1968b).

There are, however, many differences between the trained mouse and the yoke mouse in addition to learning. For example, the trained mouse has a change in cue and his attention is now directed at a stimulus that the untrained mouse probably views as benign. Also, the stresses on the trained mouse are different, as are his responses to them. Finally, the trained mouse jumps more often than the yoke mouse and there is a difference in the quality of the jump, in that the trained mouse quickly learns to organize his locomotion to reach the shelf, while the untrained mouse jumps with random purpose.

To examine some of these alternatives, a mouse was trained for two successive days with 15-min sessions in the jump box. On the third day, this mouse was injected with radioactive uridine, using the double-labeling method for polysomes, and was then required to *perform* the jump box task. The incorporation of radioactive uridine into brain polysomes was similar to that of a yoked mouse (Adair *et al.*, 1968). It was therefore concluded that the organized locomotion, the changed cue and attention, and those stress factors that operate *after* the animal has learned and is *performing* the task are not responsible for the chemical changes we observed. It is, of course, possible that the prior trained mouse had habituated to the training apparatus and the handling, and thus experienced reduced stress. This cannot be ruled out, but the animals do show fear reactions when placed into the training apparatus. Furthermore, mice previously exposed to the training situation as yoke mice (15-min sessions on two successive days) learned the task perfectly well on the third day and showed the increased incorporation into brain polysomes. Other behaviors related to the jump box were also tested and the results are clear. When the animal learned to jump to the shelf in response to a conditioned stimulus, the increased incorporation of radioactive uridine into brain polysomes was observed (Adair *et al.*, 1968b). Thus, the process of changing cue (*i.e.*, learning) seems to be relevant to the chemical change we observed (Adair *et al.*, 1968b).

Enough information is still not available to reach an unequivocal conclusion concerning cause-and-effect relationships or the biological significance of these results. Although the training experience causes both a change in behavior (learning) and in chemicals in the brain, there are no data that indicate whether either of these changes is the cause of the other, whether they might even be completely unrelated responses to two different input stimuli. This problem is common to all research on the nervous system where an experience has more than one behavioral, biological, and chemical response. Whether this chemical response has anything to do with the learning process *per se* or with a response incidental to this process, such as emotional responses, cannot be answered at this time.

Many of the ^{14}C and ^{3}H-labeled RNA mixtures from yoke and trained animals were sedimented in sucrose gradients to see if the increased radioactivity was located in a single species of RNA that might have a unique function (Zemp *et al.*, 1966). In all cases, the increased radioactivity associated with the RNA of the trained mouse was located throughout the gradient and was quite heterogenous with respect to sedimentation rate. The patterns of radioactivity were of the same general shape for RNA from brain, liver, and kidney from trained mice and untrained mice. Thus the increased incorporation in brain RNA resembled that found when RNA synthesis is stimulated in liver by hydrocortisone or in uterus by estrogen.

It was concluded that the increased radioactivity was not confined to a single species of RNA, but was distributed among many species, and that a general increase was observed in the synthesis of rapidly labeled RNA due to a metabolic stimulation of the cells involved. That there is also increased incorporation into polysomes of the brain during the training experience (Adair *et al.*, 1968 a and b) further substantiates this idea. Thus no evidence was found for an RNA with a function that does not involve protein synthesis; indeed, the RNA found was similar to RNA extracted from other tissues. Further work is needed to establish whether this RNA is involved in the amount of proteins already present.

Because hormones are among the few substances in the body that have been shown to affect RNA synthesis, it was of interest to ascertain the effect of various hormonal influences on this chemical response to experiential stimulation. In these experiments we were concerned mainly with whether the experience stimulated a chain of events which involved secretion of hormones from the adrenals or the pituitary which then led to the increased incorporation into RNA or polysomes in the brain. We have been able to show that mice adrenalectomized seven days prior to the training were able to learn the jump-box task and did show the increased incorporation into polysomes (Adair *et al.*, 1968b). Unfortunately, technical reasons prevented us from testing hypophysectomized mice in the same way. However, we have been carrying out studies on the effects of short term avoidance conditioning in the rat (Coleman, 1969). The training is similar to that used in the mice and the apparatus consisted of a runway with an escape platform at one end. The rats were hypophysectomized 7 days prior to use and were in fairly good health at the time of training. The double labeling method using [^{14}C]- and [^{3}H] uridine was used. Hypophysectomized rats resembled normal rats in that both groups showed increased incorporation of radioactive uridine into brain RNA as compared to quiet or yoked rats. We conclude that the pituitary gland and the adrenal gland play no acute role in the increased incorporation into RNA and polysomes during the 15-min experience. That is, the activity of these glands is not a necessary step prior to the change in RNA during the time of training. We have yet to explore whether secretions from these glands that are not used up in the seven days after the gland was removed might be necessary for the maintenance of proper brain function in relation to this chemical response.

REFERENCES

ADAIR, LINDA B., WILSON, J. E. AND GLASSMAN, E. (1968a) *Proc. Natl. Acad. Sci. U.S.*, **61**, 917–922

ADAIR, LINDA B., WILSON, J. E., ZEMP, J. W. AND GLASSMAN, E. (1968b) *Proc. Natl. Acad. Sci. U.S.*, 606–613.

COLEMAN, M. S., *Ph. D. Thesis, The Department of Biochemistry, University of North Carolina*, Chapel Hill, North Carolina, U.S.A., 1969

KAHAN, B., KRIGMAN, M. R., WILSON, J. E. AND GLASSMAN, E., (1970) *Proc. Natl. Acad. Sci. U.S.*, in press.

SCHLESINGER, K. AND WIMER, R. (1967) *J. Comp. Physiol. Psychol.*, **63**, 139–141.

ZEMP, J. W., WILSON, J. E., SCHLESINGER, K., BOGGAN, W. O. AND GLASSMAN, E. (1966) *Proc. Natl. Acad. Sci. U.S.*, **55**, 1423–1431.

ZEMP, J. W., WILSON, J. E. AND GLASSMAN, E. (1967) *Proc. Natl. Acad. Sci. U.S.*, **58**, 1120–1125.

DISCUSSION

SACHAR: Since there are differences between trained and yoked animals in adrenal response, have you treated animals with ACTH or corticosteroids to see if this provokes changes in uptake of radioactive uridine?

GLASSMAN: Adrenalectomy, in a large series of animals, had no effect on the ability of these animals to learn the task or on the ability to show the RNA effect. Hypophysectomy in about 6–8 pairs of rats in a related paradigm, also failed to affect learning and uridine incorporation, that is: if the animals learn, they show the RNA effect. I don't know how to reconcile this with Gispen's results, but as I was pointing out in the discussion of his paper, the peptide may be restoring the ability of the animal to learn and this in turn may affect the RNA effect. The peptide might affect the polysomes indirectly, in that the chemical response only occurs in animals that learn. I do not think there is any basic disagreement between Gispen's and my results.

Effects of ACTH and corticosteroids on animal behavior

I. A. MIRSKY

Laboratory of Clinical Sciences, University of Pittsburgh, School of Medicine, 3811 O'Hara Street, Pittsburgh, Penna. 15213 (U.S.A.)

The evaluation of the influence of any endogenous agent on the behavior of animal or man is obfuscated by our ignorance of the nature and processes involved in "behavior". The procedures employed to investigate active or passive avoidance behavior, for example, can be specified in detail and thereby defined operationally. The interrelated processes, however, that define "learning", such as changes in response effectiveness, in motivational state, in the accruing of repetitive experiences with the conditional stimuli, etc., are only indirectly measurable as the behavior of the animal during a conditioning trial. Accordingly, confusion and controversy is inevitable if different experimental models of "learning" and different "behaviors", are equated in studies on the influence of any agent. This became evident during the course of the symposium on the "Effects of ACTH and corticosteroids on animal behavior".

It would be quite redundant to review the abundant evidence that endogenous and exogenous adrenocorticotropin (ACTH) and adrenal corticosteroids can influence both the acquisition and retention of an active or psasive avoidance response; ACTH enhances the acquisition and inhibits the extinction of the response while the corticosteroids induce the reverse. These conclusions are supported rather than contradicted by the observations of McEwen and Weiss which suggest that "ACTH and corticosterone have their principle influence under conditions of mild generalized fear". As Levine, Glassman, McEwen, van Delft, Weijnen and other participants in the symposium emphasized, the effects of these hormones on the conditioned avoidance response need not apply to other types of behavior. Thus, while McEwen reported that high levels of ACTH produced accelerated rates of responding in a discrimination task with food reinforcement while corticosterone reduced this effect, published studies by Levine and Jones, and unpublished studies by Miller and Caul in my laboratory have demonstrated that in contrast to its effect on aversive conditioning, ACTH does not influence other types of appetitive learning in the rat. The contradictions which have arisen occasionally regarding specific experimental results simply emphasize the sensitivity of the experimental subjects to various situational variables which differ from one experiment to another.

In accord with the aforementioned are Delacour's observations that lesions in the centrum medianum parafascicularis complex of the thalamus impair the acquisition of some types of behavior and not of others. Thus, he found that the acquisition of two operationally different avoidance behaviors were impaired by the thalamic lesion while the acquisition of two appetitive responses were not affected.

In considering that action of any agent, it becomes pertinent to establish the molecular configuration essential to the action. Thus, the extensive studies by De Wied and his colleagues established that a fragment of the molecule of ACTH, *viz.*, the heptapeptide 4–10, is as effective as the intact ACTH molecule in normalizing the impaired acquisition of a shuttle-box avoidance response in hypophysectomized rats and in inhibiting the extinction of avoidance behavior in several active avoidance situations. This led to an exploration of the possibility that other similarly active peptides may be produced *in vivo* by the adenohypophysis. De Wied, Witter and Lande, starting with a fraction rich in MSH activity, isolated a number of smaller active subfractions. A paucity of material prevented the identification of the amino acid components of these fractions and the determination of whether the active peptides have some common amino acid sequences. Nevertheless, these studies revealed the possibility that a number of small, behaviorally active peptides may be produced by the adenohypophysis.

In contrast to the inhibitory action of ACTH — and fragments thereof — on the extinction of an avoidance response, adrenal corticosteroids facilitate the extinction of the same response. Evaluation of a variety of related steroids by Van Wimersma Greidanus led to the conclusion that only the pregnene type steroids, *i.e.*, steroids containing 21 C atoms with a double bond in A or B rings, a keto or hydroxygroup at C_3 and by preference a keto group at C_{20}, are capable of facilitating the extinction of a pole-jumping avoidance response. The same structural characteristics might be involved in a number of other effects of steroids on the CNS, *viz.*, anesthesia, facilitation of self-stimulation in some areas and inhibition of such stimulation in other areas, reduction of electroshock thresholds, etc.

The comprehensive review by Bohus on the effects of implantations of corticosteroids in the central nervous system demonstrated the involvement of the brain stem and forebrain facilitatory and inhibitory neuronal systems in determining the rate of extinction of an avoidance response. In accord with these observations was the report by McEwen and Weiss on the uptake of labeled corticosterone by various areas of the CNS. These elegant studies revealed a free and rapid exchange of the hormone between the circulating blood and the brain with the hippocampus exhibiting a pronounced tendency to retain the hormone at higher concentrations and for longer intervals than other structures. Cell fractionation studies revealed that hippocampal nuclei have the greatest tendency to bind corticosterone. The effect of such binding on the synthesis of specific enzymes suggested an interaction between the corticosteroids and biogenic amines in the CNS. These fundamental studies promise important insights on the molecular basis of neuronal activity that determine behavior. In similar vein are the studies reported by Glassman, by Gispen and Schotman on the macromolecular changes induced in the brains of animals exposed to a variety of learning experiences.

The influence of the pituitary–adrenal axis on the regulation of appetite was the subject of two reports. Denton and Nelson revealed the complexities involved in determining the regulation of the appetite for salt, while Stevenson and Franklin reviewed extensive studies on the regulation of food and water intake.

No summary can do justice to the eleven reports which consisted essentially of summaries of a mass of information relevant to various facets of the problem that comprised the subject of the symposium. As was undoubtedly anticipated, the formal presentations and the informal discussions yielded more questions than answers, and more uncertainties than certainties. Yet, the internal consistency of the data from different experimental approaches, in different laboratories in many countries encourages a more intensive pursuit of the mechanisms whereby neuro-endocrine interactions modulate normal and abnormal behaviors. This symposium revealed that the application of the concepts and tools of various disciplines can be focused to identify sites and modes of action of physiological and pharmacological agents within the central nervous system where the intricate interplay of facilitation and inhibition, of arousal and depression, mediate the motivational processes of fear and anxiety.

NOTE OF THE EDITORS

At the conference Drs. DENTON and STEVENSON presented their papers in session III; in this book their contributions have been included in the second session.

SESSION IV

Chairman: R. A. CLEGHORN

ACTH, Corticosteroids and the Brain: Clinical Studies

Department of Psychiatry, Allan Memorial Institute, McGill University, 1025 Pine Avenue West, Montreal 112, P. Quebec, Canada

Effects of ACTH on EEG Habituation in Human Subjects

E. ENDRÖCZI, K. LISSÁK, T. FEKETE

Institute of Physiology, University Medical School, Rakóczi út 80, Pécs (Hungary)

AND D. DE WIED

Rudolf Magnus Institute for Pharmacology, Medical Faculty, University for Utrecht, Vondellaan 6, Utrecht (The Netherlands)

The phenomenon of stimulus-induced alpha activity has been reported by a number of investigators (Adrian and Matthews, 1934; Bagchi, 1937; Blake and Gerard, 1937; Williams, 1939; Bjirner, 1949; Goldie and Green, 1960; Morrell, 1966; Endröczi *et al.*, 1969). An enhancement of EEG synchrony has sometimes been interpreted as a shift in the level of vigilance (Blake and Gerard, 1937; Loomis *et al.*, 1938; Oswald, 1962). Another group of investigators has noted that the activation of alpha activity by sensory stimulation is accompanied by autonomic responses which were habituated in the previous sessions (Darrow, 1947; Jung, 1954; Sokolov and Paramonova, 1961). Moreover, an enhanced alpha activity could be observed during sustained attention (Williams, 1939; Toman, 1943) and stimulus-induced alpha waves have been reported in studies on sleep-deprived persons (Armington and Mitnick, 1959).

The synchronization of EEG activity, or the enhancement of alpha rhythm, are common phenomena during differential conditioning as a response to the differential signal and during the course of the extinction of conditioned reflex activity (Motokawa and Huzimori, 1949; Iwama, 1950; Rusinov, 1960, etc.). The EEG synchrony occurring during conditioning has been considered as an electrical sign of internal inhibition.

Involvement of pituitary-adrenocortical hormones in the control of brain mechanisms has been suggested on the basis of behavioural and psychic alterations associated with adrenocortical deficiency, and by the administration of ACTH and adrenocortical steroids (Liddel *et al.*, 1935; Thorn, 1949; Cleghorn, 1957). Both ACTH and corticosteroid treatment resulted in an increased convulsive reactivity, a slowing of the EEG activity, and an increased sensitivity to hyperventilation and photic driving in human subjects (Hoefer and Glaser, 1950; Glaser, 1953; Steifler and Feldman, 1953; Woodbury, 1954, etc.). These observations have been corroborated by animal experiments (Feldman *et al.*, 1961; Lissák and Endröczi, 1962, 1965; Endröczi *et al.*, 1969; Endröczi, 1969).

A facilitatory effect of ACTH upon extinction of a fear-conditioned response has been observed by Mirsky *et al.* (1953). Since this observation, a number of data indicate the influence of pituitary-adrenocortical hormones on conditioned reflex processes (Murphy and Miller, 1955; Endröczi and Lissák, 1962; De Wied, 1966, 1967; Levine and Jones, 1965; Korányi *et al.*, 1965; Bohus and Korányi, 1969).

Concerning the effect of corticosteroids on central nervous processes, it was suggested that they facilitate "internal inhibition" and such an action is mediated via descending inhibitory influence of the basal forebrain which plays a basic role in the control of sensory input into the diencephalon (Endröczi and Lissák, 1962; Lissák and Endröczi, 1960, 1965; Endröczi et al., 1967; Endröczi, 1969).

The present paper deals with findings which were obtained during the course of electrocorticographic conditioning in 16 human subjects who were treated with ACTH and ACTH fragments.

EEG synchrony provoked by repetition of sound or flicker stimuli

Only mentally healthy men were used for the study. The observations were performed between 4 and 7 o'clock p.m. in a sound-proof room, and the electrical activity was registered with a 12-channel Hellige Neuroscript apparatus. Fifty sound or flicker stimuli, lasting for 10 sec, were given in 40-sec. intervals in a daily session. The 4 and 12 cycles per second (cps) test stimuli were presented alternately and the subjects were requested to make a handgrip reaction in response to a test stimulus of 12 cps. The motor performance was registered electromyographically on the EEG apparatus.

Repetition of the test stimulus for several hundred times resulted in the development of EEG synchrony upon presentation of the test stimulus. The synchronization of EEG activity provoked by the test stimulus showed some characteristic features which might be summarized as follows:

(i) At least 50 to 100 repetitions of the test stimulus were necessary to provoke synchronized EEG response; in some cases more than 400 presentations were required.

(ii) The frequency range of the EEG response was independent of the frequency of the test stimulus. In the majority of cases, an enhancement of alpha activity was provoked by either 4 or 12 cps test stimuli; but there were two persons who responded consistently with high amplitude slow waves of 5 to 6 cps.

(iii) When the subjects were requested to make a handgrip (which had been associated with the test stimulus of 12 cps) during the inter-signal intervals (according to the time estimation of the subject in the middle of the period), the somatic reaction was accompanied by appearance of EEG synchronization.

(iv) Memorization of words and mental tasks performed by the subject during inter-trial intervals also failed to inhibit stimulus-induced EEG synchrony.

(v) The first manifestation of stimulus-induced EEG synchrony was found in the parieto-temporal records; but in an advanced stage, frontal and occipital areas were also included.

(vi) In the majority of cases, stimulus-induced EEG synchrony appeared earlier and with greater amplitude on the dominant hemisphere as judged by the right- or left-handedness of the subject.

Influence of ACTH and two ACTH analogues on stimulus-induced EEG synchrony

Synthetic ACTH β 1-24 and two fragments of this molecule (ACTH 1-10 and 11-24)

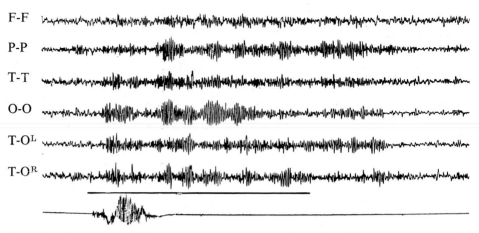

Fig. 1. Stimulus-provoked EEG synchrony; elicited by a sound stimulus of 12 cps; electromyographic response is known on the last channel. Synchronization at 6 cps frequency range is more pronounced on the dominant hemisphere. F–F: bifrontal, P–P: biparietal, T–T: bitemporal, O–O: bioccipital, T–O^L: temporo-occipital on the left, and T–O^R on the right side.

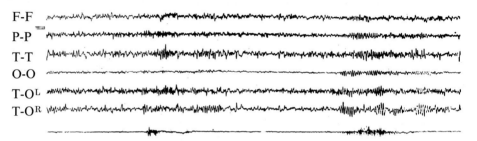

Fig. 2. Deliberate motor activity performed during intersignal interval is accompanied by appearance of an enhancement of alpha activity. The motor activity is registered on the last channel. Characteristic is the lack of synchronization in the 4th channel (O-O)

were used; the fragments were injected intravenously in amounts of 1 or 2 mg dissolved in physiological saline. ACTH 1-24 was given in a dose of 50 units, which was approximately 0.5 mg. The peptides were obtained from Organon, Oss, Holland, through one of us (de W.).

The subjects were hospitalized for reason of minor neurological symptoms during the whole observation period. The injections were given in the ward and the subjects were unaware of the relation between injection and experimental procedure.

Administration of 50 units ACTH resulted in a suppression of the number of synchronized EEG responses, and the effect lasted for at least two days. It is remarkable that the decrease in the number of positive responses was not observed during the first 1 to 2 hours following ACTH treatment, and a significant suppression of positive EEG responses developed on the day following injection. Administration of physiological saline solution did not influence stimulus-induced EEG synchronization.

The administration of ACTH 1-10 simulated the effect of the 1-24 ACTH molecule and an intravenous injection of 1 or 2 mg led to a marked suppression of the stimulus-induced EEG synchronization. The effect of ACTH 1-10 showed a faster development,

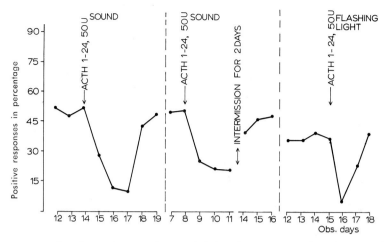

Fig. 3. The suppressive effects of ACTH β 1-24 administration on the number of synchronized EEG responses in 3 subjects. The ordinate shows the number of positive responses in per cent, the abscissa corresponds to the days of observation. In the first two cases , sound, in the third one, flashes of light were used as test stimuli.

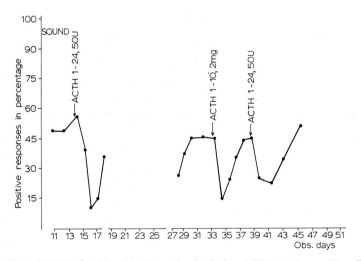

Fig. 4. The effect of ACTH β 1–24 and 1–10 on stimulus-induced EEG synchrony. The effect of interruption of the experimental procedure from 18th to 28th day is also shown.

and its duration was approximately the same as that of the ACTH β 1-24. In contrast to these observations, the administration of ACTH 11-24, in a dose of 1 or 2 mg, did not influence EEG synchrony evoked by the test stimuli.

The normalization of suppressed EEG synchrony after ACTH injection occurred on the 4th or 5th day even if the training and testing period was interrupted for 2 days. Characteristic for the stability of EEG synchrony as provoked by the test stimulus was, that an interruption of the experimental procedure for more than 8 to 10 days resulted only in a decline in the number of positive responses and additional trials were neces-

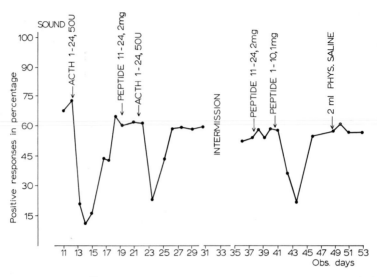

Fig. 5. The effects of ACTH$^\intercal\beta$ 1–24, 1–10 and 11–24 as well as physiological saline solution given to the same subject on stimulus-induced EEG synchrony.

TABLE I

THE EFFECTS OF ACTH AND ACTH-FRAGMENTS ON STIMULUS-PROVOKED EEG SYNCHRONY

	Treatment	No.	Maximal suppression of stimulus-provoked EEG synchrony*	Recovery period in days
Physiol. saline		6	no effect	—
ACTH 11–24	1 mg	2	no effect	—
ACTH 11–24	2 mg	4	no effect	—
ACTH β 1–24	50 U	12	60– 60– 70 70– 70– 70 70– 70– 80 90–100–100	3–4
ACTH 1–10	1 mg	5	60– 70– 70 80– 80– 80	2–3
ACTH 1–10	2 mg	3	70– 70– 90	2–3

* Percentual decrease in the number of positive responses on the day following injection.

sary to reach the previous level. An intervening disease, like influenza, also led to a suppression of stimulus-induced EEG synchronization.

It is generally known that the presentation of a novel stimulus elicits both behavioural and EEG arousal, and that the repetition of this stimulus results in the elimination of arousal reaction. This phase has been called "habituation". A prolonged repetition of the test stimulus leads to the development of a secondary phase of the habituation in which the test stimulus provokes enhancement of alpha activity or bursting slow waves (Endröczi *et al.*, 1969). The EEG synchronization elicited by the test stimulus seems to be organized within a temporal and spatial frame of the central nervous system which is unrelated to those necessary for short-term memory or task-solving processes. A predominancy of the paramount hemisphere and a pre-dilectory site on parietal and temporal cortical fields suggests a triggering role of nonspecific thalamic nuclei in the organization of stimulus-induced EEG synchronization. The EEG synchrony evoked by the test stimulus can be associated with a deliberate motor reaction and this character of electrical correlate opens up a possibility to study associative functions of the brain on the basis of objective indices.

Suppression of synchronized EEG response to the test stimulus after ACTH injection had a relatively long delay and lasted over a long period. Participation of adrenocortical steroids in this action can be excluded by the fact that the ACTH 1-10 also suppressed the stimulus-induced EEG synchronization. This finding suggests an extra-adrenal action of the ACTH molecule and emphasizes the importance of the first 10 amino acids for this effect. This assumption does not exclude the possibility that corticosteroids, secreted in excess during the first hours of ACTH β 1-24 administration, also affect or alter central nervous processes. For example, a longer latency in the action of ACTH β 1-24 than that of the decapeptide might indicate that the increased corticosteroid output counteracts or modifies the extra-adrenal influence of ACTH.

An independent action of ACTH of corticosteroids on brain processes has been noted by Wassermann et al. (1965), Ferrari et al. (1963, 1966), Korányi et al. (1965), Bohus and De Wied (1960), De Wied (1966), among others. Moreover, it has been found that fragments of the ACTH molecule, like ACTH 1-10, or ACTH analogues, like alpha- and beta-MSH possess the same activity on avoidance behaviour as the parent molecule, despite the lack of an effect of these fragments on corticosteroidogenesis (Greven and De Wied, 1967).

To understand the physiological meaning of stimulus-provoked EEG synchrony and to interpret suppression of this electrical correlate by ACTH administration, we must consider the changes which occur during repetition of a test stimulus in the excitability state of the central nervous system. Thus, a repetition of a neutral stimulus results in the development of three consecutive phases which manifest themselves in EEG activity in the form of EEG arousal (1st phase), of the elimination of arousal response (2nd phase) and in an overwhelming inhibition associated by appearance of synchronized EEG activity (3rd phase). If we assume that the habituation (2nd phase) represents a balanced, stimulus-specific control of the activatory system by the inhibitory one, and that the 3rd phase reflects a predominance of inhibitory processes, the action of ACTH upon stimulus-induced EEG synchrony can be interpreted as a kind of "dis-inhibition".

REFERENCES

ADRIAN, E. D. AND MATTHEWS, B. H. C. (1934) The Berger rhythm. Potential changes from occipital lobes in man. *Brain*, **57**, 355–385.

ARMINGTON, J. C. AND MITNICK, L. L. (1959) EEG and sleep deprivation. *J. Appl. Physiol.*, **14** 247–250.

BAGCHI, B. K. (1937) The adaptation and variability of response of the human brain wave rhythm. *J. Psychol.*, **3**, 464–485.

BJIRNER, B. (1949) Alpha depression and lowered pulse rate during delayed reactions in a serial reaction test. *Acta Physiol. Scand.*, **19**, Suppl. 65, 1–93.

BLAKE, H. AND GERARD, R. W. (1937) Brain potentials during sleep. *Amer. J. Physiol.*, **119**, 692–703.

BOHUS, B. AND DE WIED, D. (1966) Inhibitory and facilitatory effect of two related peptides on extinction of avoidance behavior. *Science*, **153**, 318–320.

BOHUS, B. AND KORÁNYI, L. (1969) Hormonal conditioning of adaptive behavioural processes. In: *Results in Neurophysiology, Neuroendocrinology, Neuropharmacology and Behaviour*, K. LISSÁK (Ed.), Akadémiai Kiadó, Budapest, pp. 50–76.

CLEGHORN, R. A. (1957) *Steroid Hormones in Relation to Neuropsychiatric Disorders*, H. Hoagland (Ed.), Academic Press, New York, pp. 3–11.

DARROW, C. W. (1947) Psychological and psychophysiological states and significance of the electroencephalogram. *Psychol. Rev.*, **54**, 157–168.

DE WIED, D. (1966) Inhibitory effect of ACTH and related peptides on extinction of conditioned avoidance behavior in rats. *Proc. Soc. Exptl. Biol. (N.Y.)*, **122**, 28–32.

DE WIED, D. (1967) Opposite effects of ACTH and glucocorticosteroids on extinction of conditioned avoidance behavior. *Proc. 2nd Intern. Congr. on Hormonal Steroids, Milan, May 1966*, Exc. Med. Intern. Congress Series, No. **132**, 945–951.

LEVINE, S. AND JONES, L. E. (1965) Adrenocorticotropic hormone (ACTH) and passive avoidance learning. *J. Comp. Physiol. Psychol.*, **59**, 357–360.

DE WIED, D. AND BOHUS, B. (1966) Long-term and short-term effects on retention of a conditioned avoidance response in rats by treatment with long acting pitressin and α-MSH. *Nature (Lond.)*, **212**, 1484–1486.

ENDRÖCZI, E. AND LISSÁK, K. (1962) Spontaneous goal-directed motor activity related to the alimentary conditioned reflex behaviour and its regulation by neural and humoral factors. *Acta Physiol. Acad. Sci. Hung.*, **21**, 265–283.

ENDRÖCZI, E., LISSÁK, K. AND HARTMANN, G. (1967) Meso-diencephalic inhibitory and activatory mechanisms. *Acta Physiol. Acad. Sci. Hung.*, **31**, 117–125.

ENDRÖCZI, E., FEKETE, T., LISSÁK, K. AND OZSVÁTH, K. (1969) Electroencephalographic studies of the habituation in humans. *Acta Physiol. Acad. Sci. Hung.*, **34**, 311–318.

ENDRÖCZI, E. (1969) Brain stem and diencephalic substrate of hormonally conditioned motivated behavioural reactions. In: *Recent Developments in Neurophysiology, Neuroendocrinology, Neuropharmacology and Behaviour*, Lissák, K. (Ed.), Akadémiai Kiadó, Budapest, p. 29–50.

FELDMAN, S., TODT, J. AND PORTER, R. W. (1961) Effect of adrenocortical hormones on evoked potentials in the brain stem, *Neurology (Minneapolis)*, **11**, 110–118.

FERRARI, W., GESSA, L. AND VAREIN, L. (1965) Behavioural effects induced by intracisternally injected ACTH and MSH. *Ann. N.Y. Acad. Sci.*, **104**, 330–345.

GLASER, G. H. (1953) On the relationship between adrenal cortical activity and the convulsive state. *Epilepsia*, **2**, 7–15.

GOLDIE, L. AND GREEN, J. M. (1960) Paradoxical blocking and arousal in the drowsy state. *Nature (Lond.)*, **187**, 952–953.

GREVEN, H. M. AND DE WIED, D. (1967) The active sequence in the ACTH molecule responsible for inhibition of the extinction of conditioned avoidance behaviour in rats. *Europ. J. Pharmacol.*, **2**, 14–16.

HOEFER, P. F. A. AND GLASER, G. H. (1950) Effects of pituitary adrenocorticotropic hormone (ACTH) therapy. Electroencephalographic and neuropsychiatric changes in 15 patients. *J. Amer. Med. Assoc.*, **143**, 620–640.

IWAMA, K. (1950) Delayed conditioned reflex in man and brain waves. *Tohoku J. Exptl. Med.*, **52**, 53–62.

JUNG, R. (1954) Correlation of bioelectrical and autonomic phenomena with alterations of consciousness and arousal in man. In: *Brain Mechanisms and Consciousness*, J. DELAFRESNAYE (Ed.), Thomas, Springfield, Ill., pp. 310–340.

KORÁNYI, L., ENDRÖCZI, E. AND TÁRNOK, F. (1965) Sexual behaviour in the course of avoidance conditioning in male rabbits. *Neuroendocrinology*, **1**, 144–157.

KORÁNYI, L. AND ENDRÖCZI, E. (1967) The effect of ACTH on nervous processes. *Neuroendocrinology*, **2**, 65–75.

KORÁNYI, L., ENDRÖCZI, E., LISSÁK, K. AND SZEPES, É. (1967) The effect of ACTH on behavioural processes motivated by fear in mice. *J. Physiol. Behaviour*, **2**, 439–445.

LIDDEL, H. S., ANDERSON, C., KOTYUKA, O. AND HARTMAN, F.A. (1935) Effect of extract of adrenal cortex on experimental neurosis in sheep. *Arch. Neurol. Psychiat. (Chic.)*, **43**, 973–993.

LISSÁK, K. AND ENDRÖCZI, E. (1960) *Die neuroendokrine Steuerung der Adaptationstätigkeit*, Akadémiai Kiadó, Budapest, p. 175.

LISSÁK, K. AND ENDRÖCZI, E. (1962) Some aspects of the effect of hippocampal stimulation on the endocrine system. In: *Physiologie de l'Hippocampe, CNRS Symposium, Montpellier*, p. 463–473.

LISSÁK, K. AND ENDRÖCZI, E. (1965) *Neuroendocrine Control of Adaptation*, Pergamon Press, Oxford, p. 193.

LOOMIS, A. L., HARVEY, E. N. AND HOBART, G. A. (1938) Distribution of disturbance patterns in the human electroencephalogram with special reference to sleep. *J. Neurophysiol.*, **1**, 413–430.

MIRSKY, I., MILLER, R. AND STEIN, M. (1953) Relation of adrenocortical activity and adaptive behavior. *Psychosom. Med.*, **15**, 574–584.

MORRELL, L. K. (1966) Some characteristics of stimulus-provoked alpha activity. *Electroencephal. Clin. Neurophysiol.*, **21**, 552–561.

MOTOKAWA, K. AND HUZIMORI, B. (1949) EEG and conditioned reflexes. *Tohoku J. Exptl. Med.*, **50**, 214–234.

MULHOLLAND, T. AND RUNNELS, S. (1962) Increased occurrence of EEG alpha during increased attention. *J. Psychol.*, **54**, 317–330.

MURPHY, J. V. AND MILLER, R. (1955) The effect of adrenocorticotrophic hormone (ACTH) on avoidance conditioning in the rat. *J. Comp. Physiol. Psychol.*, **48**, 47–49.

OSWALD, I. (1962) *Sleeping and Waking*, Elsevier, Amsterdam, p. 232.

RUSINOV, V. S. (1960) General and localized alterations in the electroencephalogram during the formation of conditioned reflexes in man. *Electroencephal. Clin. Neurophysiol.*, Suppl. **13**, 311–320.

SOKOLOV, E. N. AND PARAMONOVA, N. P. (1961) Dynamics of the orienting reflex during the development of sleep inhibition in man. *Pavlov J. Higher Nerv. Act.*, **11**, 10–17. (in Russian).

STEIFLER, M. AND FELDMAN, S. (1953) On the effect of cortisone on the electroencephalogram. *Confinia Neurol. (Basel)*, **13**, 96–114.

TOMAN, J. E. P. (1943) The electroencephalogram during mental effort. *Federation Proc.*, **2**, 49.

WASSERMAN, M. J., BELTON, N. R. AND MILLICHAP, J. C. (1965) Effect of corticotropin (ACTH) on experimental seizures. Adrenal independence and relation to intracellular brain sodium. *Neurology (Minneapolis)*, **15**, 1136–1141.

WILLIAMS, A. C. (1939) Some psychological correlates of the electroencephalogram. *Arch. Psychol.*, **240**, 1–48.

WOODBURY, D. M. (1954) Effect of hormones on brain excitability and electrolytes. *Recent Progr. Hormone Res.*, **10**, 275–357.

DISCUSSION

HENKIN: The timing of the phenomena which you have described is difficult to understand in terms of the half-life of ACTH. It is well known that the half-life of ACTH in physiological saline injected intravenously is very short. The major effects of intravenously injected ACTH in man occur either during or shortly after its administration. In fact, measurement of the effects of ACTH 8–16 hours after intravenous injection offer little in the way of observable physiological changes. The fact that the phenomena you described occurred 24–48 hours after the administration of ACTH intravenously is difficult to interpret in terms of the response to the ACTH itself. In order to obtain useful corroborative information it would be of interest to know what changes occurred in plasma eosinophils and cortisol or in the urinary excretion of 17-hydroxycorticosteroids at the same time that your observed phenomena occurred. None of that information was presented. I think that there are important unanswered questions in your study with respect to the timing of your observed response particularly with respect to its specific relationship to ACTH.

ENDRÖCZI: I suppose that the half-life of ACTH that you refer to was measured by its action on the adrenal cortex. However the half-life of the extra-adrenal action of ACTH should be much longer. As an example: the half-life of the extra-adrenal effects of ACTH on the vascular platform, measured by several researchers in Hungary, is much longer and not comparable at all with the direct adrenocortical action.

It is difficult to tell what happens in the organs after administration of these 11–24 and 1–10 peptides; the psychological situation was very complicated in our study. EEG synchrony is a situation specific response and not stimulus situation specific. We do not know what factors are involved in this kind of humoral conditioning. The sensory input might have been affected by the peptides or by the excitability level of the brain.

HENKIN: Again, all the more reason that you must be very careful. The fact that there are other significant stimuli, other influences that can alter the response you are measuring makes it all the more important to relate the effect specifically to ACTH and not other stimuli and you have not done this. By the nature of your conclusions you have related your results specifically to an ACTH effect yet you have not demonstrated these interrelationships conclusively.

ENDRÖCZI: We have shown the effects of administration of the peptide, but we do not know yet the mechanism involved in its action.

MIRSKY: You have injected ACTH-(11-24) as a control in your study of the ACTH effect and it had no effects?

ENDRÖCZI: Indeed, no effects could be observed.

MIRSKY: I agree with you that dealing with the half-lives of these peptides is difficult; most peptides disappear extremely rapidly from the circulation. The half-life of growth hormone is even much smaller than of ACTH and its effect is late.

WEIJNEN: Could you comment on the suggestive value of your data for the interpretation of the modification of animal behavior by ACTH analogues? How specific can we expect the peptide effect to be?

ENDRÖCZI: There might be some connection between the results of animal studies and the data presented in this paper. It seems that both ACTH-(1-24) and ACTH-(1-10) exert a disinhibitory influence, which manifests itself in suppression of the number of positive EEG responses and in a prolonged period of extinction of conditioned avoidance behavior in rats.

WEIJNEN: Dr. Korányi reported in his paper that ACTH-(1-10), injected intravenously, resulted in a marked diminution of evoked potentials in the young chick. The effect could be observed after 5–10 minutes following injection and lasted 40–60 minutes. The time course of the effects you observed after ACTH-(1-10) treatment is quite different. Should the blood–brain barrier be blamed for this difference? It would be very interesting to see the results of a replication of Dr. Korányi's study with older chickens in which the blood–brain barrier has developed, with your time schedule.

ENDRÖCZI: We have not performed experiments as such, on evoked potentials in older chickens; observations in these chickens on the effect of ACTH-(1-24) on extinction of a conditioned avoidance reflex revealed a facilitation of extinction on the 3rd and the 4th day of extinction after daily administration of ACTH for 3 days. The latency with which the effect of ACTH occurred may indicate that the blood–brain barrier reduced the penetration of ACTH. But the effect might also be due to corticosteroids produced after ACTH administration.

   These data were obtained in preliminary studies by Korányi *et al.* and it is clear that the effect of ACTH-(1-10) or of smaller fragments of this hormone, in older chickens remains to be elucidated.

The Effects of ACTH and Corticosteroids on Epileptiform Disorders

ROBERT KLEIN

Pediatric Clinical Center, Boston City Hospital, Boston, Mass. 02118 (U.S.A.)

I feel somewhat of a fraud discussing this material with you since I have done no active work in this field for a number of years now. In 1950, we reported the effect of short term treatment with ACTH in 6 patients with various forms of epilepsy (Klein and Livingston, 1950). We were very impressed with the dramatic improvement in the electroencephalograms associated with ACTH administration. When the hormone treatment was discontinued, the electroencephalograms reverted to their previous abnormal state rapidly and in those patients with remissions of their clinical symptoms, there was also a clinical relapse. Indeed, in one patient, there was an apparent exacerbation of symptoms upon withdrawal of treatment. These obervations were not followed up because it did not seem practical to treat anyone with long term administration of ACTH who could be managed by more conventional means (at that time no corticosteroids with fewer side effects were available for treatment).

It was not clear what the mechanism of action of ACTH was in these patients. The treatment had been tried in the first place because, in my naivité, I felt that the known effects of ACTH leading to relatively increased metabolism of fat and breakdown of protein and decreased utilization of carbohydrate might mimic the metabolic effect of a ketogenic diet. It had been known, however, that administration of desoxycorticosterone would produce amelioration of epilepsy since McQuarrie's original report in 1942. Therefore, the possibility that the effect of ACTH might be mediated through changes in electrolyte metabolism had to be considered. We did treat 2 of these patients with desoxycorticosterone with less benefit than was noted when they were given ACTH, but the dose or duration of treatment with desoxycorticosterone might not have been adequate. The overall sodium and potassium balances were similar with treatment with either ACTH or desoxycorticosterone and did not seem to correlate with clinical or EEG remissions. In this regard, it is of interest to note that in the one patient of McQuarrie's whose electrolyte balance was measured, no overall retention of sodium was found since the patient was kept on a low sodium diet.

Fig. 1 illustrates EEG of one patient after 4 days of DOC treatment, after 10 days of ACTH, and 1 month after ACTH was stopped. Similar changes in EEG's have been illustrated in many reports. Since the time of our report, approximately 179 patients with various forms of epilepsy exclusive of infantile myoclonic spasms treated with ACTH have been reported. (Gastaut *et al.*, 1959; Chieffi and Fois, 1965;

A   B   C

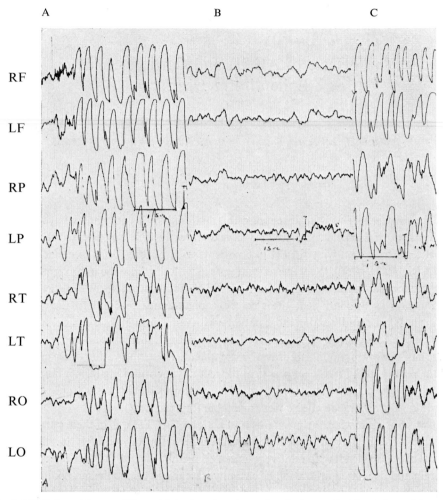

Fig. 1. EEG's from 13-year-old boy with both petit and grand mal seizures. A. After 4 days of desoxy-corticosterone. B. After 10 days of ACTH. C. One month later.
From: KLEIN, R. AND LIVINGSTON, S. (1950) The effect of adrenocorticotropic hormone in epilepsy. *J. Pediat.*, **37**, 733–742.

Lanternier, 1965; Bergamini *et al.*, 1966). Of these, 34 were adults and will not be considered further since the results were almost uniformly unsuccessful and different from the results in children. Of the 145 children treated, 23% were rendered free of seizures, 43% were markedly improved, and 34% were not helped and some of these actually became worse during treatment. The improvement in their electroencephalograms correlated in degree and duration with their clinical improvement. The benefit in nearly all cases was temporary. A few of the patients who became worse were suffering from grand mal epilepsy and had an increased number of their seizures while receiving ACTH. More commonly, however, deterioration occurred in patients with petit mal or psychomotor epilepsy who developed grand mal seizures without amelioration of their original symptoms. There were others whose original petit mal attacks ceased but who developed grand mal at the same time. In general, the authors considered these last patients to have neither deteriorated nor improved. Gastaut felt that petit mal in children responded very well to ACTH therapy. Three children in his study with petit mal were granted long term relief from fits by the injection of a single dose of ACTH. He found, however, that adults with petit mal were least likely to respond to ACTH favorably. This led him to suggest that only early treatment of petit mal afforded an opportunity for long term benefit from ACTH administration. In contradistinction, Chieffi found ACTH to be of no value in patients with pure petit mal with 3 per second spike and wave forms on electroencephalography (patients with petit mal variant with 2 per second spike and wave forms were improved, however), but he reported longer lasting benefit from treatment with ACTH in various forms of epilepsy which he felt might be the result of longer periods of therapy than those used by Gastaut. Other authors also reported less benefit in patients with pure petit mal than in other forms of epilepsy treated but none reported benefit lasting much longer than the actual period of treatment. The tendency for replacement of minor motor seizure activity with grand mal fits after ACTH treatment was also noted in the patients with infantile myoclonic spasms with hypsarrhythmia to be discussed.

In 1958 the opportunity arose to treat patients with hypsarrhythmia with prednisone*. I felt that with the availability of prednisone we might be able to avoid some of the questions about changes in sodium and potassium metabolism being the mediator of the ACTH effect. You can seen that I retained my naivité for a long time. We treated 26 patients with infantile myoclonic spasms, all but one of whom had electroencephalograms with the classic appearance of hypsarrhythmia in 1958 and 1959. While we were studying these patients, Sorel's (1958) report on the treatment of hypsarrhythmia with ACTH was published. The reason for presenting our results at this late date is that this is one of the two studies with a group of patients treated with prednisone and there are undocumented statements in the literature that the use of ACTH produces superior results to those from corticosteroid treatment. A third group of patients has been treated with hydrocortisone. Except for a few sporadic cases all the other reported patients have been treated with ACTH.

Twenty-two of our 26 patients were followed from 6 to 30 months. The other 4 were seen only while in the hospital or for 4 months or less after discharge. The EEG became normal in 14 of these patients in from 2 to 6 weeks of treatment. In 8, there was improvement in the EEG without achievement of a completely normal tracing and in 4 there was no change in EEG. Six months or more after beginning treatment, there were 11 children with normal EEG's. Seven children with either normal or improved EEG's while on therapy showed regression of their tracings although most of them no longer demonstrated hypsarrhythmia but had other abnormal patterns. Of the 4 patients whose EEG's had not changed during the course of treatment, 2 now had improved EEG patterns and 2 were further deteriorated. Clinically 20 of the 26 children had no seizures after 2–6 weeks of prednisone administration, 4 had fewer fits, and 2 were unchanged. Six months or more after initial treatment, there were still 11 children who

---

* Study done with Dr. Irving Chaimovitz, Pittsburgh, Pa.

References pp. 268–269

TABLE I

EFFECT OF ACTH AND CORTICOSTEROIDS IN CHILDREN WITH INFANTILE MYOCLONIC
SPASMS (HYPSARRHYTHMIA)

	Seizures			EEG			Developmental Status	
	No.	Controlled	Improved	No.	Normal	Improved	No.	Normal
After initial Rx.	509	45%	14%	412	30%	32%		?
6–18 mos. after Rx.	106	48%					250	14%

Results of treatment of patients with infantile myoclonic spasms (hypsarrhythmia) with ACTH or corticosteroids. Patients reported from literature (references in text) or personally observed.

were having no seizures, 7 had relapsed and were having seizures once more. The number of fits was still reduced in some of these. Generally, the infantile myoclonic spasms had been replaced by grand mal attacks in this group. Among those observed for more than a year only 4 of 17 were considered to be functioning at a normal developmental and intellectual level. It is impossible to give a valid estimate of their pre-treatment functional level. All patients were treated for at least a month. The mean duration of treatment was 7 months. In several cases as the medication was being gradually reduced before discontinuing it entirely, the patient had an exacerbation of symptoms. In these cases, the dose of prednisone was increased to the previously suppressive level and the patients were treated for 3 months more before gradual reduction in dose was once again carried out. The dose of prednisone was 30–40 mg/day for an average of 3.5 months after which the dose was gradually diminished to zero over an equal period of time.

I have reviewed reports in the literature of 509 patients with hypsarrhythmia who have been treated with ACTH or, in the case of 75 patients, with corticosteroid (Sorel, 1958, Low, 1958, Stamps, 1959, Gastaut, 1959, Pauli, 1960, Dobbs, 1960, Allen, 1961, Dummermuth, 1961, Millichap, 1962, Gastaut, 1964, Jeavons, 1964, Willoughby, 1966, Lanternier, 1965, Chieffi, 1965, Chevrie, 1968, Alvin, 1966, Danielsen, 1965, Oftedal, 1967). This survey by no means includes all patients reported in the world's literature. Table I presents the results. Forty-five percent of the patients treated had no myoclonic spasms at least during the period of therapy. In the individual series reported the percentage of patients completely controlled clinically varied between 19 and 77% with three exceptions. These exceptions were two reports involving only 6 and 2 patients, all of whom were controlled and one report of 12 patients, 4 of whom were improved but none of whom were completely controlled. In additon, 19% of the over 500 patients were improved but still had occasional seizures. Reports on later incidence of fits were adequate for only 106 patients. Forty-eight percent of these continued to be free of seizures for 6 to 18 months after the initial course of therapy. The late developmental status of the patients in these various studies was assessed by different means. Of approximately 250 patients reported, 14%

were considered to have normal motor and intellectual development. This is similar to the percentage of normal end results in patients treated with usual anticonvulsive medications or untreated. The results of electroencephalography were available for 412 patients. Thirty percent developed a normal electroencephalogram with treatment and 32% more were said to have improved but not entirely normal electroencephalograms. They usually did not have hypsarrhythmia any longer but showed other forms of dysrhythmia.

It proved impossible to evaluate the developmental status of the patients before ACTH treatment reported in the literature as it had in examining our own patients when they were having repeated seizures. In most reports those treated late in their disease and those with other cerebral abnormalities responded less well to therapy.

Grossi-Bianchi (1966) reported a striking synergistic effect of pyridoxine administration with ACTH.

The mechanisms of action of adrenal steroids and ACTH in epilepsy are obscure. The most attractive hypothesis to us at present is that these agents act directly or indirectly upon nerve membrane making it more difficult for depolarization to occur spontaneously or after various stimuli. For purposes of this discussion, let us consider that this change involves the set of increased intracellular K, increased active Na efflux and hyperpolarization of the membrane. There is some evidence to support this possibility. The evidence, however, is still far from adequate nor does it suggest whether the effect is direct or indirect. First, we have shown in unpublished work that intravenous administration of hydrocortisone or aldosterone raises muscle membrane potential although we have no measurements of nerve cell membrane resting potential. It is known that aldosterone increases active sodium transport in the toad bladder. This is supported by increased energy release as the result of increased activity of the Na- and K-dependent ATP'ase. This would be expected to increase membrane potential. Second, it has been shown by Woodbury (1957) that aldosterone increases the ratio of intracellular to extracellular potassium and lowers intracellular Na in both brain and muscle. The same author reported similar effects in brain after diphenylhydantoin administration (Woodbury, 1958). In our studies similar electrolyte changes were found in muscle after acute administration of cortisone (Klein, 1962). These effects, too, should be associated with increased resting membrane potential. Third, desoxycorticosterone, which for all practical purposes affects only electrolyte metabolism, ameliorates epilepsy. On the other hand Chieffi (1965) reported that when patients were improved by ACTH therapy they lost sodium and retained potassium. In this regard, Woodbury (1954) has also shown that sodium-retaining hormones elevated the electroshock seizure threshold in animals. The 11-oxygenated corticosteroids antagonized this effect and, when given alone, actually lowered the electroshock seizure threshold.

It is difficult to explain the lowering of the electroshock seizure threshold by 11-oxygenated corticosteroids since this same group of drugs seems to be able to prevent fits in humans with epilepsy. It is also difficult to explain why many patients with such conditions as collagen diseases developed fits for the first time when being treated with corticosteroids or ACTH. It has been postulated that the development of fits was dependent in part upon the presence of the underlying disease. Some doubt must be cast upon this explanation by the finding that in some reports of epileptic patients treated with ACTH, as many as 10 % of the patients had more frequent attacks during treatment. The problem is further complicated by the frequent antagonistic effects on cellular electrolytes produced by the direct and by the renal effects of adrenal steroids. Most of the adrenal steroids in greater or lesser degree directly affect cells so as to increase intracellular potassium and decrease intracellular sodium. Their renal effect is to cause sodium retention and potassium loss. In the long run this tends to actually increase cellular sodium and lower cellular potassium. It also produces hypochloremic, hypokalemic alkalosis. This effect, moreover, is modulated by diet. With minimal sodium intake, no increase in sodium retention follows steroid administration. Since there is less reabsorption from the renal tubule of sodium in exchange for potassium there is no potassium loss. In this situation the primary effect of the adrenal corticosteroid directly upon the cell will predominate and intracellular sodium will be lowered and potassium increased.

In conclusion I can only state that ACTH and adrenal corticosteroids frequently improve the patients with epilepsy dramatically. This effect is variable and usually is transitory. Its mechanism is unknown and its usefulness circumscribed. There is no clear difference between the therapeutic effect of ACTH and that of various corticosteroids in epileptic patients.

REFERENCES

ALLEN, R. J. (1961) An evaluation of steroid treatment in hypsarhythmia. *Electroencephalog. Clin. Neurophysiol.*, **13**, 147.

ALVIN, A., BILLING, L., HAGBERG, B., HAGNE, I., HELLSTROM, B., HERRLIN, K. M., JACOBSSON, E., KAIJSER, K., KARLSSON, B., KIRSTEIN, L., LARSSON, L. E., NORMARK, A., OBERGER, E., PETERSEN, I. AND SODERHJELM, L. (1966) Kortikotropin vid infantil spasm med hypsarytmi. *Nord. Med.*, **75**, 234–237.

BERGAMINI, L., BROGLIA, S., RICCIO, A. AND FRANCHINI, V. (1966) Résultats favorables du traitement avec ACTH en différents types d'épilepsie résistents à toute thérapie mèdicamenteuse classique. *Riv. Neurol.*, **36**, 49–62.

CHEVRIE, J. J., AICARDI, J., THIEFFRY, ST., GRISON, D. AND MISSOFFE, C. (1968) Traitement hormonal de 58 cas de spasmes infantiles. *Arch. Franc. Pediat.*, **25**, 263–276.

CHIEFFI, A. AND FOIS, A. (1965) Influence of ACTH on convulsive activity in children. Electroencephalographic and clinical observations. *Helv. Paediat. Acta*, **20**, 466–475.

DANIELSEN, J. (1965) Infantile spasms and hypsarhythmia treated with corticosteroids. *Acta Neurol. Scand.*, **13**, Suppl. 41, 489–492.

DOBBS, J. M. AND BAIRD, H. W. (1960) The use of corticotropin and a corticosteroid in patients with minor motor seizures. *Am. J. Diseases Childhood*, **100**, 584.

DUMERMUTH, G. (1961) Über das Syndrom der Blitz-Nick-Salaam-krämpfe und seine Behandlung mit ACTH und Hydrocortison. *Helv. Paediat. Acta*, **16**, 244.

GASTAUT, N., SALTIEL, J., RAYBAUD, C., PITOT, M. AND MEYNADIER, A. (1958) A propos du traitement par l'A.C.T.H. des Encéphalites myocloniques de la première enfance avec hypsarythmie. *Pédiatrie*, **14**, 35–41.

GASTAUT, H., MIRIBEL, G., FAVEL, P. AND VIGOUROUX, M. (1959) Effets cliniques et electroencéphalographiques de l'A.C.T.H. dans les différents types d'épilepsie. *Rev. Neurol.*, **101**, 753–762.

GASTAUT, H., SOULAYROL, R., ROGER, J. AND PINSARD, N. (1964) *L'encéphalopathie myoclonique infantile avec hypsarythmie*, Masson & Cie, Paris VI.

GROSSI-BIANCHI, M. L., GANDULLIA, E., PISTONE, F. M. AND SEGNI, G. (1966) Associazione di piridossina e ACTH nel trattamento dell'encefalopatia mioclonica infantile con ipsaritmia. *Minerva Pediat.*, **18**, 160–161.

JEAVONS, P. M. AND BOWER, B. D. (1964) *Infantile Spasms, Clinics in Developmental Medicine*, No. 15, William Heinemann Medical Books, Ltd., New York.

KLEIN, R. AND LIVINGSTON, S. (1950) The effect of adrenocorticotropic hormone in epilepsy. *J. Pediat.*, **37**, 733–742.

KLEIN, R., GANELIN, R., ZELKOWITZ, P., HAYS, P. AND RICHARDS, C. (1962) Effect of quinidine, ouabain, and corticosteroids on muscle sodium, potassium, and water content. *Proc. Soc. Exptl. Biol. Med.*, **110**, 280–285.

LANTERNIER, J. (1965) Les dérivés cortisoniques dans les troubles de l'épilepsie. *Rev. Neuropsychiatrie Infantile*, **13**, 477–481.

LOW, N. L. (1958) Infantile spasms with mental retardation. II. Treatment with cortisone and adreno-corticotropin. *Pediatrics*, **22**, 1165.

MCQUARRIE, I., ANDERSON, J. A. AND ZIEGLER, M. R. (1942) Observations on antagonistic effects of posterior pituitary and cortico-adrenal hormones in epileptic subject. *J. Clin. Endocrinol.*, **2**, 406.

MILLICHAP, J. G. AND BICKFORD, R. G. (1962) Infantile spasms, hypsarrhythmia, and mental retardation, response to corticotropin and its relation to age and etiology in 21 patients. *J. Amer. Med. Assoc.*, **182**, 523.

OFTEDAL, S.-I. (1967) Steroid treatment of infantile spasms with hypsarrhythmia. *Electroencephalog. Clin. Neurophysiol.*, **23**, 390–391.

PAULI, L., O'BEIL, R., YBANEZ, M. AND LIVINGSTON, S. (1960) Minor motor epilepsy. Treatment with corticotropin (ACTH) and steroid therapy. *J. Am. Med. Assoc.*, **174**, 1408.

SOREL, L. L. AND DUSAUCY-BAULOYE, A. (1958) A propos de 21 cas d'hypsarrhythmia de Gibbs: son traitement spectaculaire par l'ACTH. *Acta Neurol. Psychiat. Belg.*, **58**, 130.

STAMPS, F. W., GIBBS, E. L., ROSENTHAL, I. M. AND GIBBS, F. A. (1959) Treatment of hypsarrhythmia with ACTH. *J. Am. Med. Assoc.*, **171**, 408.

WILLOUGHBY, J. A., THURSTON, D. L. AND HOLOWACH, J. (1966) Infantile myoclonic seizures: An evaluation of ACTH and corticosteroid therapy. *J. Pediat.*, **69**, 1136–1138.

WOODBURY, D. M. (1954) Effects of hormones on brain excitability and electrolytes. *Recent Progr. Hormone Res.*, **10**, 65.

WOODBURY, D. M. AND KOCH, A. (1957) Effects of aldosterone and desoxycorticosterone on tissue electrolytes. *Proc. Soc. Exptl. Biol. Med.*, **94**, 720–723.

WOODBURY, D. M., KOCH, A. AND VERNADAKIS, A. (1958) Relation between excitability and metabolism in brain and elucidated by anticonvulsant drugs. *Neurology*, **8**, Suppl. 1, 112–116.

DISCUSSION

FELDMAN: How do you reconcile the evidence that glucocorticosteroids may improve epilepsy, with data which show epileptic effects of the same steroids in patients and animals? Is it possible that their effects on epileptic disorders is stronger than on brain excitability?

KLEIN: I have no real answer. It may be that their correction of a putative metabolic abnormality may be more important than their toxic effect of producing lowered convulsive thresholds, *e.g.*, if they produce fits in only 10%, this may be obscured by beneficial effects in a greater number.

CLEGHORN: In 1951 or 1952, when the early euphoric effects of ACTH and cortisone were reported we thought it would be a good idea to try these hormones in the treatment of depression. This turned out not to be a good idea. Actually, we had one patient going into status epilepticus which rather shocked us at the time. Fortunately, the patient recovered.

VAN DER VELDEN: Have you been able to compare children treated with ACTH only, with children treated with corticosteroids only?

KLEIN: Only in children with infantile myoclonic spasms were the numbers great enough. The results of the treatment with prednisone were not different from those with ACTH, which formed the larger group.

The Effects of Corticosteroids and ACTH on Sensory Systems

ROBERT I. HENKIN

Section of Neuroendocrinology, Experimental Therapeutics Branch, National Heart Institute, National Institutes of Health, Bethesda, Md. 20014 (U.S.A.)

INTRODUCTION

The purpose of this paper is to detail some of the relationships which exist between adrenal cortical hormone secretion and neural activity. Particular attention will be paid to the effects of these hormones on sensory detection and perception, especially in the gustatory, olfactory and auditory systems. These results will be related to the manner by which adrenocortical hormones control the detection and integration of sensory signals.

THE RELATIONSHIP BETWEEN ADRENOCORTICAL STEROIDS AND GUSTATORY DETECTION AND PERCEPTION

Taste in normal subjects and in patients with adrenocortical insufficiency

Taste detection thresholds have been studied in normal subjects and in patients with adrenocortical insufficiency. Using a three-drop, forced choice technique the median *detection threshold* was determined by a variation of the methods of limits in both normal volunteers and patients (Henkin, Gill and Bartter, 1963). The details of this procedure have been previously described (Henkin *et al.*, 1963; Henkin, 1967).

Fig. 1 illustrates detection thresholds obtained for representatives of each of four taste qualities in both normal volunteers and in patients with untreated adrenocortical insufficiency. The stimuli for these tests were various solutions of chemically pure substances. For salt, solutions of NaCl, potassium chloride (KCl) and sodium bicarbonate ($NaHCO_3$) were used; for sweet, sucrose was used; for bitter, urea, and for sour, solutions of hydrochloric acid (HCl) were used. Among the normal volunteers median detection thresholds for the three salt solutions and for sucrose were approximately the same, 12 mmoles/l. For urea there was an increase of detection threshold to 120 mmoles/l. For HCl the median detection threshold was 0.8 mmole/l, which was lower than for the salts, sucrose or urea. These thresholds are similar to those obtained in normal volunteers by other investigators (Pfaffman, 1959; Knowles and Johnson, 1941; Cameron, 1947; Schutz and Pilgrim, 1957; Cragg, 1937; Harris and Kalmus, 1949). Median detection thresholds for each salt solution among the patients with untreated adrenocortical insufficiency are approximately 0.1 mmole/l

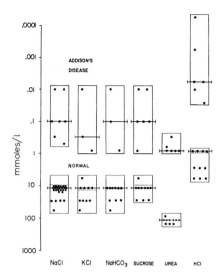

Fig. 1. Detection thresholds in normal volunteers compared with those in patients with untreated adrenocortical insufficiency for representatives of each taste quality. The lower closed circles represent the individual detection thresholds for each quality in normal volunteers. The ordinate is in mmoles/l. The large enclosure around these dots defines the upper and lower limits of the range of responses of the volunteers. The line through the enclosure represents the median detection threshold of the volunteers. The dotted lines within the lower enclosures indicate median detection thresholds determined by other investigators (Pfaffman, 1959; Knowles and Johnson, 1941; Cameron, 1947). The dots and the upper enclosure represent individual detection thresholds and the range of responses in patients with adrenocortical insufficiency, either untreated or taken off replacement therapy. The solid line through this enclosure represents the median detection threshold of the untreated patients. The detection thresholds of the patients are significantly lower than those of the normal volunteers; there is no overlap between the data obtained in each group.

which is significantly lower than that obtained in the normal volunteers. Detection thresholds for sucrose, HCl and urea are also significantly lower among patients with untreated adrenocortical insufficiency than among the normal volunteers. This phenomenon has been confirmed by several investigators (Kosowicz and Pruszewicz, 1967; Pruszewicz and Kosowicz, 1966) and has been used by physicians as an adjunctive tool in the clinical diagnosis of adrenocortical insufficiency. The pattern of responsiveness for taste detection acuity among the untreated patients is similar to that noted for the normal volunteers although at a level of responsiveness approximately 150 times greater. Detection thresholds for the three salts and sucrose were the same. There was an increase in the median detection threshold of urea while the median detection threshold for HCl was lower than for either NaCl, sucrose, or urea

Tasterdetection acuity for each of four taste qualities was also studied in patients with adrenocortical insufficiency treated with daily intramuscular injections of 20 mg of deoxycorticosterone acetate (DOCA) for periods of 2 to 7 days (Fig. 2). This hormone is a potent sodium–potassium (Na–K)-active steroid. The dose given was about 7 times that normally required for replacement therapy in these patients.

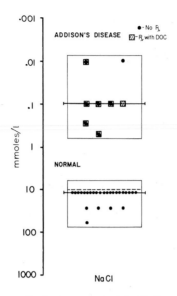

Fig. 2. Detection thresholds in normal volunteers compared with those in patients with adrenocortical insufficiency treated with deoxycorticosterone acetate (DOCA). The hatched squares indicate detection thresholds in each patient after treatment. In general, there is no alteration in the already lowered detection threshold after this treatment. These data presented here for NaCl are similar to those obtained with representatives of each of four taste qualities.

Taste detection acuity was tested at least once a day during this treatment period. Comparison of detection thresholds of the patients with those of normal volunteers revealed that the increased taste detection sensitivity observed in patients with untreated adrenocortical insufficiency persisted even though they were treated with DOCA for as long as 7 days; median detection thresholds of the patients for NaCl after treatment with DOCA or in the untreated state was 0.1 mmole/l (Fig. 2). Similar data were obtained for the detection of each of the other salts, for sucrose, HCl and urea. Thus Na–K-active steroids, although they play a significant role in the control of serum Na and K concentration and of extracellular fluid volume, do not return to normal the increased taste detection sensitivity observed in these patients.

Changes in taste detection acuity were studied in patients with adrenocortical insufficiency treated with prednisolone ($\triangle_1$F), 20 mg a day, for two or more days. This hormone is one of the more potent of the carbohydrate-active steroids and it has little, if any, Na–K activity. The dose given was about 3 times that normally required for replacement therapy. This treatment returned taste thresholds to normal in each case (Fig. 3). In the untreated state, the median detection threshold for NaCl was 0.1 mmole/l; however, after treatment with $\triangle_1$F for 2 days the median detection threshold was 12 mmoles/l. This threshold is not significantly different from those obtained in normal volunteers (Fig. 3).

The return to normal taste acuity is independent of the type of carbohydrate-active steroid used. In this study, prednisolone was used. In other studies, treatment with hydrocortisone, cortisone, and dexamethasone have also returned taste detection

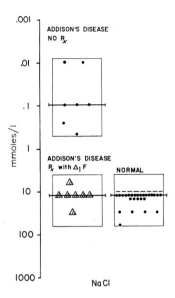

Fig. 3. Detection thresholds in normal volunteers compared with those in patients with adrenocortical insufficiency treated with prednisolone (Δ_1F). The hatched triangles indicate detection thresholds in each patient after treatment. These thresholds are not different from those obtained in normal volunteers.

acuity to normal. The return to normal acuity is also independent of the route of administration of the hormone; *i.e.*, oral, subcutaneous or intravenous administration produced a return of taste acuity to normal. However, the amount of hormone administered does influence the time required to return taste acuity to normal. After administration of a large amount of hormone less time is required to return taste acuity to normal than after administration of a small amount of hormone. Patients who were given adequate replacement doses of these hormones during maintenance therapy did not exhibit abnormalities of taste detection.

To demonstrate the manner by which increases and decreases in taste acuity occurred following stopping and starting replacement therapy with carbohydrate-active steroids, metabolic balance studies were carried out in several patients with adrenocortical insufficiency (Fig. 4). The detection acuity of the patients was tested at least once daily for representatives of each of four taste qualities. This is shown in Fig. 5 for one patient (G.I.B.) for NaCl. A similar pattern of responses occurred in each patient for representatives of each of four taste qualities. Detection thresholds were first determined approximately one week after all replacement therapy had been withdrawn. At this time the patient's detection threshold for NaCl was 0.1 mmole/l, a level significantly lower than normal. After oral treatment with Δ_1F, 20 mg a day, her taste detection thresholds returned to normal within 48 h without significant alteration in her abnormal serum Na or K concentration or extracellular fluid volume, as represented by measurements of body weight. Treatment with Δ_1F continued for 10 days. During this time taste acuity remained within normal limits. At the end of

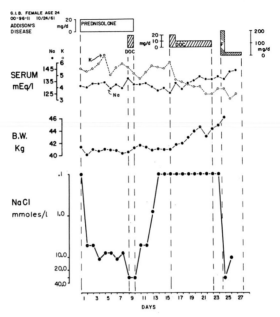

Fig. 4. Effects of Δ_1F, DOCA, hydrocortisone (F) and no treatment on serum Na and K concentrations, body weight and taste detection thresholds for NaCl in one patient with adrenocortical insufficiency. Threshold values for NaCl ranging from 6–60 mmoles/l are within normal limits. Serum concentration of Na between 135 and 145 mEq/l and of K between 3.5 and 4.5 mEq/l are considered within normal limits.

this period treatment with $\triangle_1$F was discontinued. Within 4 days her detection thresholds for NaCl fell from a normal threshold of 30 mmoles/l during treatment to a level of 0.1 mmole/l which is significantly below normal. These data demonstrate a lag period between the time treatment with carbohydrate-active steroids is stopped and the onset of increased detection acuity. Increased acuity does not occur immediately after treatment is discontinued but appears gradually over a period of 3 to 4 days. Additional experiments suggest that this lag period cannot be shortened (Henkin, unpublished observations). At the time when this patient's taste sensitivity increased to abnormal levels, there was no significant alteration either in her body weight, her hyponatremia or her hyperkalemia.

Six days after treatment with $\triangle_1$F was discontinued, the patient was given DOCA, intramuscularly, 20 mg a day for 2 days. Treatment with DOCA corrected her hyperkalemia and hyponatremia to normal and produced an increase in body weight of approximately 2 kg. In spite of these corrections to normal there was no alteration of her increased detection acuity for the taste of NaCl, or for three other taste qualities.

Within 24 h after 200 mg of hydrocortisone acetate (F) was given intravenously, taste detection thresholds for each taste quality returned to normal. This return of taste acuity to normal was not accompanied by a further increase in body weight or change in serum Na or K concentration.

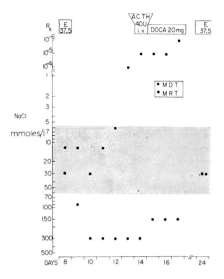

Fig. 5. Effect of cortisone acetate, DOCA, ACTH and no treatment on detection and recognition thresholds for NaCl in one patient with adrenocortical insufficiency. Threshold values for NaCl ranging from 6–60 mmoles/l are within normal limits for both sensory detection (■) and recognition (●). Note that with the termination of hormonal replacement there is a dichotomous *increase* in sensory detection acuity and a *decrease* in sensory integrative capacity. Solutions of NaCl as concentrated as 150 mmoles/l were called either sweet, bitter, sour or salty without specific pattern. Treatment with ACTH, 40 U i.v. over 8 h neither altered serum or urinary levels of carbohydrate-active steroid, nor taste detection or recognition thresholds. Treatment with DOCA, 20 mg intramuscularly, for two days did not alter this abnormal pattern. Only after treatment with carbohydrate-active steroids did both sensory phenomena return to normal. Similar results have been observed for three other taste qualities in this and other patients with this disease.

These data demonstrate the lag period not only between the termination of replacement therapy and the onset of increased taste acuity, but also between the beginning of replacement therapy with carbohydrate-active steroids and the return of taste acuity to normal. Approximately twice as much time is required for the increase in taste sensitivity to occur after treatment is discontinued as it is for sensitivity to return to normal after treatment with carbohydrate-active steroids is reinstituted.

These data also demonstrate that the return of taste sensitivity to normal is dose related, for after treatment with 20 mg of $\triangle_1F$ for 2 days taste acuity in G.I.B. returned to normal while it returned to normal within 24 h after treatment with 200 mg of F. In another patient whose daily maintenance dose of $\triangle_1F$ was 5.0 mg, treatment with 2.5 mg for 4 days did not return taste acuity to normal.

The mechanism by which these lag periods occur is not known. The period of 3–4 days before increased sensitivity occurs after carbohydrate-active steroids are discontinued varies little among the patients studied. This lag period is long if one considers that the half-life of most carbohydrate-active steroids is less than 24 h. These data suggest that even though significant carbohydrate-active steroid activity cannot be found in blood or urine of most patients 48 h after the administration of the last dose of steroid, tissue levels of hormone are still present and at least another 24 to 48 h are required before some tissue stores are depleted to a level such that

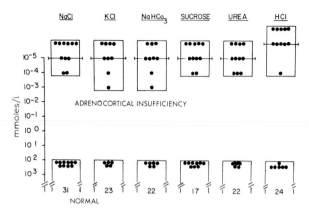

Fig. 6. Detection thresholds in normal volunteers (bottom) compared with those in patients with un-treated adrenocortical insufficiency (top) for the vapor above various solutions. The numbers at the bottom of the open enclosures indicate the number of normal volunteers who could not detect any difference between water and the vapor above the various solutions presented. The detection thresholds of the patients are significantly lower than those of the normal volunteers for each solution; there is also no overlap between the responses of each group.

increased detection sensitivity occurs. By contrast, physiological effects of Na–K-active steroids similarly evaluated demonstrate that 24 to 48 h after treatment with DOCA is discontinued in patients with adrenocortical insufficiency, some manifestations of hyperkalemia and hyponatremia can be observed. Since the half-life of these hormones is not more than 18–24 h, the onset of the effects of deficiency of these hormones seems consistent with our knowledge of the physiological chemistry of these hormones. The possible differences in tissue storage and release of Na–K-active and carbohydrate-active steroids is not well known but these observations may offer clues to some of the differences in their timing of action.

Coincident with the onset of increased taste detection acuity in patients with untreated adrenocortical insufficiency there was a significant decrease in taste recognition acuity. This manifested itself as a significant increase in median *recognition threshold** for each of 4 taste qualities at the same time that a significant decrease in each median detection threshold occurred. This is exemplified in one patient with adrenocortical insufficiency in Fig. 5. During treatment with carbohydrate-active steroids both detection and recognition thresholds for each taste quality were within normal limits. For convenience this is shown for NaCl only in Fig. 5. Following withdrawal of therapy there was the progressive decrease in median *detection threshold* shown previously. In addition there was a concomitant, progressive increase in median *recognition threshold*. Thus, at a time when detection acuity for NaCl was more than 1000 times more sensitive than normal, recognition ability, the ability to integrate sensory information about taste, was about five to ten times lower than normal. This dichotomy in responsiveness persisted as long as carbohydrate-active steroids were withheld. Treatment with DOCA, 20 mg daily for two days, altered.

---

* Median recognition threshold is the lowest concentration of solute and water appreciated as salty, sweet, bitter or sour for NaCl, sucrose, urea or HCl, respectively (Henkin *et al.*, 1963).

neither the lowered detection threshold nor the elevated recognition threshold. However, within 24 h after carbohydrate-active steroid therapy was resumed, detection and recognition thresholds for each taste quality returned to normal limits.

Taste in patients with adrenocortical hyperfunction

Since the absence of carbohydrate-active steroid has been associated with an increase in taste detection acuity it might be logical to hypothesize that excessive amounts of adrenocortical hormone produce a decrease in taste detection acuity. Indeed, taste detection acuity has been found to be below normal in each of five patients with Cushing's syndrome studied in our laboratory (Henkin, 1968). Each of these patients had excessive secretion of carbohydrate-active steroid due to the presence of adreno-cortical hyperplasia or adenoma. However, this aspect of taste–steroid relationship is not nearly as clear-cut or as well studied as that relating taste acuity to the absence of adrenocortical steroids. Treatment of normal subjects with large doses of various carbohydrate-active and/or Na–K-active steroids for periods of 5–8 days did not lower their taste detection sensitivity below normal (Henkin, unpublished). Also, endogenous secretion of excessive amounts of aldosterone from patients with aldo-steronomas or with nodular adrenocortical hyperplasia and hyperaldosteronism did not affect taste detection sensitivity significantly for any taste quality, although these patients often had marked abnormalities of serum sodium and potassium con-centration and of extracellular fluid volume (Henkin, unpublished).

The physiological role of carbohydrate-active steroid in regulation of taste detection acuity

The previous data suggest that the detection of gustatory stimuli is inversely related to the tissue concentration of carbohydrate-active steroids. Thus, these hormones normally appear to exert an inhibitory effect on taste detection sensitivity. If the concentration of carbohydrate-active steroid increases, as in Cushing's syndrome, there is a further increase in inhibition and a decrease in detection acuity. However, if the hormone is removed, this normal inhibition is removed and taste detection acuity increases to abnormally high levels.

This effect is not dissimilar in some ways to that exerted by the vagus nerve on heart rate. Normally, the vagus nerve controls heart rate through the inhibitory action of cholinergic fibers. An increase in vagal tone produces a decrease in heart rate, while removal of vagal tone produces an increase in heart rate. This inverse effect, inhibitory in nature, like that of carbohydrate-active steroid on taste acuity, is an example of a complex negative feedback system.

The regulation of taste detection sensitivity by carbohydrate-active steroid is not limited to abnormal disease states, such as adrenocortical insufficiency or Cushing's syndrome. Since adrenocortical hormones play a significant role in the control of many physiological processes, it is not surprising that they exert influences over many aspects of biochemical and physiological homeostasis which are experienced in normal as well as pathological physiology. One such role appears to be that which carbohydrate-active steroids play in association with periodic changes in the meta-bolic net. It is well known that there is a cyclic variation in the manner in which adrenocortical secretion occurs and this is reflected in cyclic changes in many of the physiological systems influenced by adrenocortical steroids. There are cyclic changes in eosinophil number, serum Na and K concentration, extracellular fluid volume and, of course, secretion of the various hormones and metabolic products of the adrenocortex itself. Since there is an intimate relationship between the se-cretion of carbohydrate-active steroid and taste detection acuity, it is not surprising that taste detection acuity varies over a 24-h period.

The peak excretion of adrenocortical hormone, as measured by urinary excretion of 17-hydroxycorticosteroids, aldosterone, or other urinary metabolites of carbo-hydrate-active steroid excretion, is approximately the same, around 3:00–4:00 a.m. These results have been confirmed by several investigators (Perkoff et al., 1959; Martin and Hellman, 1964; Wolf et al., 1966; Laatikainen and Vihko, 1968). Ex-periments to alter this timing have been performed, in which morphine, administered to normal volunteers to delay this peak, has blocked secretion of various adreno-cortical hormones for up to several hours (McDonald et al., 1959). Coincident with this increase in carbohydrate-active steroid secretion in the early morning, taste detection thresholds for NaCl have been shown to be at their highest level for the day. Later in the day there is a decrease in the secretion of carbohydrate-active steroid, accompanied by a gradual rise in taste sensitivity until a peak is reached. At this time, taste detection sensitivities, e.g., detection thresholds for NaCl, are at their lowest level of the day. Generally corresponding with the time that taste de-tection acuity is at its height is the time during which most of the population of the Western world eat their largest daily meal.*

There are indications that factors other than secretion of adrenocortical hormones may influence the circadian variation of taste detection sensitivity. When all adreno-cortical hormones are functionally absent, as in patients with untreated adreno-cortical insufficiency or after total adrenalectomy, there is little or no demonstrable circadian variation in taste detection acuity or in eosinophil number, serum sodium or potassium concentration. There may, however, be a continued variation in adreno-corticotrophin (ACTH) secretion (Martin and Hellman, 1964). After patients with adrenocortical insufficiency are treated with divided doses of exogenous carbo-hydrate-active steroid, the circadian variation in taste acuity is observed once again. These phenomena of circadian variation and the levels of organization which control the variation for taste acuity will be discussed in detail in another publication.

Other aspects of the general question of circadian variation as related to taste detection sensitivity deserve mention. Thresholds for NaCl in normal subjects vary during a 24-h period from 60 to 0.5 mmoles/l. During this time the measurements of variation in the secretion of adrenocortical hormones is relatively small, usually

---

* Reversal of the normal day–night work–sleep pattern has been associated with a reversal in the usual secretory pattern of adrenocortical hormones. Similar to this reversal there is a reversal of timing of changes in taste acuity in such patients (Henkin, unpublished).

less than a factor of 2 or 3. However, variations in taste sensitivity within each day may extend over a range as great as 100 or 2 log units. Curiously these circadian variations in taste are consistently greater for women than for men.

THE RELATIONSHIP BETWEEN ADRENOCORTICAL STEROIDS AND OLFACTION DETECTION SENSITIVITY

Olfactory detection in normal volunteers and in patients with adrenocortical insufficiency

To study olfactory acuity in normal volunteers and in patients with adrenocortical insufficiency, detection thresholds for various olfactory stimuli were obtained. In the initial experiments, the solutions used for olfactory stimuli were the same as those used as taste stimuli. Each volunteer or patient was required to sniff each of three bottles, two of which were water and one of which was an aqueous solution of a given concentration of NaCl, KCl, NaHCO₃, sucrose, urea or HCl. Median detection thresholds, *i.e.*, the least concentrated vapor detected as different from water, were obtained for each of these vapors (Henkin and Bartter, 1966).

The results of these studies carried out in patients with untreated adrenocortical insufficiency and in normal volunteers for the vapor above each of the solutions noted above are shown in Fig. 6. Most normal subjects could not discriminate between H₂O and any of the solutions while some could distinguish water from solutions as dilute as 150 mEq/l. These data also demonstrated that patients with untreated adrenocortical insufficiency, using olfactory clues alone, could detect differences between water and these various solutions at 1/10000, the concentration that normal

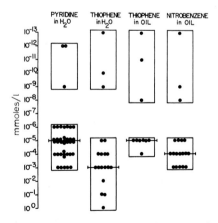

Fig. 7. Detection threshold in normal volunteers (bottom) compared with those in patients with untreated adrenocortical insufficiency (top) for the vapor above solutions of various concentrations of pyridine, thiophene and nitrobenzene. The detection thresholds of the patients are significantly lower than those of the normal volunteers for each vapor; there is also no overlap between the responses of each group.

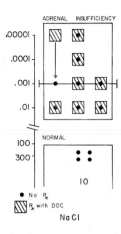

Fig. 8. Detection thresholds in normal volunteers compared with those in patients with adreno-cortical insufficiency treated with DOCA for the vapor above a solution of NaCl. The hatched squares which generally surround the detection thresholds determined in the patients indicate that there is no change in their lowered detection thresholds after this treatment. Data similar to that presented for NaCl were obtained with solutions representative of each taste quality and for pyridine, nitrobenzene and thiophene.

subjects could. There was no overlap between the responses of the normal subjects and those of the untreated patients, similar to the results shown with gustatory stimuli. The median detection threshold obtained among the untreated patients was approximately 1/100 the concentration they required to detect a difference between water and these solutions through the sense of taste.

Since detection of vapors above stimuli used to elicit taste responses are not those usually associated with olfactory detection, a further experiment was carried out in which stimuli generally considered odorous were used. Differences in the detection of vapors above water and pyridine, water and thiophene, mineral oil and thiophene and mineral oil and nitrobenzene were obtained using techniques similar to those used previously (Henkin and Bartter, 1966). As in the previous studies, patients with untreated adrenocortical insufficiency detected each solute in significantly lower concentration than did normal volunteers (Fig. 7). Differences between the acuity of patients with adrenocortical insufficiency and normal volunteers to detect vapors which have a significant vapor pressure is of the same order of magnitude as differences in their acuity to detect vapors above solutions which are not considered odoriferous and are not thought of as having significant vapor pressure. The difference in sensitivity is approximately 10^4.

Fig. 8 illustrates that increases in olfactory detection sensitivity do not return to normal after treatment of patients with adrenocortical insufficiency with Na–K-active steroids. In these experiments, daily intramuscular injections of 20 mg of DOCA were given to 7 patients with adrenocortical insufficiency for 2 to 10 days without any alteration in their olfactory detection sensitivity, although there were increases in their body weight and correction of their hyponatremia and hyperkalemia toward normal levels. This is shown in Fig. 8 for the detection of NaCl in water.

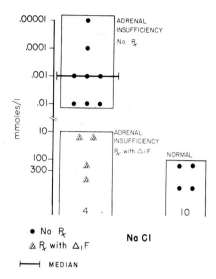

Fig. 9. Detection thresholds in normal volunteers compared with those in patients with adrenocortical insufficiency treated with Δ_1F for the vapor above a solution of NaCl. The hatched triangles indicate that after treatment thresholds obtained in the patients are not significantly different from those in normal volunteers. Four of the eight patients could no longer detect any difference between water and the vapor above a solution of NaCl. Data similar to that presented here were also obtained with solutions representative of each taste quality and for pyridine, nitrobenzene and thiophene.

Similar results occurred after presentation of each of the other solutions noted previously. There was no overlap between the responses of the patients and those of the normal subjects.

Fig. 9 illustrates that treatment of patients with adrenocortical insufficiency with carbohydrate-active steroid returned olfactory detection sensitivity to normal. Treatment with Δ_1F, 20 mg a day, returned sensitivity to the normal range within 24 h. The figure illustrates that 4 of the 7 treated patients could no longer detect any difference between a solution of NaCl as concentrated as 300 mmoles/l and two solutions of water. Thus, treatment with carbohydrate-active steroid returned taste sensitivity as well as olfactory sensitivity to normal. Similar results were obtained after the presentation of stimuli generally considered odorous as well as with those stimuli generally considered nonodorous.

Fig. 10 illustrates a detailed study carried out in one patient with adrenocortical insufficiency in whom changes in taste and olfaction were correlated with changes in serum electrolytes and body fluids after treatment with various adrenal steroid hormones. This study is representative of the type of study carried out in several patients with adrenocortical insufficiency. Taste data from a similar study previously carried out in this patient were illustrated in Fig. 4.

Treatment with a maintenance dose of 0.75 mg of dexamethasone produced normal taste and smell detection thresholds for NaCl, normal body weight and normal serum concentrations of Na and K. After treatment with dexamethasone was discontinued and treatment with DOCA, 20 mg a day was begun, there was no change observed

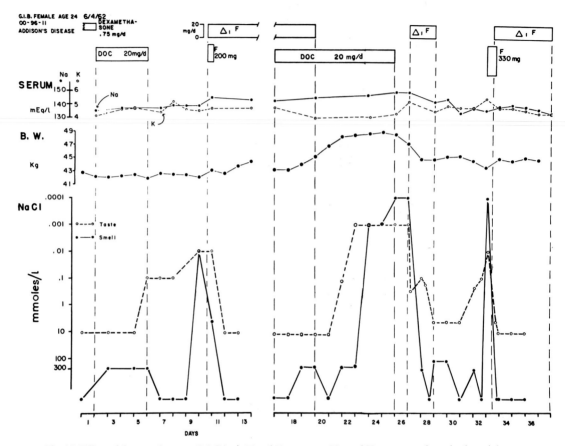

Fig. 10. Effect of dexamethasone, DOCA, Δ_1F and F on serum Na and K concentrations, body weight and taste and smell thresholds for NaCl in one patient with adrenocortical insufficiency. Threshold values for the vapor above a solution of NaCl equal to or greater than 150 mmoles/l are within normal limits.

in serum Na or K concentrations or in weight; however, within 4 days after dexa-methasone was discontinued, taste detection thresholds for NaCl decreased to the same abnormally low levels previously observed (Fig. 5). Seven days after carbo-hydrate-active steroids were discontinued there was a significant decrease in olfactory detection thresholds. Treatment with Δ_1F, 20 mg a day, returned smell sensitivity to normal within 24 h, while an additional 12 h were required before taste sensitivity returned to the normal range. This study was then repeated to document once again the timing of these changes (the second half of Fig. 10). Taste and smell thresholds were both significantly lower than normal at the beginning of this portion of the study, for the patient had been without treatment for 9 days. Treatment with carbohydrate-active steroid once again returned taste and smell detection thresholds to normal with smell detection returning to normal first, followed by a return of taste detection to normal approximately 12 h later. Withdrawal of treatment with carbohydrate-active steroids once again produced an increase in taste detection sensitivity, this time within 3 days after treatment was stopped. This was a full 24 h earlier than noted in the first part of the study. An additional 2 days without treatment with carbohydrate-active steroids were required before smell detection sensitivity increased to abnormally low levels. This time period was 24 h shorter than that observed during the first part of the study in which carbohydrate-active steroids were withdrawn. Treatment with carbohydrate-active steroids once again returned smell sensitivity to normal approximately 12 h after treatment was initiated. This was 12 h before taste sensitivity returned to normal, which was similar to that noted in the previous study.

The time required for changes in sensory acuity to occur is probably dependent upon depletion of tissue concentration of these hormones, as noted previously. Perhaps depletion of tissue stores of carbohydrate-active steroid takes place over a number of days and if tissue sites are not fully repleted, depletion might occur more quickly. The onset of increased olfactory detection acuity occurred consistently in this patient two to three days after taste detection hypersensitivity occurred. Treatment with carbohydrate-active steroids also returned olfactory detection thresholds to normal within 12 to 24 h, a shorter time than observed for the return of taste hypersensitivity to normal.

The basis for these differences in timing of changes in detection acuity is not known. However, it is possible that carbohydrate-active steroids may persist for a longer time in those tissues involved with olfaction than in those tissues which mediate taste. More time may be required for the hormone stores to be metabolized and utilized prior to the onset of increased olfactory detection sensitivity in those tissues which mediate olfaction than in those which mediate gustation. In addition, once these stores are utilized they may be replaced more readily than tissue stores of the gustatory system when carbohydrate-active steroid becomes available again. This differential sensitivity may relate to the manner by which different parts of the nervous system metabolize and bind carbohydrate-active steroid.

Although it is unusual to consider that either normal volunteers or patients with untreated adrenocortical insufficiency can detect NaCl or other substances normally considered nonodorous by olfactory cues alone, many macrosomatic animals detect various stimuli by olfactory cues. This question has been considered previously by several observers who noted the "odor" of "nonodorous" substances such as sugar (Andres, 1953) various metals (Raub, 1934) clay and rocks (Bear and Thomas, 1964) and various minerals (Halla and Van Tassel, 1956; Haler, 1954). In an effort to evaluate the physiological basis of this phenomenon, olfactory and chemical studies with two different radionuclides of NaCl were carried out. The results of these studies described in detail elsewhere (Henkin and Bartter, 1966) indicate that there is a vapor phase above a solution of NaCl and that this is made primarily of chlorine gas. It is this gas which is the stimulus for olfactory detection in both normal subjects and patients with adrenocortical insufficiency.

References pp. 292–293

THE RELATIONSHIP BETWEEN ADRENOCORTICAL STEROIDS AND AUDITORY DETECTION AND PERCEPTION

Auditory detection acuity in normal volunteers and in patients with adrenocortical insufficiency

Auditory detection acuity was measured in 15 normal subjects aged 18 to 26 (mean age, 21.6), in 10 normal subjects aged 39 to 61 (mean age, 47.1) and in 8 patients with adrenocortical insufficiency. Four of the patients, aged 19 to 52, had adrenocortical insufficiency due to Addison's disease or subsequent to adrenalectomy; four, aged 14 to 57, had adrenocortical insufficiency secondary to panhypopituitarism. Auditory sensitivity was measured in the same manner in both subjects and patients by each of two investigators, one of whom participated in the study without knowledge of the identity or the treatment given to the subjects or patients. Each subject and patient was seated alone, comfortably, in an arm chair, in an Industrial Acoustic Corporation Model 1204 double-walled sound chamber. Auditory signals were provided by a Southwestern Industrial Electronics M-2 R-C audio-oscillator attenuated by a Model 350-B Hewlett–Packard attenuator and delivered through Knight KN848 circum-aural earphones. Auditory signals were delivered in a standard manner by a variation of the method of limits. The details of this procedure have been previously presented (Henkin *et al.*, 1967).

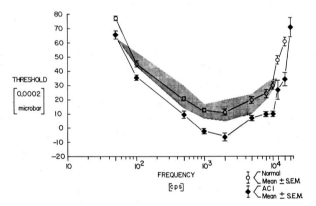

Fig. 11. Comparison of auditory detection thresholds for sinusoidal stimuli in normal subjects with those in patients with untreated adrenocortical insufficiency. The ordinate is scaled in absolute sound pressure units of microbars, referable to 0.0002 dynes/cm²; the abscissa is scaled in frequency units of cycles per sec [Hertz (Hz)]. The borders of the cross-hatched area indicate the upper and lower limits of detection responsiveness of a large number of normal subjects determined by three groups of investigators under various conditions (Sivian and White, 1933; Von Békésy, 1953; Steinberg *et al.*, 1940). The open circles within this cross-hatched area illustrate the mean detection thresholds obtained in a group of normal volunteers, under the conditions used for the present studies. The lines extending above and below these circles indicate ± 1 S.E.M. The data obtained in normal subjects in the present studies fall within the rather large variation usually considered normal. The black diamonds below the cross hatched area illustrate the mean detection thresholds obtained in 8 patients with untreated adrenocortical insufficiency and panhypopituitarism. The lines extending above and below these symbols indicate ± 1 S.E.M. The thresholds obtained in the untreated patients are significantly lower than those found in the normal subjects for all frequencies above 100 cps.

Fig. 11 shows the auditory thresholds to sinusoidal stimuli in normal volunteers and in patients with untreated adrenocortical insufficiency. The normal range of hearing acuity is shown by the hatched area. The mean lower limit of frequency response obtained in the normal subjects under the conditions used in this study was 50 Hertz (Hz); the mean upper limit of responsiveness frequency was 15 500 Hz. The most sensitive frequencies for auditory detection for the normal subjects were between 1000 and 4000 Hz. Comparison of the responses of the normal volunteers with those of the untreated patients showed that there was a significant increase in the range of frequency responsiveness of the patients. This was particularly apparent at the upper limits of the frequency range, where the patients detected a signal approximately 3500 Hz higher than the normal subjects. These responses are, of course, dependent upon the particular method used to determine these thresholds as noted previously (Henkin *et al.*, 1967). The auditory detection thresholds of the patients were also significantly below those of the normal subjects, particularly in the range where hearing sensitivity is most acute, between 1000 and 4000 Hz. However, this increase in acuity in the untreated patients extended over most of the frequency range above 5000 Hz.

Fig. 12 illustrates that treatment of the patients with adrenocortical insufficiency with DOCA, carried out in experiments similar to those previously described for the sensory modalities of taste and olfaction, neither raised their auditory detection thresholds significantly nor decreased their frequency response range, although it did return serum Na and K concentration to normal and increased extracellular fluid volume.

Treatment of the patients with adrenocortical insufficiency with carbohydrate-active steroid returned auditory detection thresholds to normal limits after treatment with 20 mg of $\triangle_1 F$ for as little as 2 days (Fig. 13). This return encompassed both a

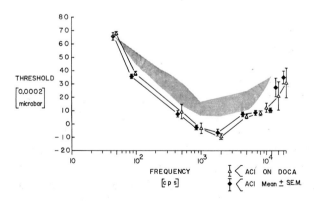

Fig. 12. Comparison of auditory detection threshold for sinusoidal stimuli in normal subjects with those in patients with adrenocortical insufficiency treated with DOCA. The presentation of the data is similar to that used in Fig. 11. The open triangles, which are generally next to the lower closed diamonds, indicate that treatment of the patients with DOCA does not alter the already lowered auditory detection acuity.

References pp. 292–293

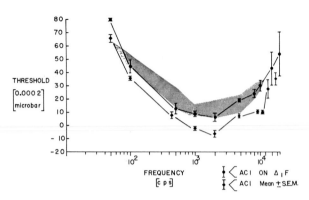

Fig. 13. Comparison of auditory detection thresholds for sinusoidal stimuli in normal subjects with those in patients with adrenocortical insufficiency treated with Δ_1F. The presentation of the data is similar to that used in Figs. 11 and 12. The closed circles within the hatched area illustrate the auditory detection thresholds obtained in the patients after treatment with Δ_1F. Note that these circles are all within the hatched area and mean values cannot be distinguished from those of normal subjects,

diminution of the range of frequency response to normal and an increase in the intensity required to detect the auditory signals.

Auditory perception in normal volunteers and in patients with adrenocortical insufficiency

These results, and those obtained in taste and in olfaction indicate that removal of carbohydrate-active steroids is associated with a better than normal detection of sensory stimuli. Clinically, however, these patients do not function better than normal. Rather, they operate at an extremely low level of efficiency with many somatic and psychic complaints. Most patients without treatment with carbohydrate-active steroid for more than 48 h complained of severe joint and muscle aching. Lights from their hospital rooms and noises from the machines which cleaned the floors in the corridors produced responses of discomfort from the patients although these same stimuli were tolerated or not even noticed during treatment with carbohydrate-active steroid. In an effort to evaluate these less favorable effects of the removal of carbohydrate-active steroid, auditory perception ability was studied in patients with adrenocortical insufficiency simultaneously with the measurement of their detection acuity.

A general effect of the withdrawal of carbohydrate-active steroid on auditory acuity is illustrated in Fig. 14 in which the entire dynamic range of auditory responsiveness in normal subjects and in patients with untreated adrenocortical insufficiency is compared. This dynamic range refers to the range of intensity of auditory sound over which humans respond. The lower limit of this range is that sound which is just detected as different from silence while the upper limit of this range is that sound which just produces an acoustical pain. In normal subjects this range extends over approximately 80 dB. Fig. 14 shows that patients with untreated adrenocortical insufficiency exhibit a compression of this dynamic range of hearing. They exhibit a significant increase in hearing sensitivity at the lower or threshold end of the sensitivity

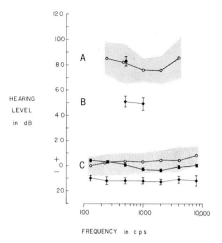

Fig. 14. Comparison of audiometric thresholds and contralateral threshold shifts (CTS) in normal subjects with those in patients with adrenocortical insufficiency, off treatment. A, open circles; mean CTS determined in 44 normal subjects, aged 15–34, by Jepson (1963); the upper and lower limits of the upper gray area represent the range of these responses (*ibid.*). The closed circle within the upper gray area represents the CTS determined in the 20 normal subjects of this study. The lines above and below this closed circle represent ± 1 S.E.M. Data for the CTS at 500 cps in the subjects of this study are similar to that obtained by Jepson. B, closed diamonds: mean CTS obtained in this study of 12 patients with adrenocortical insufficiency, off treatment, aged 19–57; the lines above and below these rectangles represents ± 1 S.E.M. C, open circles: mean audiometric thresholds in normal subjects obtained by Jepson (1963), the lower gray area, the range of these thresholds. Closed blocks within the lower gray area: audiometric thresholds obtained in the normal subjects of this study, closed diamonds below the lower gray area: audiometric thresholds obtained in patients with adrenocortical insufficiency, off treatment, with ± 1 S.E.M. At each frequency, both mean audiometric threshold and CTS for the patients with adrenocortical insufficiency were significantly below those of either group of normal subjects.

scale but there is a more than compensatory decrease in sensitivity at the upper limit of hearing which restricts rather than expands their sensitivity range. The increase in sensitivity at detection threshold is approximately 10 to 12 dB while the decrease in sensitivity at the pain threshold is approximately 20 dB. Thus the total dynamic range over which auditory activity occurs in patients with untreated adrenocortical insufficiency is approximately 70 dB compared to the range of 80 dB in normal volunteers. Thus, in the untreated patients, the dynamic auditory range was decreased by approximately 10 dB or a factor of 2. This indicates that while auditory detection sensitivity is significantly greater than normal in patients with adrenocortical insufficiency, their responsiveness is less than normal over the entire auditory spectrum.

An example of another type of abnormality which these patients exhibit after treatment with carbohydrate-active steroid is withdrawn is an impairment of integration of auditory information. To study these abnormalities standardized lists of 50 phonetically balanced (PB) words were presented to patients with untreated cortical insufficiency 40 and 60 dB above each patient's detection threshold at 1000 Hz under standardized conditions. These conditions have been described elsewhere in detail (Henkin and Daly, 1968). These words were also presented to the patients after they were treated with DOCA and with $\triangle_1$F. The results of these experiments ex-

TABLE I

SPEECH DISCRIMINATION ABILITY IN NORMAL VOLUNTEERS AND IN PATIENTS WITH
ADRENOCORTICAL INSUFFICIENCY

Comparison of responses to PB and LPFS lists of words in normal volunteers and in patients with untreated adrenocortical insufficiency and panhypopituitarism, and after treatment with DOCA, Δ_1F and ACTH. The results recorded after treatment with carbohydrate-active steroids among patients with panhypopituitarism are the same as those obtained in normal subjects.

Subjects	*PB Words*		*LPFS words*	
	40	*60*	*40*	*60*
		% correct		
Normal volunteers	92 ± 1.2*	97 ± 0.6	31 ± 1.7	54 ± 1.6
Adrenocortical insufficiency, untreated	63 ± 5.2†	88 ± 2.8††	6 ± 1.6†	23 ± 2.5†
Adrenocortical insufficiency, treated with DOCA	64 ± 5.2†	89 ± 1.3††	7 ± 2.2†	23 ± 3.6†
Adrenocortical insufficiency, treated with carbohydrate-active steroid	89 ± 3.0	96 ± 3.1	31 ± 2.0	56 ± 3.3
Addison's disease (partial) or panhypopituitarism after treatment with ACTH, 40 U/day, 4th day	86 ± 4.2	95 ± 0.7	28 ± 4.2	47 ± 10.1

PB, phonetically balanced word lists presented 40 and 60 dB above detection threshold determined at 1000 cps.
LPFS, low pass filtered speech word lists presented 40 and 60 dB above detection threshold determined at 1000 cps.
* Mean ± S.E.M.
ACTH, adrenocorticotrophin.
† $P < 0.01$ with respect to results of normal volunteers or after treatment with carbohydrate-active steroids.
†† $P < 0.01$ with respect to results of normal volunteers; $P < 0.02$ with respect to results after treatment with carbohydrate-active steroids.

pressed in terms of the per cent of the number of words each patient was able to recognize correctly are shown in Table I. Under similar conditions other sets of standardized lists of words from which frequencies above 500 cps had been selectively filtered out (Von Békesy, 1953) were also presented. These lists, called the low pass filtered speech (LPFS) were also presented 40 dB and 60 dB above each patient's detection threshold at 1000 Hz in a standard manner (Henkin and Daly, 1968).

The untreated patients correctly recognized approximately 60% of the words from the PB lists presented 40 dB above threshold and only 89% when presented 60 dB above threshold. After treatment with DOCA, there was no significant change in responsiveness at either loudness level. However, after treatment with Δ_1F, 20 mg daily for 48 h, responsiveness increased to 89% and 96% for the lists presented 40 and 60 dB above thresholds, respectively. These responses are not significantly different from those obtained in normal subjects (Henkin and Daly, 1968). Intravenous therapy for 5 days with 40 units of ACTH to two patients with panhypopituitarism and to one with relative adrenocortical insufficiency also returned word recognition and adrenocortical function to normal (Table I). These results demonstrate that without treatment, the patients were less able to recognize words than were normal subjects, that treatment with DOCA did not improve their ability and that only treatment with carbohydrate-active steroid returned auditory integration to normal.

A response pattern even more strikingly abnormal than that for the PB words occurred following the presentation of the LPFS words. In the untreated and the DOCA-treated condition there was a more significant impairment in word recognition ability of the patients with adrenocortical insufficiency when compared to the ability of normal subjects. Treatment with DOCA did not improve this severe disability although treatment with $\triangle_1 F$ returned responsiveness to normal.

This inability to recognize words occurred at the same time that other recognition or "integrative" abnormalities occurred. These patients were unable to localize sound stimuli when presented more than 30 degrees from either side of the midline; however, they made correct localization judgments if the stimuli were presented in the midline (Henkin and Daly, 1968). They had difficulty in judgement of the time at which an amplitude-modulated tone changed its character as it was amplified over a range of just noticeable increments from 1 to 5 dB (Henkin and Daly, 1968). Their ability to judge the loudness of tones presented alternately to each ear was also severely impaired when untreated, but returned to normal after treatment with carbohydrate-active steroid was resumed (Henkin and Daly, 1968).

These data indicate that patients with untreated adrenocortical insufficiency exhibit a significant impairment in their ability to recognize or "integrate" auditory information. Although off treatment they can detect auditory signals at significantly lower levels than can normal subjects, they fail to integrate this information normally.

The increase in sensory detection acuity after the removal of carbohydrate-active steroid is associated with a consistent decrease in sensory perception or integration ability for several sensory stimuli. Associated with the return to normal sensory detection acuity after the reinstitution of carbohydrate-active steroid, is a consistent increase in sensory integration ability for these same diverse sensory signals. These phenomena describe in behavioral terms some important aspects of a general mechanism of nervous system function.

These data suggest that a specific relationship exists at all times between sensory detection and perception. Detection is normally set at a "low gain" in man to allow maximal integration of all incoming sensory stimuli. This is one of the important features which distinguishes man from lower animals. Many other species can detect various sensory signals more acutely than man by taste, smell, hearing, seeing, and feeling. However, none operate on the signals more efficiently than does man. Thus, if carbohydrate-active steroids play a significant role in the control of the input of sensory stimuli through a negative feedback mechanism, then removal of carbohydrate-active steroid would significantly alter the normal gain control mechanism; the nervous system would literally be bombarded with sensory stimuli which normally would be rejected. This would occur in the nervous system at the expense of stimulus integration.

A reinterpretation of the data obtained from studies dealing with sensory deprivation (Schultz, 1965) or various forms of "schizophrenia" (Silverman, 1964) suggest that a similar dissociation between sensory detection and integration may be inferred. Various steroid abnormalities have been hypothesized as one of the causes of some "schizophrenias" (Hoagland *et al.*, 1953). Conversely, one small class of patients who have been called "schizophrenic" have in reality suffered from untreated adrenocortical insufficiency. These patients almost uniformly returned to normal mental function after treatment with carbohydrate-active steroids has been instituted. Similarly, the psychotomimetic-like effects of LSD have been shown to be associated with increases in the ability to detect sensory signals yet decreases in the ability to integrate these signals (Henkin *et al.*, 1967).

SUMMARY

Sensory detection and integration are regulated by a complex feedback system involving the interaction of the endocrine and the nervous system. Studies in man and in other animals have demonstrated that after removal of all adrenocortical hormone activity there is a significant increase in ability to detect sensory signals through the modalities of taste, olfaction, audition and proprioception. For taste, detection of each of four qualities is increased by a factor of at least 100; for olfaction, detection of various odorants, some previously considered to be without significant vapor pressure, is increased by a factor of at least 1000. For audition, detection of sinusoidal signals is increased by at least 13 decibels, particularly between 1000 Hz and 4000 Hz, in the most sensitive region of auditory acuity. Treatment of patients with adrenocortical insufficiency with Na–K-active steroids such as DOCA does not alter this increased sensory detection acuity although it does reverse the abnormal electrolyte balance present. Thus, the hyperkalemia, hyponatremia and decreased extracellular fluid concentration observed in patients with untreated adrenocortical insufficiency returns to normal without any alteration in their increased sensory acuity. Treatment with carbohydrate-active steroids alone returns sensory detection acuity to normal for each sensory modality.

Studies of patients with Cushing's syndrome, who exhibit excessive adrenal secretion of carbohydrate-active steroids, reveal a significant decrease in sensory detection acuity for the sensory modalities of taste, olfaction, audition and proprioception. Suppression of endogenous carbohydrate-active steroid secretion by treatment with exogenous steroid hormones, aminoglutethamide, or by removing the adrenal glands surgically followed by adequate steroid replacement results in a return to normal sensory detection acuity.

These studies indicate that removal of carbohydrate-active steroids allows an increase in sensory detection acuity to occur, while excessive carbohydrate-active steroid production produces a decrease in sensory detection acuity. Further studies indicate that coincident with the removal of carbohydrate-active steroids there is a significant decrease in sensory integration for the sensory modalities of taste and audition. For taste, recognition of each of four qualities is decreased by a factor of 100; for audition, recognition of various signals is markedly impaired. For audition, this impairment involves losses of ability to understand speech, changes in tonal quality, localization of tonal stimuli, and judgment of bilateral equal loudness. Treatment with Na–K-active steroids does not alter these decreases in sensory perception ability, similar to its failure to alter increases in sensory detection acuity. However, treatment with this class of steroids does return the abnormal electrolyte balance to normal, as previously observed. Treatment with carbohydrate-active steroids returns sensory perception ability to normal for taste and audition at a time when sensory detection acuity also returns to normal.

These reciprocal changes in sensory detection and perception occur in physiological as well as pathological conditions. There is a circadian pattern of change in taste detection and recognition acuity in normal subjects such that when carbohydrate-active steroid secretion is at its lowest level, taste detection acuity is at its highest and taste recognition is at its lowest. When carbohydrate-active steroid secretion is at its highest level, taste detection acuity is at its lowest while taste recognition is at its highest.

These reciprocal changes in sensory detection and perception have been related to changes in the manner by which carbohydrate-active steroids influence the metabolism of neural tissue. Carbohydrate-active steroids are a normal component of neural tissue. Following adrenalectomy, the concentration of these steroids in tissues of the central and peripheral nervous systems decreases significantly. This decrease is associated with an alteration in the manner by which neural impulses are conducted along axons and across synapses; conduction velocity along peripheral axons is significantly increased above normal while conduction across synapses is significantly prolonged. This results in a marked change in the timing by which neural stimuli from the periphery reach the higher integrative centers of the nervous system. It is this alteration in perception of the timed arrival of the sensory signals from the periphery that is hypothesized as the mechanism for the loss of perceptual ability observed in adrenocortical insufficiency. Associated with this alteration in timing is an alteration in excitability of the nervous system such that stimuli which normally would be rejected as subthreshold produce depolarizations of neurons. This increase in neural excitability by which normally subthreshold stimuli are appreciated, albeit in an abnormal manner, is hypothesized as the mechanism for the increase of sensory detection acuity observed in adrenocortical insufficiency.

These results indicate that carbohydrate-active steroids play a significant role in the manner by which sensation and perception occur. Normally, carbohydrate-active steroids act in an inhibitory manner in both the central and peripheral nervous systems; their presence inhibits both the detection and perception of incoming sensory signals. Their removal releases this inhibition and sensory detection and perception change in the manner described above. It appears that reciprocal changes in detection acuity and perceptual ability are related such that increases in detection acuity are always associated with decreases in perceptual ability.

Further studies have confirmed these hypotheses. Administration of various drugs, such as lysergic acid diethylamide (LSD-25), is associated with increases in sensory detection acuity and decreases in perceptual ability, a result which is in keeping with our subjective knowledge of the action of this drug. Coincident with these results there are changes in the urinary excretion of various steroid hormones.

These studies demonstrate that sensory detection and perception are regulated by a complex feedback system involving the interaction of the endocrine and the nervous system.

REFERENCES

ANDRES, P. (1953) Beitrag zur Frage: Kann Zucker riechen? *Z. Zuckerindust.*, **78**, 319–320.

BEAR, I. B. AND THOMAS, R. G. (1964) Nature of argillaceous odour. *Nature*, **201**, 993–995.

BOTT, E., DENTON, D. A. AND WELLERS, S. (1967) The innate appetite for salt exhibited by sodium-deficient sheep. In *Olfaction and Taste*, Vol. II, T. HAYASHI (Ed.), Pergamon Press, London.

CAMERON, A. T. (1947) The taste sense and the relative sweetness of sugars and other sweet substances. *Sugar Res. Found., Sci. Rept. Ser.*, No. 9.

CRAGG, L. H. (1937) The sour taste; threshold values and accuracy, the effects of saltiness and sweetness. *Trans Roy. Soc. Can.*, Sect. III, 31 (3), 131.

HALER, D. (1954) Does iron smell? *Lancet*, **267**, 143.

HALLA, F. AND VAN TASSEL, R. (1956) Geruch von Gesteinsfunken. *Naturwiss.*, **43**, 344.

HARRIS, H. AND KALMUS, H. (1949) Genetical differences in taste sensitivity to phenylthiourea and to anti-thyroid substances. *Nature*, **163**, 878.

HENKIN, R. I. (1967) Taste and Disease. In *The Chemical Senses and Nutrition*, M. R. KARE AND O. MALLER (Ed.), Johns Hopkins University Press, Baltimore, Md.

HENKIN, R. I. (1968) The neuroendocrine control of perception. In *Perception*, D. HAMBURG (Ed.), *Proc. Assoc. Res. Nervous Mental Disease*, 32, William & Wilkins Co., Baltimore.

HENKIN, R. I. AND BARTTER, F. C. (1966) Studies on olfactory thresholds in normal man and in patients with adrenal insufficiency: the role of adrenal cortical steroids and of serum sodium concentration, *J. Clin. Invest.*, **45**, 1631.

HENKIN, R. I., BUCHSBAUM, M., WELPTON, D., ZAHN, T., SCOTT, W., WYNNE, L. AND SILVERMAN, J. (1967) Physiological and psychological effects of LSD in chronic users. *Clin. Res.*, 484.

HENKIN, R. I. AND DALY, R. L. (1968) Auditory detection and perception in normal man and in patients with adrenal cortical insufficiency. *J. Clin. Invest.*, **47**, 1259.

HENKIN, R. I., GILL, JR., J. R. AND BARTTER, F. C. (1963) Studies on taste thresholds in normal man and in patients with adrenal cortical insufficiency: the role of adrenal cortical steroids and of serum sodium concentration. *J. Clin. Invest.*, **42**, 727.

HENKIN, R. I., McGLONE, R. E., DALY, R. L. AND BARTTER, F. C. (1967) Studies on auditory thresholds in normal man and in patients with adrenal cortical insufficiency: The role of adrenal cortical steroids, *J. Clin. Invest.*, **46**, 429,

HOAGLAND, H., BERGEN, J. R., SLOCOMBE, A. G. AND HUNT, C. A. (1953) Studies of adrenocortical physiology in relation to the nervous system in metabolic and toxic diseases of the nervous system, *Proc. Assoc. Res. Nervous Mental Disease*, 32, William & Wilkins Co., Baltimore.

JEPSON, O. (1963) Middle-ear muscle reflexes in man. In *Modern Developments in Audiology*, J. JERGER (Ed.), Academic Press, Inc., New York, p. 193.

KNOWLES, D. AND JOHNSON, P. E. (1941) A study of the sensitivities of prospective judges to the primary tastes. *Food Res.*, **6**, 207.

KOSOWICZ, J. AND PRUSZEWICZ, A. (1967) The "taste" test in adrenal insufficiency. *J. Clin. Endocrinol.*, **27**, 214.

LAATIKAINEN, T. AND VIHKO, R. (1968) Diurnal variation in the concentrations of solvalyzable steroids in human plasma. *J. Clin. Endocrinol. Metab.*, **28**, 1356–1360.

MARTIN, M. AND HELLMAN, D. E. (1964) Temporal variations in SU-4885 responsiveness in man: Evidence in support of circadian variation in ACTH secretion. *J. Clin. Endocrinol. Metab.*, **24**, 253–260.

McDONALD, R. K., EVANS, F. T., WEISE, V. K. AND PATRICK, R. W. (1959) Effect of morphine and nalorphine on plasma hydrocortisone levels in man. *J. Pharm. Exptl. Therap.*, **125**, 241–247.

PERKOFF, G. T., EIK-NES, K., NUGENT, C. A., FRED, H. L., NIMER, R. A., RUSH, L., SAMUELS, L. T.

AND TYLER, F. H. (1959) Studies of the diurnal variations of plasma 17-hydroxycorticosteroids in man. *J. Clin. Endocrinol. Metab.*, **19**, 432–443.

PFAFFMAN, C. (1959) The sense of taste. In *Handbook of Physiology, Neurophysiology*, vol. 1, American Physiological Assoc., Washington, D.C.

PRUSZEWICZ, A. AND KOSOWICZ, J. (1966) Quantitative and qualitative studies of the taste and smell in adrenal insufficiency. *Endokrynol. Polska*, **17**, 321–327. (Pol.).

RAUB, E. (1934) Die Entstehung des Metallgeruchs und Geschmacks. *Z. Angew. Chem.*, **47**, 673–675.

SCHULTZ, D. P. (1965) *Sensory Restriction: Effects on Behavior*, Academic Press, Inc., New York.

SCHUTZ, H. G. AND PILGRIM, J. F. (1957) Sweetness of various compounds and its measurement. *Food Res.*, **22**, 206.

SILVERMAN, J. (1964) Perceptual control of stimulus intensity in paranoid and nonparanoid schizophrenia. *J. Nervous Mental Disease*, **139**, 545.

SIVIAN, L. J. AND WHITE, S. D. (1933) On minimum audible sound fields. *J. Acoust. Soc. Amer.*, **4**, 288.

STEINBERG, J. C., MONTGOMERY, H. C. AND GARDNER, M. B. (1940) Results of the World's Fair hearing tests. *J. Acoust. Soc. Amer.*, **12**, 291.

VON BÉKÉSY, G., cited in H. FLETCHER (1953) *Speech and Hearing in Communication*, Van Nostrand, New York, p. 132.

WOLF, L. K., GORDON, R. K., ISLAND, D. P. AND LIDDLE, G. W. (1966) An analysis of factors determining the circadian pattern of aldosterone excretion, *J. Clin. Endocrinol. Metab.*, **26**, 1261.

DISCUSSION

SACHAR: Could you elaborate more on the sensory responses seen in Cushing's patients?

HENKIN: The administration of exogenous steroids to normal volunteers, as much as 50 mg of prednisone for as long as 5 days, did not significantly affect detection or recognition thresholds for any sensory modality. However, patients with Cushing's syndrome who have been exposed to the elevated levels of their own endogenous steroid hormones for a long time respond in a different manner: *i.e.*, their ability to detect and recognize sensory signals is markedly altered. Instead of exhibiting a detection threshold of 10^{-4} or 10^{-2} mM/l, their thresholds were 150–300 mM/l. In addition, they exhibit an inability to integrate these sensory signals, as do patients with Addison's disease. In patients with Cushing's syndrome axonal conduction velocity is slower than normal and the time across the synapse is also altered. They exhibit the same kind of information loss as do Addisonian's and therefore you would expect them to have the same kind of abnormality in terms of their integration of sensory signals, and they do. Patients with Cushing's syndrome add a great deal of sugar and salt to their food in order to get the taste of sweet or salt. This inability to taste or smell can be among the very first clues that the patient has Cushing's syndrome.

LARON: Did you test various cortisone analogues? I would like to know how they correlate in their action on the sensory system as we might expect differences in kind and degree of effect. And have you tested patients with other mono-hormone deficiencies, like GH or TSH deficiency?

HENKIN: We have looked at a number of cortisone analogues such as dexamethasone, hydrocortisone and prednisolone. It seems to be irrelevant as to which carbohydrate-active steroid is used, because all carbohydrate-active steroids seem to act in the same manner with respect to altering sensory detection and perception. The only difference among these analogues lies in the timing with which thresholds return to normal and this seems to be correlated with the carbohydrate activity of the steroid; *i.e.*, the more potent the carbohydrate activity, the faster the return to normal. Each sodium–potassium-active steroid used had no effect in returning thresholds to normal. To answer your second question, patients with other hormonal defects do exhibit sensory abnormalities. Patients with acromegaly have decreased taste acuity for the detection and recognition of each taste quality. The mechanism of this defect probably differs from that observed in patients with Cushing's syndrome and this phenomenon will be discussed in full in a paper to be published soon. Patients with thyroid disease may exhibit decreased taste acuity of a specific type; *e.g.*, some patients with athyreotic cretinism have been found to exhibit an inability to taste phenylthiourea (PTU) as bitter. However, this observation has not been well studied in terms of their ability or inability to detect or recognize other taste qualities.

McClure: Do you feel that the conduction responses that you refer to, are due in any way to the interaction of cortisol with biogenic amines at the synapses?

Henkin: I am sure that the phenomenon is very complex and it is impossible to say that any of these symptoms are due to carbohydrate-active steroids alone. You raise a very important point, one that we are concerned with and pursuing at the present time.

Denton: In relation to your very fascinating data, there is one point on which I would like to hear your comment. You will recall that subsequent to Richter's original observation that the preference threshold for NaCl in the rat was lowered by adrenalectomy, the electrophysiological investigations showed that there was no change in electric threshold as determined by single fibre recording (Pfaffman).

Henkin: That is a complex story. First of all, the rat is very different from the human in terms of his taste, neural and adrenal responses. By that I mean, an adrenalectomized rat can be maintained for as long as you wish by giving him salt water while a human can not. The nerve of an adrenalectomized rat shows increased excitability. This can be returned to normal by administration of DOCA, salt or hydrocortisone. In this sense, the rat is a poor specimen to compare with man for the situation is not analogous. There are other points we could raise. But it is enough for the moment to say that the animals Richter and Pfaffman have studied were all treated with large doses of salt during the time they were adrenalectomized. It is therefore impossible to evaluate their data without considering these physiological species differences.

Mirsky: Since both olfactory and a number of other modalities have a direct relationship to age, in terms of a rise of the threshold with age, have you controlled your data for the age effect?

Henkin: Each patient in these studies was used as his own control. In general, I do not think that one can say unequivocally that taste and smell thresholds are altered by age.

Klein: Do you have any measurements of synapses, other than nerve-to-muscle?

Henkin: We have looked at only one synapse other than the myoneural junction, that of the spinal cord in cat. Conduction across this single synapse was altered in the adrenalectomized cat when compared to the normal, intact cat.

Pituitary-Adrenal and Related Syndromes of Childhood: Effects on IQ and Learning *

JOHN MONEY

Department of Psychiatry and Behavioral Sciences and Department of Pediatrics, The Johns Hopkins University and Hospital, Baltimore, Md. 21205 (U.S.A.)

Whereas animals can be forced to submit to the contingencies of experimental design in order to test the influence of adrenocortical or other steroids on cognition and learning, human beings cannot. Whatever information one may obtain about these steroidal influences in man must be from clinical syndromes, that is from so-called experiments of nature, or from clinical investigative research with a therapeutic intention.

I propose in this paper to examine several clinical syndromes in which one may expect to find evidence, if such there be, of a relationship between intelligence and hormones, in particular those produced by the pituitary and adrenal cortex, especially in fetal life when the central nervous system is actively differentiating. I have, with many different colleagues over the years, been studying and following patients with these conditions since 1951 in the psychohormonal research unit at The Johns Hopkins Hospital.

CONGENITAL ADRENOGENITAL SYNDROME

This well known syndrome occurs in both males and females, the latter being genitally hermaphroditic. It has its origins initially in genetics, as an autosomal recessive, then in erroneous fetal hormonal functioning of the adrenal cortices, and finally in continuation of this same hormonal error postnatally. The postnatal error can be corrected by cortisone therapy, as was discovered in 1950. Since then a generation of patients has grown up without precocious and virilizing maturation of the physique. They constitute an important contrast group to compare with the older generation whose physical development was accelerated and virilized, irrespective of genetic sex.

To be able to compare these two groups is of value because of the overall finding of a tendency toward high IQ in the adrenogenital syndrome (Fig. 1 and Table 1). A comparison of 17 patients treated from infancy onward with 11 first treated after the age of 18 years showed no significant IQ difference between the two groups (Money and Lewis, 1966). Thus, one cannot ascribe the tendency to IQ elevation to premature somatic maturation alone.

* Supported in Research by Grants 2-K3-HD-18653 and 5-RD1-HD-00325, United States Public Health Service.

References p. 303

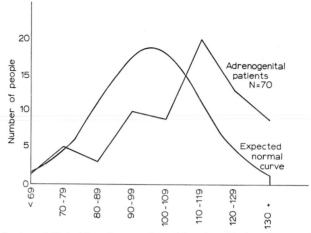

Fig. 1. Distribution of IQ in 70 patients, male and female, with the adrenogenital syndrome.

TABLE 1

DISTRIBUTION OF WECHSLER IQS, EXPECTED AND OBSERVED, IN 70 CASES OF THE ADRENO-
GENITAL SYNDROME

IQ Level	Expected Percentage	Observed Percentage	Expected Number	Observed Number	Expected Cumulative Percentage	Observed Cumulative Percentage
130+	2.2	*12.9*	1.5	9	2.2	*12.9*
120–129	6.7	*18.6*	5.0	13	8.9	*31.5*
110–119	16.1	*28.6*	11.0	20	25.0	*60.1*
100–109	25.0	12.8	17.5	9	50.0	72.9
90– 99	25.0	14.3	17.5	10	75.0	87.2
80– 89	16.1	4.3	11.0	3	91.1	91.5
70– 79	6.7	7.1	5.0	5	97.8	98.6
< 69	2.2	1.4	1.5	1	100.0	100.0

Italics show increased incidence of IQs above 110.

Various other comparisons of subgroups from among the total of 70 were carried out to give support to the conclusion that the finding of IQ elevation is not an artifact of sampling or other bias. Nor can it be ascribed to differential elevation of verbal *versus* nonverbal IQ (Lewis, Money and Epstein, 1968). Further support was forthcoming from Leningrad in Russia: Dr. L. Lieberman wrote in a personal communication that his patients showed higher than average educational status. At Duke University in North Carolina (personal communication), there is some doubt as to the status of IQ in their adrenogenital patients, so that one obviously needs at least one additional survey of a large, unselected number of patients.

As matters now stand, it is possible that the tendency to IQ elevation is in some way a direct product of genetics, related to the genetic determinant of the adreno-

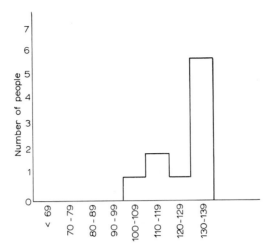

Fig. 2. Distribution of IQ in 10 cases of progestin-induced hermaphroditism.

cortical anomaly itself. Alternatively, it is a direct product of the effect on the brain of excessively high levels of fetal adrenocortical androgens.

PROGESTIN-INDUCED HERMAPHRODITISM IN FEMALES

The hypothesis of a favorable intellectual effect of fetal androgenic steroids on the developing cerebral cortex gains some support from the study of girls exogenously masculinized in utero (Ehrhardt and Money, 1967). In the type of case in question, prenatal masculinization of the female external genitalia was brought about as a side effect of the administration of synthetic progestin to the mother to prevent threatened miscarriage.

Ten girls born with this type of masculinization, all accurately diagnosed and sex-assigned at birth, were surgically corrected early in life, as needed. Subsequently they returned for psychologic study. No known sampling bias could be ascertained to account for the fact that 60% had an IQ of 130 or higher (Fig. 2). One concludes, therefore, that the hormone administered to the mother crossed the placenta and had a favorable influence on the cerebral cortex of the fetus as well as a masculinizing effect on the genitalia. It is, perhaps, not fortuitous that two similar patients, virilized in utero from unknown causes, and now adult, both have a Ph. D. and hold responsible professional positions of leadership.

Ten, or even twelve, cases are too few on which to confirm a hypothesis of a favorable influence of fetal steroids on intelligence. There is, however, additional supportive evidence from the study of Katharina Dalton (1968) in London.

Dalton was able to trace and obtain schoolteachers' ratings on 79 children whose antenatal care she had been responsible for 9 to 10 years earlier. Dalton, but not the teachers, knew the pregnancy histories of these 79 children. The pregnancy histories and the numbers of children traced fell into three groups as follows:

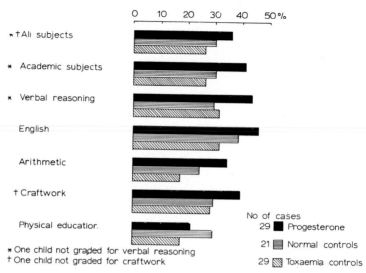

Fig. 3. Percentages of children rated above average by school teachers at age 9–10 years, relative to fetal-hormonal history. $N = 79$.

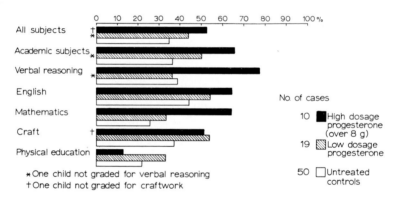

Fig. 4. Percentages of children rated above average by school teachers at age 9–10 years, relative to dosage of progesterone in fetal-hormonal history. $N = 79$.

toxemia treated with progesterone	29
toxemia untreated	29
uncomplicated, normal pregnancy	21

Dalton's findings are reproduced in Figs. 3, 4 and 5. These findings show that the children of progesterone-treated pregnancies were rated as above average more often than their matched controls; and the children of toxemic untreated pregnancies were so rated least often. In the progesterone-treated group, the proportion of above-average achievers correlates positively with a higher total dosage (800 mg or more) of progesterone from the 24th week to delivery, as compared with a lower total dosage of less than 800 mg (Fig. 4). There is a similar positive correlation between above-average achievers and the earliness of onset of progesterone therapy, the dividing line being set at the 16th week (Fig. 5).

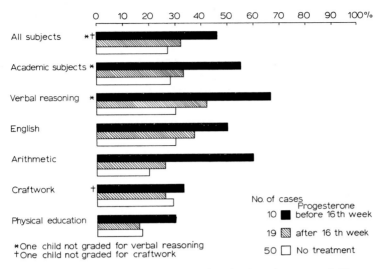

Fig. 5. Percentages of children rated above average by school teachers at age 9–10 years, relative to timing of progesterone in fetal-hormonal history. $N = 79$.

The timing of treatment had a specific effect on achievement in physical education and craftwork, for it was only in the early-treated group that progesterone treatment produced an excess of above-average achievers. Thus, one may conjecture that for a favorable progesterone effect on the organization of the motor nervous system, the critical period is earlier than for a favorable effect on the cognitional nervous system and learning. There is confirmation of sorts for this conjecture in that the hermaphroditic girls I studied with Ehrhardt were tomboys who excelled in sports, and were much given to the expenditure of physical energy, as well as being superior in IQ and school achievement. They had a fetal-hormonal history of very early treatment with synthetic progestin — early enough to affect the morphology of the external sex organs.

ANDROGEN INSENSITIVITY SYNDROME

In the adrenogenital syndrome, if the trend toward elevation of IQ is, indeed, a product of fetal hormonal levels, then the hormone responsible is a virilizing hormone, an androgen; and it is one which is not produced, at least not in such vast amounts, by the normal adrenal cortex. Likewise, in the progestin-induced hermaphroditic syndrome, if the elevation of IQ is hormone-induced, then one presumes that the responsible hormone is also an androgen, and the same one as induces masculinization of the external genitals. Alternatively, the responsible hormone may be a precursor-form of this masculinizing androgen, capable of affecting the central nervous system. Whatever its structure, the hormone concerned must be, if not the one injected, namely a natural or synthetic progestin, then an androgenic substance derived from it after its entry into the body.

References p. 303

TABLE 2

DISTRIBUTION OF WECHSLER IQs, EXPECTED AND OBSERVED, IN 15 CASES OF THE ANDROGEN-
INSENSITIVITY SYNDROME

Scores	Expected percentage	Observed percentage
$\geq$ 130	2.2	0
120–129	6.7	13
110–119	16.1	20
100–109	25.0	47
90– 99	25.0	13
80– 89	16.1	7
70– 79	6.7	0
$\leq$ 69	2.2	0

If a fetal androgen or androgen-related substance might be responsible for an enhancement of IQ then the opposite effect might, by the ordinary laws of logic, be produced by lack of androgen. The syndrome most likely to supply the needed evidence is that of androgen insensitivity, also known as the syndrome of testicular feminization.

The androgen-insensitivity syndrome is the product of a genetic error that affects chromosomal males, depriving the body at the cellular level of biologically active androgen. The fetus, in consequence, differentiates as a female, despite testes in the place of ovaries, except for deformity of the uterus. At puberty, development is as for a normal female, physically and mentally, except for amenorrhea and sterility.

We have had an opportunity to study and test for intelligence 15 patients with the androgen-insensitivity syndrome (Masica, Money, Ehrhardt and Lewis, 1969). The IQs of these patients are distributed as shown in Table 2. Allowing that there is no accidental bias of sampling, then it appears that no tendency to elevation of IQ occurs when androgen is not utilized. Conversely, the defect in androgen utilization does not predispose to low IQ or mental deficiency.

Although it is a digression from the main purpose of this paper, it is well worth pointing out that the lack of a fetal androgenic effect on a chromosomal male leaves the central nervous system, as well as the genital anatomy, consistent with psycho-sexual differentiation and gender-identity development as a normal female. The experimental analogue of this phenomenon can be produced by injecting a pregnant animal with antiandrogen (Neumann and Elger, 1966; Doerner, 1969). The developmental behavior of males subject to fetal antiandrogenization may be characterized as homosexual. The experimental antithesis occurs in investigations in which the pregnant female is androgen injected, so that the fetal female is masculinized. The clitoris becomes a penis and behavioral development shows a masculinized trend.

HYPOPITUITARY DWARFISM

There is no way of measuring to what extent, if any, an infant who will later be diagnosed as a hypopituitary dwarf may have been fetally deficient in any of the

TABLE 3

DISTRIBUTION OF 34 WECHSLER AND 2 STANFORD-BINET IQs IN 36 CASES OF HYPO-
PITUITARY DWARFISM

Scores	Expected percentage	Observed percentage
≧ 130	2.2	5.6
120–129	6.7	5.6
110–119	16.1	19.4
100–109	25.0	16.7
90– 99	25.0	27.8
80– 89	16.1	13.9
70– 79	6.7	8.3
≦ 69	2.2	2.8

TABLE 4

IQ IN ADDISON'S DISEASE: 4 CASES OF JUVENILE ONSET

Case No.	Sex	Age tested	Verbal IQ	Performance IQ	Full IQ	Test
1.	M	9–10	101	103	102	WISC
2.	F	10– 4	125	104	117	WISC
3.	M	14– 4	110	110	111	WISC
4.	M	15– 5	123	107	117	WISC

pituitary hormones. So far as the development of intellect is concerned, however, the question is academic: the IQ in hypopituitary dwarfism with growth hormone deficiency is not affected adversely either pre- or postnatally, as can be seen in the normal distribution in Table 3 (Money, Drash and Lewis, 1967).

ADDISON'S DISEASE

The complete adrenocortical failure of Addison's disease does not occur prenatally. Should there be any effect on the central nervous system, when a child manifests the condition, it cannot, therefore, be attributed to the period of fetal development. The onset of complete adrenocortical failure in childhood is rare, so there are few cases on which to report. I have studied four cases. The IQs are listed in Table 4.

The patients were regulated on cortisone substitution therapy at the time of testing. Untreated, an Addisonian patient is likely to be so debilitated somatically as to be unable to perform well, but there is no evidence of a long-term adverse effect of the treated disease on IQ. Its effect on personality and psychopathology is secondary and not the result of a direct influence on the nervous system, since it ranges from negligible to disastrous denial of illness and delinquent acting out. In other words, the personality effect is in response to chronic illness and dependency on daily medication for survival.

References p. 303

TABLE 5

IQ IN CUSHING'S SYNDROME: 4 CASES OF JUVENILE ONSET

Case No.	Sex	Age tested	Verbal IQ	Performance IQ	Full IQ	Test
1.	F	7–10	104	96	100	WISC
2.	F	12– 3	118	117	119	WISC
3.	F	17	108	119	117	W-B,I
4.	M	17	140	*	*	WAIS

* Did not return for completion of test.

CUSHING'S SYNDROME

Insofar as the adrenocortices are overproductive, Cushing's syndrome is to a certain extent the antithesis of Addison's disease. Since adrenal failure in Addison's disease does not have a direct effect on IQ, one would logically expect that the converse, namely adrenal excess in Cushing's syndrome, would be also without IQ effect. Such does appear to be the case, if one may judge from the evidence of the only four cases (Table 5) I have seen of the rare juvenile form of Cushing's syndrome.

Disorders of personality, including frank psychopathology, may or may not accompany Cushing's syndrome. These disorders may be a toxic by-product of elevated corticosteroid production; or they may emanate more directly from changes in the brain, in proximity to the neurohumoral releasers responsible for the pituitary–adrenal malfunction of the syndrome, in the first place. In either case they may be augmented by a secondary reaction to the disfigurement of physique and appearance induced by the disease and the social handicaps resulting therefrom.

DISCUSSION

From the foregoing review of syndromes, it is evident that whatever correlation there may be between hormonal functions of the pituitary and adrenal, on the one hand, and cognition and learning in human beings, on the other, timing is an important variable. There is a critical period in fetal life, possibly extended into early postnatal life, before the central nervous system is fully differentiated, when hormones may exert a selective permanent organizing influence on the brain. Subsequently, the influence of hormones on brain cells is more likely to be transient and reversible, and also to be disruptive and adverse in its effects.

The syndromes of pituitary–adrenal dysfunction prenatally and in infancy are such that they demonstrate the pre-eminence of androgenic steroids in influencing the brain. These androgenic steroids may be of adrenocortical origin, but they may be of gonadal or exogenous origin also. If other adrenal and pituitary hormones are capable of exerting a direct effect on the differentiating nervous system of the fetus, then either they are incompatible with fetal viability or they do not demonstrate their effects clinically (though they may be discovered to do so experimentally).

The present state of knowledge is such that one may attribute to fetal androgenizing steroids three functions. The first is a masculinizing influence on external genital differentiation. The second is a masculinizing influence on the brain so as to produce tomboyish energy expenditure and interests, but not lesbianism (Ehrhardt and Money, 1967; Ehrhardt, Epstein and Money, 1968; Ehrhardt, Evers and Money, 1968; Money, Ehrhardt and Masica, 1968). The third is a favorable influence on intelligence and learning.

The antithesis of fetal androgenization is not estrogenization but the absence of androgenization.

SUMMARY

The congenital adrenogenital syndrome has been found to be associated with elevation of IQ. The same association has been found in girls with progestin-induced hermaphroditism; and children with a fetal-hormonal history of progesterone therapy have been found to be above average in school achievement at age 9 or 10. By contrast, in the androgen-insensitivity syndrome, no trend to IQ elevation has been found, nor, conversely, to IQ lowering. The pituitary effect in hypopituitary dwarfism has been found to be without effect on IQ level, as compared with random expectancy. The adrenocortical deficit in Addison's disease, and the excess in Cushing's syndrome in childhood appear not to affect IQ, though the CNS complications of Cushing's syndrome may induce psychopathology, over and above secondary reaction to illness.

REFERENCES

DALTON, K. (1968) Antenatal progesterone and intelligence. *Brit. J. Psychiat.*, **114**, 1377–1382.

DOERNER, G. (1969) Zur Frage einer neuroendokrinen Pathogenese, Prophylaxe und Therapie angeborener Sexualdeviationen. *Deut. Med. Wochschr.*, **94**, 390–396.

EHRHARDT, A. A., EPSTEIN, R. AND MONEY, J. (1968) Fetal androgens and female gender identity in the early-treated adrenogenital syndrome. *Johns Hopkins Med. J.*, **122**, 160–167.

EHRHARDT, A. A., EVERS, K. AND MONEY, J. (1968) Influence of androgen and some aspects of sexually dimorphic behavior in women with the late-treated adrenogenital syndrome. *Johns Hopkins Med. J.*, **123**, 115–122.

EHRHARDT, A. A. AND MONEY, J. (1967) Progestin-induced hermaphroditism: IQ and psychosexual identity in a study of ten girls. *J. Sex. Res*, **3**, 83–100.

LEWIS, V. G., MONEY, J. AND EPSTEIN, R. (1968) Concordance of verbal and nonverbal ability in the adrenogenital syndrome. *Johns Hopkins Med. J.*, **122**, 192–195.

MASICA, D. N., MONEY, J., EHRHARDT, A. A. AND LEWIS, V. G. (1969) IQ, fetal sex hormones and cognitive patterns: Studies in the testicular feminizing syndrome of androgen insensitivity. *Johns Hopkins Med. J.*, **124**, 34–43.

MONEY, J., DRASH, P. W. AND LEWIS, V. G. (1967) Dwarfism and hypopituitarism: Statural retardation without mental retardation. *Am. J. Mental Deficiency*, **72**, 122–126.

MONEY, J., EHRHARDT, A. A. AND MASICA, D. N. (1968) Fetal feminization induced by androgen insensitivity in the testicular feminizing syndrome: Effect on marriage and maternalism. *Johns Hopkins Med. J.*, **123**, 105–114.

MONEY, J. AND LEWIS, V. G. (1966) IQ, genetics and accelerated growth: Adrenogenital syndrome. *Bull. Johns Hopkins Hosp.*, **118**, 365–373.

NEUMANN, F. AND ELGER, W. (1966) Permanent changes in gonadal function and sexual behavior as a result of early feminization of male rats by treatment with an antiandrogenic steroid. *Endokrinologie*, **50**, 209–225.

DISCUSSION

LARON: Does the high IQ of patients with adrenogenital syndrome go down after treatment has been instituted? And is there any difference depending on the age at which the treatment was started?

MONEY: We compared early-treated *vs.* late-treated patients and we did not find a difference; nor a difference between treated and untreated patients.

LARON: Have you found differences between the various kinds of adrenogenital syndrome as far as the IQ is concerned? We have several children of the "salt-losing" type whose IQ's are lower than normal.

MONEY: We made subdivisions by diagnostic type and none of them turned out to be very significant. Salt-losers and hypertensives did not constitute special IQ groups.

RINGOLD: Do you know which of the progestational agents were involved in your 10-patient study and in the 79-patient study? It would be of interest to know if the synthetic 19-nor steroids, the 17*a*-acetoxy-progesterone derivates and natural progesterone all have the same type of activity.

MONEY: In our study the mothers had received 17 ethinyltestosterone or 19-nor-17-ethinyltestosterone. Dalton specified only that she used "progesterone". *(Brit. J. Psychiatry, 1968, 114, 1377–1382.)*

HENKIN: There are many interesting differences between patients with salt-losing hypertensive congenital adrenal hyperplasia and nonsalt-losing virilizing congenital adrenal hyperplasia. The 21-hydroxylase deficiency in the salt-losers may be almost complete. In the nonsalt-losers there may be either a partial block of 21-hydroxylation, or, as Bartter, Bryan and I recently published, the presence of another iso-enzyme of 21-hydroxylase. This latter hypothesis means that actually the 21-hydroxylase activity would be increased in amount. This would explain the elevated levels of aldosterone in this group of patients.

DE WIED: Did you ever treat psychosocial dwarfs with ACTH and could you observe a change in behavior?

MONEY: After getting out of the home and being admitted to the hospital, pituitary function recovers rapidly. No drug treatment is necessary. I have no experience with ACTH administration relative to behavior change in psychosocial dwarfism, therefore.

MIRSKY: The rapidity with which the return of growth hormone production occurs in psychosocial dwarfs precludes the use of other therapeutic agents.

COPPEN: Do you have the IQ of the parents and the 1st degree relatives of the adrenogenital children? There might be a bias in the selection of patients in that parents of superior IQ might tend to get their children treated.

MONEY: By and large, I have not had the time nor the personnel to do all the testing of relatives that needs to be done. We checked for the bias you mentioned by comparing local patients, many of lower socioeconomic class with the out-of-state group who were mainly upper socioeconomic. The IQ's of the two groups were not statistically different.

SACHAR: That might also be of extreme interest in the adrenogenital patients, considering the possibility that the IQ is genetically linked. There may be a genetic link-up between passage of adrenogenital trait and IQ.

MONEY: The present state of knowledge does not allow us to make a clear statement as to the one or the other. It was for that reason that I turned to the evidence of progesterone in the progestin-induced group, which suggests a fetal hormonal effect rather than a direct genetic effect.

ACTH Deficiency in Children and Adolescents (Clinical and Psychological Aspects)

ZVI LARON, MOSHE KARP, ATHALIA PERTZELAN AND JACOB FRANKEL*

Paediatric Metabolic and Endocrine Service and Rogoff–Wellcome Medical Research Institute, Division of Paediatrics, Beilinson Hospital, Tel Aviv University Medical School (Israel)

Although a method for the direct measurement of blood ACTH has been described in recent years (Demura, West, Nugent, Nakagawa and Tyler, 1966), the technique is very difficult and therefore cannot be used routinely for clinical purposes. However, for daily clinical routine, a series of indirect tests are available to appraise the degree of corticotrophin-releasing factor (CRF) or ACTH secretion (Laron, 1969).

Complete lack of ACTH results in shock and, if not immediately diagnosed and treated, is incompatible with life. Incomplete ACTH deficiency does exist, but is rare, especially in the paediatric age group. The hypothalamic centers secreting CRF or the pituitary cells secreting ACTH seem to be less vulnerable than the cells secreting other hormones, since the ACTH activity is usually the last to disappear in progressive pituitary insufficiency.

Isolated ACTH deficiency has been described only in adults (Odell, 1966). The only case reported of an adolescent girl (Cleveland, Green and Migeon, 1960) appeared to us to present an HGH deficiency as well. The clinical picture of ACTH deficiency in the paediatric age group can only be inferred from signs of adrenal insufficiency, but there is evidence which indicates that, clinically, primary CRF or ACTH deficiency is not completely identical with primary adrenal insufficiency.

In the present report, we shall analyse the clinical and psychological aspects of 14 adolescents with partial ACTH deficiency of hypothalamic or pituitary origin which were followed in our clinic.

METHODS

The regulation of ACTH secretion is shown in Fig. 1. An assessment of ACTH secretory activity based on this scheme was measured by the following tests, which were performed as described in detail by us elsewhere (Laron, 1969):

1. Insulin hypoglycaemia stress: Regular insulin in a dose of 0.1 U/kg was injected intravenously and the rise of the plasma 11-OHCS was measured before and 1 h after the injection. A normal response was considered to have a peak value of over

---

* Also at Psychology Department, Bar-Ilan University.

References pp. 314–315

TABLE 1

PERTINENT CLINICAL DATA OF 14 PATIENTS WITH ACTH DEFICIENCY

No.	Name	Sex	Diagnosis	Other hormone deficiencies	CA	HA	BA
	Subject		*Diagnosis*			*years/months*	
1	P.S.	M	Craniopharyngioma	HGH, TSH, FSH, ICSH, ADH,	12^2	7^5	5^6
2	J.S.	M	Craniopharyngioma	HGH, TSH,	17	13^6	15^7
3	A.E.	M	Craniopharyngioma	HGH, TSH, FSH, ICSH	17^5	13^5	15^4
4	Ch.A.	M	Craniopharyngioma	HGH, TSH, FSH, ICSH, ADH	19^8	11^4	15^8
5	G.B.	M	Idiopathic Pituitary insufficiency	HGH*, TSH	11^9	10^7	8
6	S.M.D.	F	Idiopathic Pituitary insufficiency	HGH, TSH	12	4^8	5
7	A.A.	M	Idiopathic Pituitary insufficiency	HGH, TSH, FSH, ICSH	15^{10}	6^{11}	7^8
8	Y.H.L.	M	Idiopathic Pituitary insufficiency	HGH, TSH, FSH, ICSH	16^4	11^{10}	12^9
9	S.D.	M	Idiopathic pituitary insufficiency	HGH, TSH, FSH, ICSH	17	7	7
10	D.G.	F	Idiopathic pituitary insufficiency	HGH, TSH, FSH, LH	17^2	10^5	13^3
11	J.L.	M	Idiopathic pituitary insufficiency	HGH, TSH, FSH, ICSH	17^2	9^8	8^6
12	S.E.	M	Idiopathic pituitary insufficiency	HGH. TSH, FSH, ICSH	17^{11}	14^9	16
13	A.B.D.	M	Idiopathic pituitary insufficiency	HGH, TSH, FSH, ICSH	18^3	11	11^6
14	R.I.	F	Idiopathic pituitary insufficiency	HGH, TSH, FSH, LH	23	12	15

CA = Chronological age;
BA = Bone age (determined according to the Atlas of Greulich and Pyle, 1959);
HA = Height age = the age at which the measured height corresponds to the 50th percentile;

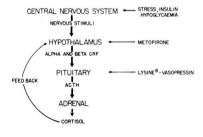

Fig. 1. Regulation of ACTH secretion.

Clinical details	Therapy
Signs of intracranial pressure at age 11. Operation at age 11[3]; At present: growth retardation, retarded sexual development. EEG pattern: irregular. Eye fundus: optic atrophy.	(—)Thyroxine Hydrocortisone 5 mg × 3/day
Operation for ASD at age 10 y. Signs of intracranial pressure at age 11 y. Operation at age 12 y.	(—)Thyroxine Prednisone 2.5 mg × 2 /day.
Signs of intracranial pressure. Operation at age 6. At present: Growth retardation and retarded sexual development.	(—)Thyroxine Durasteron
Signs of intracranial pressure at age 7[6] y. Operation at age 8 y. At present: growth retardation and retarded sexual development. Eye fundus: optic atrophy.	(—)Thyroxine Hydrocortisone 5 mg × 3/day.
Obesity since age 3 y. Growth within normal limits.	(—)Thyroxine
Growth retardation since age 4 y.	(—)Thyroxine; HGH
Growth retardation and retarded sexual development.	(—)Thyroxine; HGH
Growth retardation since age 9[9] y. Retarded sexual development.	(—)Thyroxine; HGH
Growth retardation since age 5 y. Signs of adrenal insufficiency at age 14[6] y. Retarded sexual development. Mental retardation. Deafness.	(—)Thyroxine Prednisone 2.5 mg × 2/day
Growth retardation since age 5 y. Retarded sexual development.	(—)Thyroxine
Growth retardation and retarded sexual development.	(—)Thyroxine
Delayed and retarded sexual development. Eunuchoid body build. Growth within normal limits.	(—)Thyroxine Durasteron
Growth retardation since age 12 y. Retarded sexual development.	(—)Thyroxine
Growth retardation since early childhood (7 y–?). Retarded sexual development.	(—)Thyroxine Ethinyl oestradiol; Progesterone

All body measurements represent the last visit to the clinic.
HGH* = partial deficiency.

20 μg/100 ml; a moderate, subnormal response — a peak value of 10–19 μg/100 ml; a definite abnormal response — a peak value of below 10 μg/100 ml (Laron, Karp, Nitzan and Pertzelan, 1969).

2. *Metopyrone test* (3 g given orally in 4 equal doses every 6 h). Total urinary 17-OHCS were measured the day before, the day of, and the day after, metopyrone administration. The response was considered to be normal when the total urinary 17–OHCS rose more than 2 mg/24 h, before age 10; 3 mg, between 11–13 years; more than 4 mg/day between 14–16 years, and at least 6 mg after the age of 17 years.

Whenever hypoglycaemic stress and/or metopyrone tests showed a subnormal ACTH secretion, the lysine vasopressin test was performed as follows: 5 to 10 U were administered intramuscularly and the rise in plasma 11-OHCS was then measured 1 h after the injection (Karp, Pertzelan, Doron, Kowadlo-Silbergeld and Laron,

TABLE 2

ACTH SECRETION TESTS IN 14 HYPOPITUITARY SUBJECTS

No.	Name	Sex	ITT Plasma 11-OHCS µg/100 ml	Metopyrone Urine 17-OHCS mg/100 ml	Vasopressin Plasma 11-OHCS µg/100 ml	Urine 17-OHCS mg/24 h	Urine 17-KS mg/24 h	Site of lesion
3	A.E.	M	—	13§ 1.2 → 3.8	4.0 → 6.0	17^4 2.4	1.9	P
4	Ch.A.*	M	—	15 1.2 → 4.3	3.5 → 10.3	15^5 1.8	0.6	P
8	Y.H.L.	M	7.1 → 4.8	15 2.0 → 2.5	6.0 → 11.8	15^9 2.2	1.0	P
12	S.E.	M	4.3 → 7.4	14^6 3.8 → 5.3	4.3 → 13.8	17^4 4.65	2.7	P
13	A.B.D.	M	3.3 → 6.2	—	5.2 → 12.2	18 1.9	1.1	P
2	J.S.*	M	7.0 → 8.9	16 +2.3 → 4.0	6.2 → 16.6	15^5 4.2	2.3	HP
10	D.G.	F	5.3 → 12.5	16 1.9 → 1.1	4.5 → 18.5	—	—	HP
11	J.L.	M	9.0 → 10.4	16 1.7 → 4.3	5.8 → 18.0	16 1.7		HP
1	P.S.*	M	+4.1 → 9.2		+5.5 → 26.9	11^6 1.4		H**
5	G.B.	M	7.0 → 7.5 8.1 → 7.6	9^9 2.8 → 4.8	→ 26.4	9^6 2.8	0.85	H
6	S.M.D.	F	6.8 → 8.2		6.7 → 32.0	11^7 2.3		H
7	A.A.	M	6.5 → 12.0	13 (i.v.) 0.8 → 1.7 13 (p.o.) 2.4 → 2.4 13^2 2.4 → 4.8	10.0 → 20.0	13^6 0.7	0.75	H
9	S.D.*	M	1.2 → 2.0	15^1 2.5 → 3.2	→ 55.0	15^1 2.5	1.0	H
14	R.I.	F	—	18 2.5 → 7.1 21^1 3.1 → 5.3	6.7 → 24.0	21^1 3.1	1.0	H

ITT = Insulin tolerance test.
§ = Age at testing: years — months.
* = Receiving corticosteroid replacement therapy.
+ = Test performed before operation.

P = Pituitary lesion; possibly involving also the hypothalamus.
H = Hypothalamic lesion; pituitary function within normal limits.
HP = Probably partial lesion in both hypothalamus and pituitary.
** = Before operation pituitary function normal. After operation not

TABLE 3

INCIDENCE OF CLINICAL SIGNS OF ADRENAL INSUFFICIENCY IN 14 CHILDREN AND ADOLESCENTS WITH ACTH DEFICIENCY

No.	Subject Name	Sex	Weakness	Anorexia, vomiting	Adrenal crisis	BP	Blood TRS mg/100 ml	Serum Na	Serum K Emq/l	Corticosteroid replacement therapy
			Some time during follow-up			During last year of follow-up				
1	P.S.	M	–	–	–	90/65	78	136	4.5	Hydrocortisone
2	J.S.	M	–	–	–	90/55	96	139	4.0	Prednisone
3	A.E.	M	±	–	–	90/45	86	134	3.8	–
4	Ch.A.	M	–	–	–	85/55	88	130	4.75	Hydrocortisone
5	G.B.	M	–	–	–		96			–
6	S.M.D.	F	±+	–	–	80/55	78	139	4.2	–
7	A.A.	M	++	–	–	105/55	82	130	4.5	–
8	Y.H.L.	M	++	±	–	95/65	94	134	3.4	–
9	S.D.	M	±+	–	+	90/60		134		Prednisone
10	D.G.	F	–	–	–	95/60	86			–
11	J.L.	M	–	–	–	75/40	87	135	4.1	–
12	S.E.	M	+	–	–	105/65	90	138	4.0	–
13	A.B.D.	M	±	–	–	90/40	75	133	3.8	–
14	R.I.	F				80/60	84	135	4.15	–

TRS = Total reducing substances (sugar)

1968). The interpretation of the test was identical with that in hypoglycaemia stress.

A subnormal response after hypoglycaemia and metopyrone test and a positive (normal) response to vasopressin was considered to indicate that the primary lesion was in the hypothalamus and that the pituitary ACTH insufficiency was secondary.

A negative vasopressin test with a positive ACTH test were considered to be evidence of primary pituitary lesion. The ACTH test was performed by injecting 25 U intravenously and measuring the rise of plasma 11-OHCS 1 and 2 h after injection, or by administering Depot-ACTH 20 U, twice daily for 3 days and measuring the rise of the urinary 17-OHCS and 17-KS.

Further evidence for low ACTH secretion was a low basal urinary excretion of total 17-OHCS and 17-KS.

The psychometric tests were given in the course of routine clinical follow-up and included an evaluation of intelligence based on either the Wechsler Intelligence Scale for Children (WISC) (Wechsler, 1949), or the Wechsler Adult Intelligence Scale (WAIS) (Wechsler, 1955); the Bender Visual Motor Gestalt Test (Bender, 1948); Human Figures Drawings (Harris, 1963) and the Money Map Test (Money, 1965).

RESULTS AND DISCUSSION

Clinical endocrinological aspects

On the basis of the afore-noted laboratory tests and the previously outlined criteria, 14 of the 109 children and adolescents with hypothalamic–pituitary insufficiency followed by us, were found to have an inadequate ACTH secretion. Of these, 11 were male and 3 were female. All had associated pituitary hormone deficiencies of varying number and extent.

Table 1 summarizes the pertinent clinical data, including diagnosis, age at onset of symptoms, and present therapy. The incidence encountered is less than that reported by Brasel, Wright, Wilkins and Blizzard (1965), who, however, used different criteria.

Table 2 shows the abnormal response obtained by the indirect tests of ACTH secretion. Judging from the response of the plasma 11-OHCS after vasopressin, most ACTH deficiencies were secondary to CRF deficiency. The lowest ACTH secretion has been observed in two patients with craniopharyngioma, after operation.

The ACTH test was within normal limits in all instances tested. It was also found that the basic urinary excretion of 17-OHCS and 17 KS was always low for age.

Table 3 summarizes the incidence of clinical signs of adrenal insufficiency encountered in the patients with ACTH deficiency, their blood pressure and their requirement for replacement therapy.

It is seen that only seven of fourteen patients showed any clinical signs of ACTH deficiency. One of these was a post-operative case of craniopharyngioma. Only one patient had gone through an adrenal crisis. Blood pressure was low in most patients. Serum sodium was found to be low in only four patients. Blood sugar level was below normal in only two patients.

There were four patients who required replacement therapy with hydrocortisone or one of its analogues. An attempt at withdrawal in two patients (S.D. and A.H.)

TABLE 4

PERTINENT PSYCHOMETRIC DATA FOR 13 PATIENTS WITH ACTH DEFICIENCY

Patient			Site of lesion	Age at testing yrs.–mo.	Wechsler Intelligence Scale		
No.	Name	Sex			Verbal IQ	Performance IQ	Full Scale IQ
5	G.B.	M	Hypothalamus	11	105	106	106
6	S.M.D.	F	Hypothalamus	11	92	90	91
7	A.A.	M	Hypothalamus	13^6	85	80	81
9	D.S.	M	Hypothalamus	13^{10}	63	78	67
14	R.J.	F	Hypothalamus	20^6	65	75	67
1	P.S.	M	Hypothalamus* + Pituitary	11^4	75	104	88
2	J.S.	M	H + P	14^8	91	101	99
11	J.L.	M	H + P	15^5	103	76	89
3	A.E.	M	Pituitary	14^7	60	47	49
4	Ch.A.	M	Pituitary	17^8	69	66	66
8	Y.H.L.	M	Pituitary	14^8	71	64	64
12	S.E.	M	Pituitary	16^7	81	55	66
13	A.B.D.	M	Pituitary	18^6	73	62	66

* = Craniopharyngioma post operation and irradiation.

TABLE 5

WECHSLER INTELLIGENCE SCORES* FOR TWO SUBGROUPS OF ACTH DEFICIENCY

Site of lesion	No. of patients	Verbal IQ	Performance IQ	Full Scale IQ
Hypothalamic	6	85.50 (18.19)	84.17 (11.97)	83.50 (15.12)
Pituitary	7	74.28 (9.75)	71.43 (22.23)	71.28 (16.67)

* IQs given as means, SD given in parentheses.

showed that they did not feel well without the drug. The other two were patients with craniopharyngioma after operation, and withdrawal of the drug has not yet been attempted. It is noteworthy that a few other patients who were equally deficient in ACTH and cortisone, seemed to get along well clinically, without corticosteroids.

Psychological aspects

Thirteen of the fourteen subjects with ACTH deficiency were subjected to a battery of neuropsychological tests on an individual basis. The present report deals only with the results of the intelligence tests. Table 4 shows the pertinent psychometric data for the 13 patients tested.

All three IQ scores of the Wechsler test show wide scatter, from 60 to 105, 47 to 106, and 49 to 106 for the Verbal, Performance and Full Scale IQs respectively. It is obvious that the intellectual functioning for the group as a whole is distinctly lower than the "Average" category of 90–110 IQ (Wechsler, 1949). These two findings

TABLE 6

COMPARATIVE INTELLIGENCE DATA FOR SEVERAL SUBGROUPS
OF PITUITARY INSUFFICIENCY

Diagnostic classification	No. of patients	IQ*
IR — biologically inactive HGH (hereditary)	11	73.54 (18.09)
Isolated lack of HGH (hereditary)	6	89.33 (11.36)
Isolated lack of HGH (sporadic)	6	97.00 (16.76)
Panhypopituitarism including ACTH deficiency	13	77.39 (15.90)

* IQs given as means, SD in parentheses; consists of Full Scale
Wechsler, Binet, or Cattel tests of intelligence.

are clear from Table 5, where both subgroups of the ACTH deficiency, lesions of the
hypothalamus and/or pituitary, are below the lower limits of the Average. While
the hypothalamic groups shows distinctly better scores than the pituitary group for
all three IQs, the differences lack statistical significance due to the wide scatter and
the standard deviations. As for the pituitary group, it may well be argued that the
inclusion of four cases of craniopharyngioma — combining the undetermined effects
of surgery and irradiation — reduces the average of this small group of seven cases.
A separate analysis of the four craniopharyngioma cases compared to the three pituitary non-craniopharyngioma cases shows that, contrary to expectation, the former
are superior to the latter (see Table 4). The craniopharyngioma cases have Verbal,
Performance and Full Scale IQs of 73.75, 79.75, and 75.75, compared with 75.00,
60.33, and 65.33 respectively for the three remaining pituitary patients. Thus it
appears that a factor common to both subgroups, other than the surgical intervention
and consequent irradiation, is responsible for the low IQs. While the additional
factor — or cluster of factors — can only be assumed at this time, it is nonetheless
revealing, as shown in Table 6, that low intelligence is fairly typical in patients with
hypothalamic–pituitary insufficiency as a whole. This is in contrast to findings reported by Pollitt and Money (1964) and Rosenbloom, Smith and Loeb (1966).
The lowest IQ (73.54 — Borderline category) is found for the group of IR — biologically inactive HGH (Laron, Pertzelan and Karp, 1968), followed by an IQ just short
of the Average category (89.33) for the group with isolated lack of HGH (hereditary),
and with the best performance (IQ 97.00) by the group with sporadic isolated lack
of HGH.

In view of the fact that the patients lacking ACTH also lack other hypothalamic

TABLE 7

WECHSLER FOLLOW-UP DATA FOR 4 PATIENTS WITH ACTH DEFICIENCY RECEIVING CORTICOSTEROIDS REPLACEMENT THERAPY

No.	Name	Sex	Age at testing yr–mth	V	P	FS	Replacement therapy concomitant with testing
1*	P.S.	M	11^4	69	100	82	Before operation – No treatment
			11^7	75	104	88	Post operation; Irradiation
							(–)Thyroxine + Hydrocortisone
			11^{10}	85	104	93	(–)Thyroxine + Hydrocortisone
2*	J.S.	M	14^8	91	71	80	(–)Thyroxine + Prednisone + Luminal
			15^9	101	72	86	(–)Thyroxine + Prednisone + Luminal
			16^3	99	79	88	(–)Thyroxine stopped for 2 weeks Prednisone + Luminal
			16^7	106	94	98	(–)Thyroxine + Prednisone + Luminal
4*	Ch.A.	M	17^8	69	66	66	(–)Thyroxine + Medrol + Pitressin + HCG
			18^{11}	67	75	69	(–)Thyroxine + ACTH + Pitressin + Testosterone
			19^3	67	82	72	(–)Thyroxine + ACTH + Pitressin + Testosterone
			19^{10}	—**	88	—**	(–)Thyroxine + Hydrocortisone + Pitressin + Testosterone
9	S.D.	M	13^{10}	63	78	67	Without any treatment
			15^6	80	64	70	(–)Thyroxine + Prednisone
			16^1	81	83	80	(–)Thyroxine + Prednisone
			16^{10}	76	79	74	(–)Thyroxine + Prednisone + Dianabol

Wechsler Intelligence, IQ

* Craniopharyngioma; ** Not administered at the time.
V = Verbal; P = Performance; FS = Full scale.

References pp. 314–315

and/or pituitary hormones, it would seem difficult to attribute the psychological deficits to any one or a combination of specific hormones.

It has been shown by us previously (Laron, Pertzelan and Frankel, 1969) that prenatal HGH deficiency will cause delay in mental and motor development. This is less obvious with acquired HGH deficiency, as probably examplified by most or all the sporadic HGH deficiency cases.

An attempt to correlate ACTH deficiency with mental functioning has been made in the patients receiving replacement therapy with corticosteroids (Table 7). In these four patients, there is a common upward trend in IQs. Part of the gain is probably due to the effect of the corticosteroid therapy, but in part, it may have resulted also from practice acquired by repeating the tests.

SUMMARY

Using hypoglycaemic stress, metopyrone and vasopressin tests for the indirect assessment of ACTH secretion, we found that 14 out of 109 children and adolescents with pituitary insufficiency have a partial CRF and/or ACTH deficiency associated with other hormone deficiencies. Eleven of these patients were males. Seven had, at some time, shown clinical signs of adrenocortical insufficiency, but only four seemed to require continued cortisol replacement therapy.

Most of our patients with pituitary insufficiency had distinctly below average intelligence quotients. Wide fluctuations were noted in this group, with the ACTH-deficient subjects ranking in IQ between the group with hereditary IR — biologically inactive HGH at the lower extreme, and the group with sporadic (most probably acquired) lack of HGH having highest ratings.

Replacement therapy with corticosteroids has been associated with a distinct gain in IQ, though it is not possible to establish a causal relationship due to the small number of subjects studied.

ACKNOWLEDGEMENT

Thanks are given to: Mrs. Dalia Greenberg, R. N., for her assistance in the clinical tests; and Mrs. Leah Amit, Psychological Examiner, for performing the psychological tests.

REFERENCES

BENDER, L. (1948) *Instruction for the Use of Visual Motor Gestalt Test.* American Orthopsychiatric Assoc. and Psychological Corp., New York.

BRASEL, J. A., WRIGHT, J. C., WILKINS, L. AND BLIZZARD, R. M. (1965) An evaluation of seventy-five patients with hypopituitarism beginning in childhood. *Amer. J. Med.*, **38**, 484–498.

CLEVELAND, W. W., GREEN, D. C. AND MIGEON, C. J. (1960) A case of proved adrenocorticotropin deficiency. *J. Pediat.*, **57**, 376–380.

DEMURA, H., WEST, C. D., NUGENT, C. A., NAKAGAWA, K. AND TYLER, F. H. (1966) A sensitive radioimmunoassay for plasma ACTH levels. *J. Clin. Endocrinol.*, **27**, 1297–1302.

HARRIS, D. B. (1963) *Children's Drawings as Measures of Intellectual Maturity*, Harcourt, Brace & World, Inc., New York.

KARP, M., PERTZELAN, A., DORON, M., KOWADLO-SILBERGELD, A. AND LARON, Z. (1968) Changes in blood glucose and plasma insulin, free fatty acids, growth hormone and 11-hydroxycorticosteroids during intramuscular vasopressin tests in children and adolescents. *Acta Endocrinol.*, **58**, 545–557.

LARON, Z., PERTZELAN, A. AND KARP, M. (1968) Pituitary dwarfism with high serum levels of growth hormone. *Israel J. Med. Sci.*, **4**, 883–894.

LARON, Z. (1969) The hypothalamus and the pituitary gland (hypophysis). In: *Paediatric Endocrinology*, D. HUBBLE (Ed.), Blackwell, Oxford, pp. 35–111.

LARON, Z., KARP, M., NITZAN, M. AND PERTZELAN, A. (1969) The plasma 11-hydroxycorticosteroids response to insulin-induced hypoglycaemia in children and adolescents. *Acta Endocrinol.*, **69**, 451–462.

LARON, Z., PERTZELAN, A. AND FRANKEL, J. (1969) Growth and development in the syndromes of "Familial isolated absence of HGH" or "Pituitary dwarfism with high serum concentration of an immunoreactive but biologically inactive HGH". In: HAMBURGH, M. AND BARRINGTON, E. J. W. (Eds.), *Hormones in Development*, National Foundation, New York. In press.

MONEY, J. A. (1965) *A Standardized Road-Map Test of Direction Sense*, The Johns Hopkins Press, Baltimore.

ODELL, W. D. (1966) Isolated deficiencies of anterior pituitary hormones. *J. Am. Med. Assoc.*, **197**, 1006–1016.

POLLITT, E. AND MONEY, J. (1964) Studies in the psychology of dwarfism. I. Intelligence quotient and school achievement. *J. Pediat.*, **64**, 415–421.

ROSENBLOOM, A. L., SMITH, D. W. AND LOEB, D. G. (1966) Scholastic performance of short-statured children with hypopituitarism. *J. Pediat.*, **69**, 1131–1133.

WECHSLER, D. (1949) *Wechsler Intelligence Scale for Children*, Psychological Corp., New York.

WECHSLER, D. (1955) *Wechsler Adult Intelligence Scale*, Psychological Corp., New York.

DISCUSSION

HODGES: If the scheme you outlined in one of your slides for the control of ACTH secretion is correct and if the tests you have performed to investigate the functional integrity of the hypothalamo–pituitary–adrenal system are founded on reliable theoretical concepts, it would be impossible theoretically to have a patient with, for example, a positive response to insulin and a negative response to metropyrone. Have you any such instances?

LARON: No, the metopyrone test relates well with the insulin tolerance test (ITT). So that we usually perform only the ITT test; and if this test gives negative results, we perform a lysine–vasopressin test.

MONEY: Might there be a cultural difference in some of your patient sample *versus* mine that would contribute to the observed IQ difference? I note also that you included craniopharyngioma, which I excluded, as I did also the so-called intrauterine dwarfs.

LARON: Some of the differences in results between your and our patients may be due to cultural differences — we have tested siblings as well — but I think that most differences are due to the type of patient material. I would guess that most of your patients belong to the acquired type of pituitary insufficiency and compare to some of our patients with acquired hypopituitarism and the sporadic isolated HGH-deficient patients, most of whom are of the acquired type. We found that patients who have an early intrauterine growth hormone deficiency, have the lowest intellectual performance. We are interested to know whether this intrauterine hormone deficiency inflicts a permanent damage.

HENKIN: If there were some inability to integrate sensory information in patients with adrenocortical insufficiency, then your data are perfectly consistent with the thought that these people would have trouble in doing the tasks that you gave them, resulting in their low IQ. Treatment should correct this abnormality and this concept goes along very well with their increased intellectual ability, as you showed.

Psychological Factors Relating to Activation and Inhibition of the Adrenocortical Stress Response in Man: A Review

EDWARD J. SACHAR

Montefiore Hospital and Medical Center, Bronx, N.Y. (U.S.A.)

One of the most interesting aspects of psychoendocrine research during the past decade has been the delineation of the ways in which the animal model of psychological stress has to be modified when studying the human situation. In the animal paradigm a group of rats or monkeys are exposed to a noxious psychological stimulus, and a substantial adrenocortical response generally occurs. For example, during a 24-hour period of Sidman avoidance a monkey typically puts out over three times as much urinary corticosteroids as on control days (Mason, 1968). In men exposed to stress, however, it appears that the situation is more complex. The animal model fails to take into account the elaborate system of psychological coping mechanisms, highly developed in man, which process and evaluate threatening stimuli, serving to minimize their emotional impact and inhibiting the associated adrenocortical response. This psychological buffering system can be studied systematically, however, as I will attempt to describe by reviewing some studies previously published as well as some work currently in progress.

An example of the way psychological coping mechanisms can affect the emotional and adrenocortical response to stress is a recent study we carried out at Montefiore Hospital, with Dr. Katz and other members of the Psychiatry Department, and Drs. Hellman and Gallagher of the Institute for Steroid Research (Katz *et al.*, 1969). We studied psychologically and endocrinologically a group of women awaiting surgery for nodules in the breast. The women were faced with the severe stresses of possibly having cancer, possibly losing their breasts, possibly having a fatal illness. Yet, on evaluating and rating these women psychologically, it was found that the great majority were coping remarkably well with these stresses. Some used religious faith, some denied the likelihood of any danger, some occupied themselves with much more trivial concerns, and others intellectualized the whole experience. Only a few seemed really to confront the danger and to be very distressed emotionally. At the same time as the psychological evaluations were being conducted, cortisol production rate was determined for each woman by isotopic methods. The prediction was that scores for psychological distress would correlate with cortisol production expressed in mg/g of creatinine.

Fig. 1 shows the psychological and endocrine data as a scattergram. Note that there was indeed a rather good correlation between psychiatric distress score and

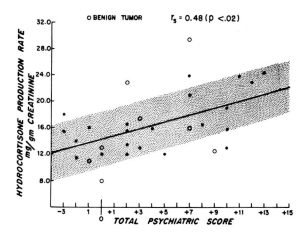

Fig. 1. Psychological distress and cortical production rate in women awaiting biopsy of breast tumors.

cortisol production rate ($p < 0.02$). Note also that most of the women had low psychiatric distress scores and low cortisol production rates, despite the severity of the situational stress. Only a few women had elevated production rates, and these were, in general, the women who were rated as showing signs of marked distress. Even in these women, however, the degree of elevation was not very great — approximately 25–35% above the mean. Although this may seem surprising, it is absolutely typical of the findings of a whole series of studies of adrenocortical activity in normal humans under stress. These include studies of college students dealing with the stress of hospitalization on a research ward (Mason *et al.*, 1965), of the parents of children dying of leukemia (Wolff *et al.*, 1964), of soldiers coping with the stress of basic training (Rose *et al.*, 1968), and of helicopter pilots under attack in Vietnam (Bourne *et al.*, 1967). In all of these investigations, most subjects showed little urinary corticosteroid elevations, and only a few showed a substantial response. The psychiatrists have been quite successful in predicting those few who will show an adrenal response, but the degree of the response has generally been only about 25–35% above basal levels. Indeed, I would guess that the same findings could also be shown for the astronauts — that they, too, would show little adrenocortical response despite the stress of the situation, due to their remarkable ability to concentrate on the technical details of the mission rather than the danger inherent in it.

It does seem then that as long as this buffer system of psychological coping mechanisms remains intact, emotional "pH" is kept within a narrow range, and the adrenocortical response is relatively slight, albeit predictable. Presumably, these psychological control mechanisms operate through neurophysiological inhibitory pathways, and hopefully, we may learn in the future something about the nature of these pathways.

As we have said, this buffer system of psychological coping mechanisms usually functions very well in normal people. But when this system is shattered, as in certain

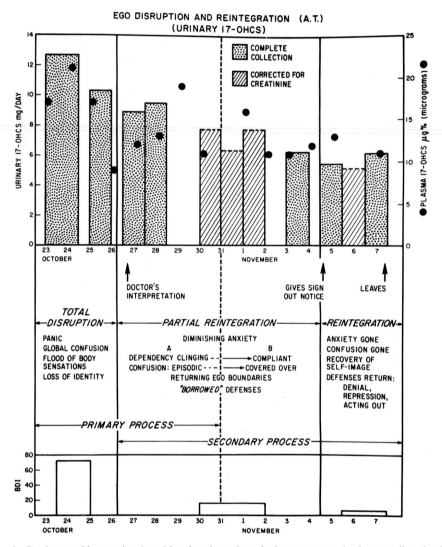

Fig. 2. Corticosteroid excretion in schizophrenic patient during acute psychotic turmoil and subsequent ego reintegration.

psychotic states, it is then possible to observe intense emotional crises and adrenocortical responses of a massive, drastic type, similar to magnitude of responses seen in the experimental animal.

This can be illustrated by longitudinal studies of acutely schizophrenic patients in states of severe psychotic turmoil. This is the period of acute confusion and panic which frequently initiates schizophrenic episodes and is associated with profound fears of dying, mental disorganization, hyperstimulability, and loss of a sense of identity. Fig. 2 shows that urinary corticosteroid excretion during this period reaches levels over twice the subsequent recovery values. This degree of adrenocortical

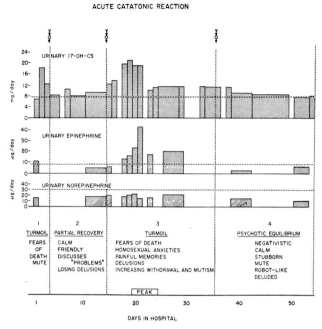

ACUTE CATATONIC REACTION

Fig. 3. Corticosteroid excretion in schizophrenic patient during acute psychotic turmoil and subsequent formation of an organized psychotic system.

activation far exceeds what is seen in normals under stress. As the patient gradually
recompensates, corticosteroid excretion gradually subsides, but it is only when the
patient's ego is almost reintegrated, with a return of his premorbid coping mechanisms,
that he reaches the range seen in stressed normals, about 25 % above his final recovery
values. These results are typical of what we have seen in a series of acute schizophrenic patients (Sachar *et al.*, 1963, 1969a).

However, it should be emphasized that such profound emotional and endocrine
upheaval is only a transient phenomenon even in schizophrenia. After the patient
forms an organized delusional system, which is associated with a subsidence of
emotional distress, corticosteroids also fall back to normal levels. This can be seen
in Fig. 3.

Following an acute episode of panic with disorganization and confusion, this
patient retreated into a catatonic shell, with a fixed delusional system and essentially
had readied a psychotic solution to his difficulties. Note that the intense elevations
in corticosteroid excretion promptly subside in association with the formation of an
organized psychotic system.

These endocrine observations, which we have made on a number of patients,
seem to support the view of the dynamic school of psychiatry which argues that the
organized delusional system serves as a kind of psychotic solution for the patient,
consoling him and buffering him from anxiety. In this respect, the fixed delusion of
the schizophrenic might be seen as a pathological psychological coping mechanism

or defense, helping him to minimize anxiety in the same way that the profound religious faith of some of our women awaiting breast surgery helped them to maintain tranquility. Indeed, as the schizophrenic patient in therapy gives up his delusions and faces painful reality again, he often reexperiences emotional distress and adrenal activation before he makes a full recovery.

I think these data also illustrate that acute schizophrenia is not a static entity, psychologically or endocrinologically, and that endocrine research must take into account the rapidly shifting phases of this illness with alternating periods of emotional equilibrium and disequilibrium. Certainly the diagnosis of schizophrenia alone will not tell us whether the adrenal cortex is activated or not. In these patients it is necessary to isolate specifically the clinical dimensions of emotional arousal and disorganization of the ego's buffering mechanism.

I would now like to show that the same is true for depressive illness, as well. Initially, endocrine researchers assumed that melancholia must be associated with profound emotional distress and adrenal activation, since the patients complained so bitterly and were so incapacitated. Initially, measurements of adrenocortical function in depressed patients seemed to confirm this idea. However, as research in this area continued, the reports have been in conflict with each other, some reporting elevated levels of corticosteroids, others reporting normal levels, and so forth.

In a recent paper (Sachar, 1967a), I pointed out some necessary controls required properly to interpret adrenocortical data from depressed patients, such as omitting phenothiazines and barbiturates, drugs which are known to interfere with the release of ACTH; giving the patient time to get over the stress of hospital admission; studying all patients both before and after recovery, in order to eliminate as far as possible factors affecting adrenal function which may have little to do with psychological state or depressive illness *per se*.

We then embarked on a series of studies of adrenocortical function in depressed patients (Sachar, 1967b). I would like to describe the most recent of these, which is presently being completed at Montefiore, in collaboration with Drs. Hellman, Gallagher and Fukushima of the Institute for Steroid Research (Sachar *et al.*, 1969b). It was undertaken with two main aims: first, to assess adrenocortical activity in depressions by the best available method, that is measurement of cortisol production by isotopic techniques. Secondly, to clarify further the precise clinical features of depressive illness which are associated with adrenocortical activation.

To elaborate on the clinical problem, progress in psychoendocrine research in depressive illness has been impeded, I believe, by ambiguous and cloudy psychiatric terminology. For example, if we believe that emotional arousal is an important factor in adrenal activation, then it is vital to assess anxiety levels in depressed patients. Simply classifying depressions in the traditional categories of involutional, reactive, endogenous and so forth, does not tell us whether the patient is anxious or not. Again, the term agitation is often used synonymously with anxiety, but they are not the same thing. Agitation is a specific symptom of motor restlessness which may or may not be associated with anxiety.

Another stressful emotion is sadness or grief. Again, this is often not present in depressed patients the way it is in the depressive experiences of everyday life. Many ⸴ depressed patients do not experience true sadness or grief and complain instead of numbness or the inability to feel.

Finally, if we believe that psychotic disorganization is an important factor in adrenal activation as it is in schizophrenics, it is very important to identify this phenomenon in depressions. Unfortunately, psychiatrists use the term "psychotic depression" in several different ways, and it is very difficult to tell from the literature in this field just what kind of patient is being described.

Using a symptom rating scale derived from the Hamilton Depression Scale, we assessed depressive symptomatology in a series of depressed patients, before and after recovery. We hypothesized that change in cortisol production from illness to recovery would correlate with scores on a small group of core psychiatric items related to emotional arousal and psychotic disorganization. Included in this core group of items were symptoms of anxiety, sadness, feelings of loss of control, feelings of body disintegration, and depersonalization.

Our results strikingly supported the hypothesis as can be seen in Fig. 4. Patients who scored low on this group of clinical items could be termed "apathetic" depressives. While they had lost their energy, appetite, libido, drive, and interest, and considered themselves worthless, they had little anxiety and emotional arousal. As can be seen, they also showed little change in cortisol production from illness to recovery.

Those scoring in the moderate range on these items could be termed "anxious" depressives. In addition to other symptoms of depression, they also were apprehensive and tearful. Usually they were very aware and concerned with the loss or disappointment which had led to their illness. As can be seen, they generally showed moderate elevations in cortisol production, about 25% above their recovery levels. In this respect, the adrenal response in these patients is very similar to stressed normals who cope poorly and experience anxiety.

Those depressed patients who scored very high on this core group of psychiatric

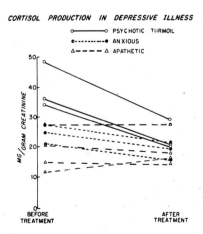

Fig. 4. Cortisol production rate in 3 types of depressed patients before and after recovery.

References pp. 323–324

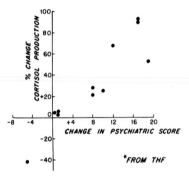

CORRELATION BETWEEN
CHANGE IN CORTISOL PRODUCTION*
AND CHANGE IN PSYCHIATRIC SCORE

Fig. 5. Correlation between % change in cortisol production during illness as compared with recovery and change in psychiatric score during illness as compared with recovery in 11 depressed
patients. Note that psychiatric scores are for emotional arousal and psychotic disorganization only,
disregarding all other symptoms of depressive illness.

items could be termed "Psychotically Disorganized". These patients showed very
striking changes in cortisol production, from 50–90% increased above their recovery
levels, far beyond what is seen in the anxious normal. In this respect they are very
similar to schizophrenic patients in states of acute psychotic turmoil. It should be
emphasized that this last group of patients are rather rare among depressed patients.
They tend to appear in disproportionately large numbers in psychoendocrine studies
because of special interest in them, but in fact they probably are less than 10% of the
population of even hospitalized depressives.

Fig. 5 shows a scattergram of the per cent change in cortisol production plotted
against change in psychiatric scores for these core items. Rank order correlation was
a striking 0.9 $p < 0.001$.

To summarize the work thus far, it appears that there are certain psychoendocrine
observations which can be made about normals, schizophrenics, and depressives.
Under stress, the normal person generally copes well, and is able to use psychological
mechanisms to preserve emotional and endocrine homeostasis, and there is little
or no enduring activation of the adrenal. The minority who cannot cope well experience anxiety, and urinary measures of adrenocortical activity are generally raised
about 25%. Depressed patients experiencing anxiety without psychotic disorganization,
show adrenal activation similar to the anxious normal.

It is only in the presence of psychotic disorganization with disintegrative anxiety
failure of all coping mechanisms that very large increases in cortisol production occur
and this may sometimes occur in the course of schizophrenic or depressive illness.
There also appear to be striking differences in the intensity of the adrenal response
in psychotic disintegrative anxiety as compared with normal or neurotic anxiety.

Thus far I have discussed only 24-hour urinary measures of adrenocortical activity.
What about the behavior of plasma cortisol, and particularly, the circadian rhythm

of plasma cortisol? Recent evidence indicates that plasma cortisol is a much more labile system than was previously appreciated. Rapid rises and falls in plasma cortisol in response to stress can be regularly observed in the normal person, as Dr. Jones's paper indicates. These plasma cortisol changes are usually of short duration, however, and do not often significantly affect the 24-hour cortisol production rate. This lability of plasma cortisol can also be seen in studies of the circadian curve, which appears to be much less smooth even in the normal than was originally thought. This is evident if frequent blood samples are taken every 15 min during the night's sleep through an indwelling cannula, without disturbing the subject. This work is being done at Montefiore Hospital by Dr. Roffwarg of the Psychiatry Department and Drs. Hellman, Gallagher and colleagues of the Institute for Steroid Research. Their observations indicate that in the normal person, plasma cortisol levels remain quite low until about 4 a.m., at which time the adrenal cortex begins to secrete in a series of bursts over several hours, with a spiking response in plasma cortisol level.

In collaboration with this group of investigators, we have begun similar studies of depressed patients before and after recovery, simultaneously monitoring sleep EEG and plasma cortisol levels via the indwelling cannula. This is an especially useful way of studying the intrinsic circadian rhythm of plasma cortisol, since it captures the segment of the day when plasma cortisol moves from its nadir to its zenith. Furthermore, since the observations are made during sleep, it offers the opportunity to study intrinsic adrenocortical activity in the patient relatively removed from environmental influences. Our preliminary observations are that as long as the patient remains asleep, the fundamental normal circadian pattern of cortisol is not altered, but every time the patient awakens during the night, there is a prompt sharp rise in plasma cortisol, which drops as soon as the patient falls asleep again. This is typical of several patients we have studied, whose sleep pattern has been disrupted in the way typical of depressive illness. It is too early to draw conclusions, except to note that because of the lability of the plasma cortisol system, circadian rhythm cannot be properly studied unless there is very detailed sampling of blood cortisol levels without disturbing the subject and with concomitant sleep records. It does appear thus far that adrenocortical activation in a depressed patient is a function of being awake and anxious.

In summary, I have reviewed the behavior of the adrenal cortex in normals under stress, and during the course of schizophrenic and depressive illnesses. I have described some psychological factors which are associated with increases in adrenocortical activity in these conditions, but I have also attempted to call attention to the very impressive psychological functions which usually serve to maintain emotional and endocrine homeostasis.

REFERENCES

BOURNE, P. G., ROSE, R. M. AND MASON, J. W. (1967) Urinary 17-OHCS levels: Data on seven helicopter ambulance medics in combat. *Arch. Gen. Psychiat.*, **17**, 104.
KATZ, J. L., GALLAGHER, T. F., HELLMAN, L., ACKMAN, P., ROTHWAX, Y., SACHAR, E. J. AND WEINER, H. (1969) Psychoendocrine aspects of cancer of the breast. *Psychosom. Med.*, in press.

MASON, J. W. (1968) The organization of psychoendocrine responses. *Psychosom. Med.*, **23**, 565.
MASON, J. W., SACHAR, E. J., FISHMAN, J. R., HAMBURG, D. A. AND HANDLON, J. H. (1965) Corticosteroid responses to hospital admission. *Arch. Gen. Psychiat.*, **13**, 1.
ROSE, R. M., POE, R. O. AND MASON, J. W. (1968) Psychological state and body size as determinants
of 17-OHCS excretion. *Arch. Internal Med.*, **121**, 406.
SACHAR, E. J. (1967a) Corticosteroids in depressive illness. I: A reevaluation of control issues and
the literature. *Arch. Gen. Psychiat.*, **17**, 544.
SACHAR, E. J. (1967b) Corticosteroids in depressive illness. II: A longitudinal psychoendocrine
study. *Arch. Gen. Psychiat.*, **17**, 554.
SACHAR, E. J., HELLMAN, L., GALLAGHER, T. F. AND FUKUSHIMA, D. (1969) Endocrinology of depression. I: Cortisol production in depressions. Presented to *NIMH Workshop on Recent Advances
in the Psychobiology of Depressive Illnesses, April.*
SACHAR, E. J., KANTER, S. S., BUIE, D., ENGLE, R. AND MEHLMAN, R. (1969a) Psychoendocrinology
of ego disintegration. *Amer. J. Psychiat.*, in press.
SACHAR, E. J., MASON, J. W., KOLMER, H. S., JR. AND ARTISS, K. L. (1963) Psychoendocrine aspects
of acute schizophrenic reactions. *Psychosom. Med.*, **25**, 510.
WOLFF, C. T., HOFER, M. A. AND MASON, J. W., (1964) Relationship between psychological defenses
and mean urinary 17-hydroxycorticosteroid excretion rates. *Psychosom. Med.*, **26**, 576.

DISCUSSION

MIRSKY: I have never met Dr. Sachar before, but I felt grateful to him after reading his fairly recent
publication where he took this mass of material which confused many of us and approached it from
a truly scientific angle, to evaluate the psychiatric aspects together with the biochemical results.
It has provided tremendous clarification in a most obscure area, and I do want to congratulate him
on his efforts to quantitate and correlate the psychological data with the biochemical ones.

NIJDAM: Could you elaborate on the relation between high cortisol levels and psychotic states?

SACHAR: High cortisol levels appear to be related to the disintegrative anxiety seen in psychotic
disorganization. There do appear to be real differences in the adrenal response in psychotic anxiety
and normal neurotic anxiety. However, as soon as the psychotic withdraws from stressful reality
by developing an organized delusional system the cortisol levels return to normal.

NIJDAM: Do you think that being unable to cope with stress is the only factor responsible for high
cortisol levels in psychotics?

SACHAR: This is a tough question to study. If there is an intrinsic abnormality of the hypothalamo-
pituitary-adrenal function in the acute psychotic, it may be possible to study this during sleep when
subjective experience and environmental influences can be minimized.

MIRSKY: In your normal as well as in your disturbed patients the increase in cortisol occurred
relatively late; whereas in similar subjects there is a marked increase in growth hormone levels very
early in sleep. This shows again that we deal with more than mere arousal. The release of growth
hormone and of ACTH appears to be dissociated.

SACHAR: These sleep studies were carried out in collaboration with Drs. Roffwarg, Hellman, Gallagher, Finkelstein and other members of the Institute for Steroid Research. Whereas elevations of
cortisol typically occur beginning 3:30 to 4:30 a.m., as part of the normal circadian rhythm, the spike
in growth hormone occurs earlier in the night associated with stage 4 sleep. We measured growth
hormone concurrently with plasma cortisol, and it is interesting that in some depressed patients this
growth hormone peak is absent. The response of growth hormone to insulin infusion is also absent
in some cases. We are at present attempting to evaluate the significance of these findings.

McCLURE: Would you, please, comment on some recent findings we have obtained at McGill
University showing that cortisol levels in the cerebrospinal fluid (CFS) of normal control subjects
were higher than those of psychiatrically depressed patients.

SACHAR: I am not sure of the significance of the low CSF cortisol levels observed in your patients.
Presumably it reflects diffusion from blood. It would be interesting to know which group of depressed patients showed such low levels.

Correlation Between Psychic and Endocrinological Responses to Emotional Stress

M. T. JONES, P. K. BRIDGES AND D. LEAK

Sherrington School of Physiology, St. Thomas' Hospital, London, S.E. 1
Department of Psychological Medicine, Royal Free Hospital, London, W.C. 1
and Department of Medicine, McGregor Clinic and St. Joseph's Hospital, Hamilton, Ontario (Canada)
(Formerly King's College Hospital, London, U.K.)

There are a number of methodological and theoretical problems involved when studying the influence of emotional stress in man. Firstly, it is not easy to define the emotion induced by stress and it is even more difficult to ensure that subjects undergoing a common stress are experiencing qualitatively similar emotions, which in any case are likely to vary in intensity between individuals. Secondly, there is the problem of choosing a stress which is sufficiently realistic to ensure reliable responses in the subjects. A wide variety of stresses have been used, some of which might be considered relatively unreliable stimuli which possibly produce alertness while not necessarily provoking anxiety. These include, for example, one minute's unpleasant noise (Goldstein, 1964), sorting metal balls in a disagreeable environment (Levi, 1963) and carrying out psychological tests (Frankenhaeuser and Post, 1962). Subjects have also been investigated in more disturbing conditions such as paratroop training (Bloom, von Euler and Frankenhaeuser, 1963), watching horrific films (Lazarus, Speisman and Mordkoff, 1963), among those accompanying patients to hospital Emergency Department (Bliss, Migeon, Branch and Samuels, 1956) and students undergoing University examinations (Hodges, Jones and Stockham, 1962). In the present work, the effect of a University examination was studied since it is a stress in which the subjects are personally involved in the situation and their future is affected by the outcome.

Thirdly, there is the problem of how indicative are the changes in the particular physiological parameter used in the study of the subject's psychological response to the stress. A wide spectrum of physiological parameters have been employed in various studies and include changes in heart rate and blood pressure (Glickstein, 1960; Hickam, Cargill and Golden, 1948), palmar skin resistance (Harrison, 1964), and gastric motility, eye blink, finger pulse volume and respiratory rate (Sternbach, 1962; Wing, 1963). In addition, measurements of plasma and urinary 17-hydroxycorticosteroids (Bliss *et al.*, 1956; Persky, Hamburg, Basowitz, Grinker, Sabshin, Kovchin, Herz, Board and Heath, 1958) and of urinary catecholamines (Elmajian, Hope and Lawson, 1958, Levi, 1963) have been included in a number of studies. The multiplicity of bodily effects that accompany emotional stress illustrate the complexity of the stress response and it is not known to what extent these responses are intercorrelated. Therefore, it is questionable which are the best indices of emotional response and whether work which employs one parameter can be compared with studies using a different parameter. In the present work several parameters have been used, *i.e.* plasma 11-hydroxycorticosteroid concentrations, blood pressure, pulse rate, and urinary catecholamine excretion rates. The intercorrelations between those parameters have been investigated.

Though it is not easy to define the state of anxiety induced by stress, it is possible to assess some psychological and physical variables which might be related to the way individuals respond to stress. The personality was assessed by the Eysenck Personality Inventory (Eysenck and Eysenck, 1964). This includes two scales, giving results in the dimensions of Neuroticism (N scale) and Extraversion (E scale). Physique was assessed by the method of Parnell (1958) which gives a seven point scale for each of three physical components; Fat, Muscularity and Linearity.

The volunteers used in the present experiments were male medical students, aged about 20 years, taking the second M.B. Anatomy oral examination. Data from 80 students are included in the plasma 11-hydroxycorticosteroid studies but only those from 48 students are in the studies on blood pressure changes and catecholamine excretion rates. Each subject was asked to empty his bladder shortly before the examination which lasted 15 min. Immediately afterwards the heart rate and blood pressure were taken by the auscultation method, the students sitting with the arm at heart level. The diastolic pressure was taken as the changing of the sounds from phase III to phase IV on the Korotkov scale. Each student then drank 250 ml of water and rested in the sitting position until the bladder was again emptied 1 h after the examination was begun. All urine was collected into containers with sodium metabisulphite and sodium fluoride and stored at —20°C for subsequent estimation of catecholamines. Thirty minutes after the beginning of the examination a 5-ml of venous blood was collected in a tube containing heparin. The specimen was centrifuged at once and the plasma stored at —20°C.

Two months later the students attended for similar collections of specimens to provide control results during resting conditions. The subjects were asked to avoid exercise and to refrain from smoking and from drinking tea, coffee or alcohol before the control observations although it was felt unreasonable to insist on this before the examination. All estimations of blood pressure were made by the same observer.

Plasma 11-hydroxycorticosteroids was measured fluorimetrically by the method of Zenker and Bernstein (1958), but the fluorescence intensity was measured 15 min after addition of the fluorescent reagent and not at $1\frac{1}{2}$ h as in the original method. This was done at 15 min so as to minimise the large non-specific fluorescence which occurs if the fluorescence is read at later times.

Urinary adrenaline and noradrenaline were measured by differential fluorimetry as described by Leak, Brunjes, Johns and Starr (1962).

Table 1 shows mean values for blood pressure and pulse rates, urinary volume, catecholamine excretion rates and plasma 11-hydroxycorticosteroid concentrations

TABLE 1

MEANS OF PHYSIOLOGICAL VARIABLES IN 48 SUBJECTS

	Control		Stress		Significance of differences p
	Mean ($\pm$ S.D.)				
Systolic pressure (mm Hg)	122	$\pm$ 12	144	$\pm$ 21	< .001
Diastolic pressure (mm Hg)	79	$\pm$ 8	92	$\pm$ 11	< .001
Pulse pressure (mm Hg)	43	$\pm$ 9	52	$\pm$ 18	< .001
Heart rate (beats/min)	72	$\pm$ 11	103	$\pm$ 19	< .001
Plasma 11-OHCS (μg/100 ml)	19.72	$\pm$ 5.40	32.81	$\pm$ 9.51	< .001
Urine volume (ml)	74.18	$\pm$ 44.41	49.75	$\pm$ 33.12	< .01
Total catecholamines (μg per h)	2.70	$\pm$ 1.96	4.92	$\pm$ 2.97	< .001
Adrenaline (μg per h)	0.52	$\pm$ 0.32	1.21	$\pm$ 0.90	< .001
Noradrenaline (μg per h)	2.19	$\pm$ 2.01	3.71	$\pm$ 3.09	< .01

during control and examination conditions in 48 students. Stress caused a highly significant rise in all the parameters and a marked anti-diuresis.

An examination of the individual data for the various candidates showed a marked variation in the way individuals reacted to the stress. Thus, some showed marked elevations in their plasma 11-hydroxycorticosteroids but little change in B.P. or catecholamine excretion rates and *vice versa*. In order, therefore, to assess the relationships between the physiological indices of the psychological stress, four parameters were compared as measures of the anxiety response. The indices examined were heart rate, systolic blood pressure, urinary adrenaline excretion and plasma 11-hydroxycorticosteroids. The product–moment correlation coefficients between the results for the variables are given in Table 2 and none are statistically significant under the stress conditions.

The rank order of the subjects' responses in each parameter might offer a better assessment of the comparative relationships between the measures of anxiety. Therefore, the subjects were ranked from the one with the highest result to the one with

TABLE 2

PRODUCT–MOMENT CORRELATION COEFFICIENTS

	Control				Stress		
	Heart rate	Systolic B.P.	Plasma cortisol		Heart rate	Systolic B.P.	Plasma cortisol
Systolic B.P.	0.178			Systolic B.P.	0.236		
Plasma cortisol	−0.012	−0.053		Plasma cortisol	0.142	0.251	
Adrenaline excretion	0.038	0.141	0.113	Adrenaline excretion	0.135	0.278	−0.118

($p \leqslant 0.05$ when $r \geqslant 0.288$)

References pp. 334–335

the lowest result for each parameter. In this way each subject was placed in rank order for each parameter. Clearly, the agreement between the four rank orders gives an estimate of similarity between the four variables. Thus perfect concordance would be shown if each candidate had the same rank order for each parameter, *e.g.*, if a candidate had the 10th highest plasma 11-hydroxycorticosteroid level he would have the 10th highest adrenaline excretion rate etc. Kendall's coefficient of concordance (Siegel, 1956) was calculated, and includes all four groups of ranks together. The Kendall coefficient for the control results was 0.315 ($\chi^2 = 58.14$, $p < 0.1$) and for the results after the stress was 0.362 ($\chi^2 = 68.06$, $p < 0.05$). Thus, the rank orders are significantly concordant after the stress but not in the case of control observations.

The rank order correlation coefficients between the increment rises produced by stress for each parameter did not show a higher concordance for the four parameters than did the results using the stress levels alone.

The low level of concordance, even under stress conditions, confirms that responses to stress are individual in their nature. Not only do the individuals vary in their intensity of their response within a given physiological parameter, they also show varying degrees of responsiveness between different physiological parameters. So caution is necessary when comparing different experiments in which different psychological parameters are used to assess the stress response.

Why the correlation between these four parameters is low is difficult to assess. It is possible that different individuals react to anxiety in different ways. Some may activate primarily the pituitary-adrenocortical axis whilst others may activate primarily adrenal medullary activity, etc. However, there are other possible explanations. Plasma 11-hydroxycorticosteroid concentrations assess pituitary-adrenocortical activity only at one point in time, whilst urinary catecholamine levels assess the stress response over a longer period. This difference alone may account for the lack of higher concordance between these two parameters. The blood pressure was measured at the end of the examination and it is possible that the level of anxiety had decreased by this time and hence also the blood pressure response. It is quite likely that anxiety is at its highest before entering the examination. Blood pressure was not measured before the examination since permission was not granted for this in the preliminary experiment. A higher concordance may therefore be found in an experiment now in progress in which urinary corticosteroid concentration is used as the index of pituitary–adrenocortical activity and blood pressure is recorded before entering the examination.

The low correlation between the four parameters can also be explained by the fact that each parameter is modified by several factors particular to itself. Thus, the B.P. response is modified by baroreceptor reflexes, the plasma cortisol level is dependent not only on the amount of ACTH secreted and the responsiveness of the adrenal cortex but also on the rate of removal from the blood, and the urinary catecholamine levels may be modified by the renal handling of these amines.

To estimate the part played by the variables of personality and body build on the degree and nature of the stress responses, the personality and physique were assessed as described earlier. The mean scores for 80 students were neuroticism 9.08 $\pm$ 4.44

and for extraversion 11.98 ± 4.10. These compare with 10.006 ± 5.0 and 11.09 ± 4.5 reported as the mean for 347 university students by Eysenck and Eysenck, 1964. None of the students had abnormally high scores for neuroticism. Indeed, the range of extraversion and neuroticism scores is much narrower than would be found in the general population. Phenotypes were classified on a seven-point scale for the three characteristics of Fatness (F), Muscularity (M) and Linearity (L). The phenotypes may be grouped by primary and secondary traits, for example, the primary linear group includes those with secondary muscularity (Lm), secondary fat (Lf) and both secondary components equal (L). These results and the resting and stress plasma 11-hydroxycorticosteroid levels are shown in Table 3. Those with primary high muscular components had a significantly lower stress level of plasma 11-hydroxy-corticosteroids than those of a primary linear type of body build. When correlation coefficients were determined between the various parameters a negative coefficient of 0.225 ($p < 0.05$) was found between muscularity and stress levels of 11-hydroxy-corticosteroids. Additionally, a significant correlation coefficient of 0.219 ($p < 0.05$) was found between the neuroticism score and the control plasma 11-hydroxycorti-costeroids. It is possible that the control values were influenced by the mild anticipatory anxiety induced by the taking of blood samples. Since no significant correlation exists between stress levels of plasma adrenocortical hormones and the neuroticism score, it is likely that neuroticism relates only to psychological sensitivity to mild stress and is not important when stress is severe.

TABLE 3

MEAN RESULTS

Phenotype group	No.	E.P.I.		Phenotype			Plasma cortisol ($\mu g/100$ ml)	
		E. Score	N. Score	F	M	L	Control	Stress
L, Lm, Lf	21	11.6 ± 4.6	8.1 ± 3.8	2.6	3.4	5.0	17.6 ± 4.8	37.7 ± 12.5*
M, Ml, Mf	37	11.9 ± 3.7	10.1 ± 4.5	3.1	5.1	2.9	20.0 ± 4.3	31.0 ± 9.4*
F, Fl, Fm	8	13.0 ± 4.2	11.5 ± 3.6	5.3	3.1	2.5	17.6 ± 5.9	33.0 ± 9.8
All subjects	80	11.9 ± 4.1	9.4 ± 4.5	3.2	4.2	3.6	19.4 ± 4.7	33.7 ± 10.2

* $p < 0.05$

The data on rates of urinary noradrenaline excretion was collected on only 48 subjects, and in these the muscular group had higher levels than the linear group but the difference does not reach significance level (Table 4) but as the number of students in the linear groups was not large, it is possible that with more data the differences might have reached significance. As would be expected, the correlation coefficient between various types of body build and urinary catecholamine excretion rates was not significant.

In another part of the study no significant correlation was found between pheno-types and the blood pressure and pulse rates, though the resting diastolic blood pres-

TABLE 4

EFFECT OF PHENOTYPE GROUP ON URINE VOLUME AND CATECHOLAMINE RESPONSE TO STRESS

Phenotype group	No.	Urine volume ml	Total catechols μg/100 ml	Adrenaline μg/100 ml	Noradrenaline μg/100 ml	% Adrenaline	Total catechols μg/h	Adrenaline μg/h	Noradrenaline μg/h	Weight (lbs)
Control										
Linear	9	80.1*	2.82	0.92	1.92	38.5	1.95	0.65	1.33	151.7*
Muscular	22	65.8	4.80	0.99	3.80	32.7	3.04	0.56	2.49	155.3†
Fat	6	59.0	4.10	0.53	3.57	18.0	2.18	0.33	1.85	177.8†
Stress										
Linear	9	35.1*	10.56	2.77	6.85	30.3	3.68	1.17	2.52	
Muscular	22	48.1	14.30	2.79	11.52	32.1	6.01	1.25	4.76	
Fat	6	45.8	9.48	3.32	6.17	29.0	4.13	1.37	2.77	

* = $P < 0.01$
† = $P < 0.02$

sure correlated significantly with the degree of fatness. This correlation between the degree of fatness and control diastolic blood pressure is of interest since it is well-known that there is a connection between obesity and hypertension (Smirk, 1957). In the present study weight correlates significantly with fatness but an association between weight and diastolic blood pressure is not found. Thus, it may be that a predisposition to hypertension in young adults can be recognised by their fat component before the weight increase is obvious.

The Eysenck Personality Inventory scores showed no significant correlation with catecholamine excretion rate or the blood pressure and pulse rates.

No correlation was found between performance of the candidates at the examination and any of the physiological responses studied nor with the characteristics of physique or personality.

The present study was aimed, in part, at constructing a classification of the physiological responses resulting from the stress situation and their relation to individual characteristics. For this purpose, in addition to the above correlation coefficient matrix, a cluster analysis was carried out employing the classification program (CLASP) written for the Orion computer. Of the various methods of clustering a matrix of coefficients, that of median sorting has been employed here, which is similar

TABLE 5

MEANS OF PERSONAL DATA BY GROUPS

		Group		p
E.P.I.	N. score	A	7.6	
		B	9.7	
		R	10.6	
	E. score	A	11.2	
		B	11.9	
		R	12.7	
Phenotype	F	A	3.4	⎰ 0.02
		B	2.4	⎱
		R	3.3	} 0.01
	M	A	3.6	⎰ 0.001 ⎰
		B	4.9	⎱ } 0.001
		R	4.4	
	L	A	4.2	⎰ 0.02 ⎰
		B	3.4	⎱ } 0.01
		R	3.0	
	Height ins.	A	72.3	} 0.001 ⎰
		B	68.3	⎱ } 0.01
		R	70.5	} 0.01
	Weight lbs.	A	161.8	} 0.01
		B	143.8	⎱
		R	162.1	} 0.01

Group A ($n = 18$)   Group B ($n = 9$)   Remainder ($n = 21$)

References pp. 334–335

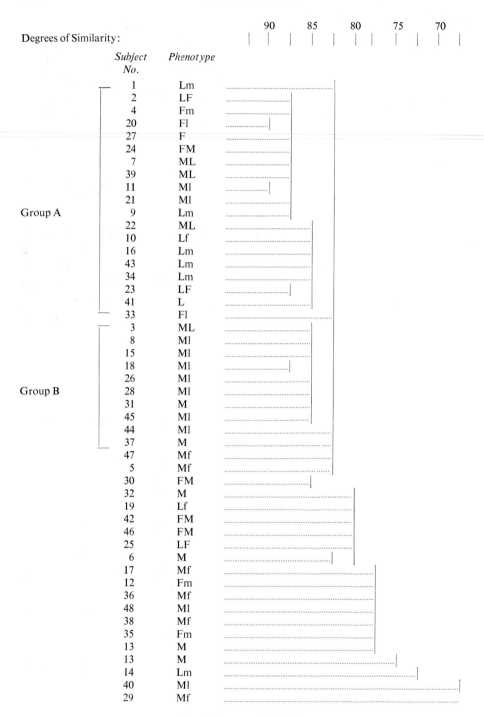

Fig. 1. Degrees of similarity.

TABLE 6

MEANS OF PHYSIOLOGICAL VARIABLES BY GROUPS

	Group	Control	p		Stress	p
Heart rate	A	70			100	
beats/min	B	66	} 0.05	} 0.05	96	
	R	77			108	
Plasma cortisol	A	17.6			34.1	
μg/100 ml	B	21.3			30.3	
	R	20.9			32.8	
Total catecholamines	A	3.2			3.8	} 0.001
μg/h	B	3.8	} 0.01	} 0.05	7.5	
	R	1.9			4.9	} 0.05
Adrenaline	A	0.5			1.1	
μg/h	B	0.5			1.2	
	R	0.5			1.3	
Noradrenaline	A	2.7			2.7	} 0.001
μg/h	B	3.3	} 0.01	} 0.05	6.3	
	R	1.4			3.7	} 0.05

Group A ($n = 18$)   Group B ($n = 9$)   Remainder ($n = 21$)

to the centroid method of Sokal and Michener (1958). Statistical significance is not given to the similarity coefficients as the magnitude of the individual coefficient is less important than the average level at which groups are formed. The measures of body build and personality together with the physiological variables after stress were included in the cluster analysis for 48 subjects, and the resulting dendrogram is shown in Fig. 1. Two main groups emerge whose levels of similarity were 85% or over One contained 18 subjects (group A) and the other 9 subjects (group B), leaving a remainder of 21 (group R). The phenotypes are given in Table 5 and it can be seen that group B consists exclusively of primarily muscular subjects, nearly all of whom had linearity as the secondary characteristics. Group A contains mainly subjects with primary linear or fat physiques. Of the total of 16 subjects with a major linear component (L, Lm, Lf, LF, ML), 11 appear in this group. The groups differ significantly in their physiques but not in relation to personality. The cluster analysis was based only on the stress values but the mean control values are shown as well in Table 6. The groups A and B differ in relation to the control heart rates, and also in relation to noradrenaline excretion in both control and stress conditions. The adrenaline excretion rates were almost identical in the two groups, both before and after stress. Group A in response to stress showed no increase in the noradrenaline excretion rate above the control value whilst group B was responsible for most of the noradrenaline response to stress.

Thus, group B which had the highest muscularity and lowest fat component showed the most marked noradrenaline response to stress; whilst group A, characterised by predominant linearity with the lowest muscular component, produced no noradrenaline response. These findings are of interest because of several reports that there is a differential catecholamine response on the basis of the evoking experience. Noradrenaline output has been stated to be particularly associated with active, aggressive behaviour whilst adrenaline excretion is more related to anxiety and tension (Elmajian, 1957; Schildkraut and Kety, 1967). Of course, mucular subjects may tend to respond to certain situations with anger rather than anxiety although it was not felt possible to assess the precise subjective experience at the time of the examination. The linear group A had the highest plasma cortisol level, whilst the mainly muscular group B had the lowest. These differences were not significant but, as stated earlier, when these results on 48 students were combined with the data on 32 other students, a significant negative correlation was found between muscularity and the stress plasma 11-hydroxycortisteroid levels. We are at present assessing the adrenocortical responsiveness of these 44 students to injected ACTH in an attempt to determine whether muscularity is associated with a reduced plasma 11-hydroxycorticosteroid response as a result of some peripheral mechanism.

In conclusion, it appears that a University oral examination is suitable for the investigation of the effects of stress since it is a realistic situation in which the subject's future is involved. There is a highly significant increase in pulse rate, blood pressure, plasma 11-hydroxycorticosteroids and in urinary adrenaline and noradrenaline excretion. The degree of concordance between these various parameters is low and there are several possible explanations for this. Physique with a high muscular component appears to be associated with a smaller plasma 11-hydroxycorticosteroid rise and a greater noradrenaline excretion rate in response to emotional stress than those with a different kind of body build. The mechanisms responsible for these particular associations between body build and the degree of plasma 11-hydroxycorticosteroid and urinary noradrenaline responses to stress have not been evaluated.

REFERENCES

BLISS, E. L., MIGEON, C. J., BRANCH, C. H. H. AND SAMUELS, L. T. (1956) Reaction of the adrenal cortex to emotional stress. *Psychosom. Med.*, **18**, 56–76.

BLOOM, G., VON EULER, U. S. AND FRANKENHAEUSER, M. (1963) Catecholamine excretion and personality traits in paratroop trainees. *Acta Physiol. Scand.*, **58**, 77–89.

ELMAJIAN, F. (1957) Excretion of epinephrine and norepinephrine in various emotional states. *J. Clin. Endocrinol.*, **17**, 608.

ELMAJIAN, F., HOPE, J. M. AND LAWSON, E. T. (1958) Excretion of epinephrine and norepinephrine under stress. *Recent Progr. Hormone Res.*, **14**, 513–553.

EYSENCK, H. J. AND EYSENCK, S. B. G. (1964) *Manual of the Eysenck Personality Inventory*, University of London Press, London.

FRANKENHAEUSER, M. AND POST, B. (1962) Catecholamine excretion during mental work as modified by centrally acting drugs. *Acta Physiol. Scand.*, **55**, 74–81.

GLICKSTEIN, M. (1960) Temporal patterns of cardiovascular response. *Arch. Gen. Psychiat.*, **2**, 12–21.

GOLDSTEIN, I. B. (1964) Physiological responses in anxious women patients: A study of autonomic activity and muscle tension. *Arch. Gen. Psychiat.*, **10**, 382–388.

HARRISON, J. (1964) The behaviour of the palmar sweat glands in stress. *J. Psychosom. Res.*, **8**, 187–191.

HICKAM, J. B., CARGILL, W. H. AND GOLDEN, A. (1948) Cardiovascular reactions to emotional stimuli: Effect on the cardiac output, arteriovenous oxygen difference, arterial pressure and peripheral resistance. *J. Clin. Invest.*, **27**, 290–298.

HODGES, J. R., JONES, M. T. AND STOCKHAM, M. A. (1962) Effect of emotion on blood corticotrophin and cortisol concentrations in man. *Nature*, **193**, 1187.

LAZARUS, R. S., SPEISMAN, J. C. AND MORDKOFF, A. M. (1963) The relationship between autonomic indicators of psychological stress: Heart rate and skin conductance. *Psychosom. Med.*, **25**, 19–30.

Leak, D., Brunjes, S., Johns, V. J. and Starr, P. (1962) Adrenal medullary response to insulin hypoglycaemia in hypothyroid patients. *J. Lab. Clin. Med.*, **60**, 811–817.

Levi, L. (1963) The urinary output of adrenaline and noradrenaline during experimentally induced emotional stress in clinically different groups. *Acta Psychotherap.*, **11**, 218–227 (No. 3–4).

Parnell, R. W. (1958) *Behaviour and Physique*, Arnold, London.

Persky, H. *et al.* (1958) Relation of emotional responses and changes in plasma hydrocortisone level after stressful interview. *Arch. Neurol. Psychiat.*, **79**, 434–447.

Schildkraut, J. J. and Kety, S. S. (1967) Biogenic amines and emotion. *Science*, **156**, 21.

Siegel, S. (1956) *Nonparametric Statistics*, McGraw-Hill Book Co., Inc., New York.

Smirk, F. H. (1957) *High Arterial Pressure*, Blackwell, Oxford.

Sokal, R. R. and Michener, C. D. (1958) A statistical method for evaluating systematic relationships. *Univ. Kansas Sci. Bull.*, **38**, 1409.

Sternbach, R. A. (1962) Assessing differential autonomic patterns in emotions. *J. Psychosom. Res.*, **6**, 87–91.

Wing, L. (1963) Physiological effects of performing a difficult task in patients with anxiety states. *J. Psychosom. Res.*, **7**, 283–294.

Zenker, N. and Bernstein, D. E. (1958) The estimation of small amounts of corticosterone in rat plasma. *J. Biol. Chem.*, **231**, 695–701.

DISCUSSION

De Wied: Quite some variation can be seen in your data. Did the results depend on the character of the professor, or on the result of the examination?

Jones: There are two professors as examiners. An internal examiner, who is the same each year, and an external one, who changes. We have not seen any striking differences between one year and the next. As far as the relation between examination results and physiological responses is concerned, we have found no significant correlation between the results and any of the physiological data.

Laron: Did you measure skin-fold thickness, as we know there is a correlation between cortisol secretion and degree of obesity.

Jones: Yes we have measured skin-fold thickness. However, the number of subjects with a high primary fat component in our studies was small so that we are unable to say much about any correlation between obesity and adrenocortical responsiveness. However, the mean stress value for plasma 11-hydroxycorticosteroids was lower in the group with a high primary fat content.

Hodges: I need hardly remind you of our earliest experiment in this field when we showed very high plasma cortisol levels indeed in the blood of female students in a similar stressful situation.

Jones: Certainly, some students did show very high plasma cortisol levels after the examination. When you and I first looked at the effects of examinations, I think we were lucky to have as volunteers the ones who showed very marked responses. But at that time we had data only on a handful of students. When the number was increased, however, a very wide scatter of responsiveness was seen.

Pituitary-Adrenal Activity During Psychosis and Depression

ALEC COPPEN

M.R.C. Neuropsychiatric Research Unit. Carshalton, and West Park Hospital, Epsom, Surrey, England

During the past decade there have been numerous investigations into the chemical pathology of the major psychoses and I think it true to say that no area has been more fully investigated than the pituitary–adrenal axis, particularly in the affective disorders. These investigations have to be seen in the light of our knowledge of the peculiar sensitivity of the pituitary–adrenal axis to any psychological stress in normal subjects. Indeed, it would be very surprising if mentally ill patients, suffering acute psychological turmoil were not to show considerable changes in adrenocortical function. The problem has been to determine the changes that occur in psychoses and to see if these changes are in any way specific to the condition, and to see if there is a causal relationship between the illness and the endocrine change.

One incentive to the intensive investigation of adrenocortical activity in mental illness has been the common occurrence of severe psychiatric symptoms in both hyper- and hypoadrenalism. There are many descriptions of the psychiatric sequelae of Cushing's syndrome, which occur to some extent in about half the patients and to a severe extent in about one-fifth of them (see review by Michael and Gibbons, 1963; Coppen, 1967). The most common reaction is a depressive reaction and the psychiatric symptoms almost always remit with successful treatment of the condition. In Addison's disease, psychiatric symptoms are also prominent and depression, apathy and irritability are amongst the most common symptoms. These symptoms also improve with adequate therapy. These findings of disturbances of mood in adrenocortical disease and also on the administration of high doses of ACTH or cortisol for therapeutic purposes have naturally encouraged many investigations of adrenocortical function in the affective disorders and it is these that I will now describe.

The problems involved with these investigations are formidable, as mostly, they are carried out on acutely disturbed patients admitted, often in circumstances of great distress, to a psychiatric hospital where they are confronted by other patients who are often threatening or hostile. It is known that normal subjects, admitted to a tranquil investigation ward show increased adrenocortical activity (see review by Gibbons, 1968) so patients admitted in these much more disturbing circumstances are very likely to show a similar change in adrenocortical activity. Table I illustrates the position very well. Acutely depressed patients had their plasma 11-hydroxycorticosteroid (11-OHCS) concentration at 8 a.m. estimated on the first day of admission, and on subsequent days after admission to a quiet, tranquil metabolic ward. It will be seen

TABLE 1

8 A.M. PLASMA 11-OHCS IN DEPRESSED PATIENTS DURING FIRST WEEK AFTER ADMISSION
AND ON DISCHARGE

	Days following admission					Discharge
	0–1	1–2	2–3	3+	7	
11-OHCS (μg/100 ml)	28.4	25.9	18.9	20.6	20.0	17.9
Depression score	26.3				21.0	5.1

that depressed patients behave very much like normal subjects. There is initially an increased 11-OHCS concentration which decreased slowly for several days. This was in a quiet metabolic ward and it is noteworthy that Anderson and Dawson (1965) found that there was a strikingly high plasma 17-hydroxycorticosteroids in depressed patients on admission to a general psychiatric ward as opposed to a research metabolic ward, and these differences overshadowed the changes that followed successful treatment and clinical recovery. It is clear, therefore, that single estimates of adrenocortical activity in patients recently admitted to hospital will tell little about the relationship of the illness, *per se*, to any abnormalities that may be observed and indeed may be positively misleading. There are other difficulties in assessing adrenocortical activity in mental illness; commonly used drugs in psychiatry, such as barbiturates, may alter corticosteroid secretion, or, like imipramine, may interfere with the chemical assays (Sachar, 1967). Electroconvulsive therapy also raises plasma cortisol but only for an hour or two (Hodges, Jones, Elithorn and Bridges, 1964).

Although many steroids are produced by the adrenal cortex, *i.e.*, corticosterone, aldosterone, oestrogens and androgens — it is mainly cortisol and its metabolites that has been studied in the affective disorders. As new techniques for measuring adrenocortical activity have emerged so they have been applied to the study of these patients. Plasma 17-hydroxycorticosteroid concentrations were studied by Board, Wadeson and Persky (1957) in patients suffering from depression, newly admitted to hospital, and they found considerably raised levels of 23.7 μg per 100 ml compared to 12.3 μg per 100 ml in controls. This approach was applied in a more sophisticated way by Gibbons and McHugh (1962) who measured morning plasma 17-hydroxycorticosteroid at weekly intervals in patients receiving treatment in hospital. After one week in hospital, before the commencement of treatment, the average level was 20.8 μg per 100 ml. The average levels found in these patients after successful treatment, just before discharge from hospital, was 10.8 μg per 100 ml. The correlation between mood and plasma 17-OHCS was 0.67 although it was found that in about 30% of cases, improvement occurred with no change in plasma cortisol levels. One patient who swung from normality to mania showed no change in plasma 17-OHCS levels. In a larger series of 29 depressed patients, morning and evening plasma 11-OHCS were estimated, before, during and after recovery (Brooksbank and Coppen, 1967). Table 1 shows that there is a steep decline in morning plasma 11-OHCS concentration during the first week after admission when, clinically, there

References p. 341

TABLE 2

PLASMA 11-OHCS SOON AFTER ADMISSION, ONE WEEK AFTER ADMISSION AND ON DISCHARGE

	Time sample taken	n	Admission		Week 1		Discharge	
			Plasma 11-OHCS (μg/100 ml) mean	Depression inventory score mean	Plasma 11-OHCS (μg/100 ml) mean	Depression inventory score mean	Plasma 11-OHCS (μg/100 ml) mean	Depression inventory score mean
Depression	8 a.m.	29	22.1	26.3	20.0	21.0	17.9	5.1
Depression	9 p.m.	17	11.9	26.0	13.5	19.8	8.6	2.6

was little change in the patients' condition. Table II shows the average values obtained after one week, in hospital, before treatment had commenced and when there was really little change in the patient's clinical state, and then the results at discharge after an average of about 5 to 6 weeks in hospital when the patients had clinically recovered. It will be seen that depressed patients behave very much like normal subjects: hospital admission produces an elevation in adrenocortical activity which soon subsides to a level found in normal subjects or in patients just after clinical recovery. Much smaller changes were found than by Gibbons and McHugh and this may be because these patients were studied in a very quiet metabolic ward with an absence of acute disturbance.

Fourteen of the twenty-nine patients had serum plasma levels estimated more than six times during their stay in hospital and in these, the correlation between plasma levels and clinical state was calculated. Only 5 out of 14 had a significant positive correlation and one had a significant negative correlation. The evening plasma levels, taken at 9 p.m. showed a similar trend but correlated better with clinical state. There was no disturbance of the usual diurnal rhythm. In the same investigation 8 manic patients were also studied and were found to have normal morning plasma concentrations.

There have been numerous investigations of urinary steroid excretion and, on the whole, they seem to reflect the changes that were found with plasma levels. After allowance has been made for the initial increase occasioned by admission to hospital, depressed patients, on average, show but a modest increase in urinary steroid excretion (Sachar, 1967; Kurland, 1964; Stenbäck, Jakobson and Rimon, 1966; Coppen, Julian, Fry and Marks, 1967). Bunney, Mason and Hamburg (1965) made serial estimates of urinary 17-OHCS in a group of 17 depressed patients, not treated by physical methods. The majority of patients had normal urinary excretion rates and a positive correlation was found between clinical rating of the severity of the illness and urinary excretion rates. In another study Bunney and Fawcett (1965) found high 17-OHCS excretion in 3 patients who subsequently committed suicide.

Gibbons (1968) has measured cortisol secretion rates in a series of 25 patients made before and after clinical recovery. The estimations were carried out at least 4 days after admission. The average for the 12 who were assessed as being severely ill was 30.9 mg per 24 h; for those judged be to moderately ill the average was 19.5 mg. In 23 patients the cortisol secretion rate was retested after clinical recovery and was found to be 14.4 mg; the normal range is approximately 15 mg per 24 h. In these 23 patients a significant decrease in cortisol secretion rate occurred in 70% of the patients. In 6 patients, corticosterone secretion was also measured and a significant decline occurred in 5 of them (Gibbons, 1966).

Few other steroids have been studied in depression. Ferguson, Bartram, Fowlie, Cathro, Birchall and Mitchell (1964) found low levels of 11-deoxy- and 17-oxosteroid excretion in 5 depressed female patients and reported that the excretion rates returned to normal after clinical recovery. However, the single 24-h urine sample during the illness period was collected within the first three days after admission to hospital and their reports of changes in urinary steroid excretion with recovery from depression must, therefore, be interpreted with caution. In our laboratory (Coppen, Julian, Fry and Marks, 1967) we could not confirm these findings in a series of male patients suffering from depression. In the same investigation, the urinary excretion of oestrogens was measured and it was found that the excretion of oestrone and oestradiol was significantly decreased during depression. In view of the considerable disturbance in electrolyte distribution found in depressive illness (Coppen, 1965) studies of aldosterone secretion would be useful although to date there are few available. Goodwin, Murphy and Bunney (1968) in a small series of depressed patients found lower than normal excretion rates of aldosterone which increased when the patients swung to mania.

The mechanism of the increased adrenocortical activity has been studied by the administration of dexamethasone. Gibbons and Fahy (1966) reported that the intramuscular injection of 2 mg of dexamethasone caused a prompt decline in plasma cortisol of both depressed patients and control subjects. They found that although the levels were higher in the patients throughout the three hours of the experiment, the rate of fall was the same in the two groups. This they interpreted as indicating that the feedback mechanism still operates in depressed patients. They also found that a smaller dose, 1 mg, which is nearer to physiological conditions, caused a significant fall in 9 a.m. plasma cortisol level of a small group of depressives. However, these results have not been repeated in other investigations. Fawcett and Bunney (1967) found that some of their severe depressives failed to respond to dexamethasone. Carroll, Martin and Davies (1968) reported that the morning plasma 11-OHCS level did not undergo its normal reduction in 14 out of 27 patients with severe depression. The resistance to dexamethasone correlated with the clinical rating of the severity of the depression. Recovery from depression was associated with return of normal responsivenesss to dexamethasone. It should be noted that in these patients the average morning plasma cortisol level (before dexamethasone) was only slightly elevated above normal. Carroll (1969), in a further series, found that the plasma cortisol response to hypoglycaemia was significantly impaired before treatment, particularly in the patients who also showed resistance to dexamethasone. He concluded that the results were consistent with a hypothalamic–pituitary insensitivity to hypoglycaemia in these subjects.

In conclusion, there is evidence of a small increase in adrenocortical activity in depressive illness but not in mania, and usually, the increase is of the same order as the increase occasioned by admission to a psychiatric hospital. Some patients show little change during recovery from a depressive illness and a marked increase in adrenocortical activity is by no means an invariable accompaniment of a depressive illness. There are also reports that adrenalectomized patients on fixed doses of steroids may suffer depression which will respond to electroconvulsive treatment or antidepressant medication (Crisp and Roberts, 1963; Lindqvist and Lindqvist, 1964). It seems, therefore, unlikely that changes in adrenocortical function have a primary place in the aetiology of most cases of affective disorders.

REFERENCES

ANDERSON, W. McC. AND DAWSON, J. (1965) The variability of plasma 17-OHCS levels in affective illness and schizophrenia. *J. Psychosomat. Res.*, **9**, 237–239.

BOARD, F., WADESON, R. AND PERSKY, H. (1957) Depressive affect and endocrine functions. *A.M.A. Arch. Neurol. Psychiat.*, **78**, 612–620.

BROOKSBANK, B. W. L. AND COPPEN, A. (1967) Plasma 11-hydroxycorticosteroids in affective disorders. *Brit. J. Psychiat.*, **113**, 395–404.

BUNNEY, W. E. AND FAWCETT, J. A. (1965) Possibility of a biochemical test for suicidal potential. *Arch. Gen. Psychiat.*, **13**, 232–239.

BUNNEY, W. E., MASON, J. W. AND HAMBURG, D. A. (1965) Correlations between behavioural variables and urinary 17-hydroxycorticosteroids in depressed patients. *Psychosomat. Med.*, **27**, 299–308.

CARROLL, B. J., MARTIN, F. I. R. AND DAVIES, B. (1968) Resistance to suppression by dexamethasone of plasma 11-OHCS levels in severe depressive illness. *Brit. Med. J.*, ii, 285–287.

CARROLL, B. J. (1969) Hypothalamic-pituitary function in depressive illness: Insensitivity to hypoglycaemia. *Brit. Med. J.*, **11**, 27–28.

COPPEN, A. (1965) Mineral metabolism in the affective disorders. *Brit. J. Psychiat.*, **111**, 1133–1138.

COPPEN, A. (1967) The biochemistry of the affective disorders. *Brit. J. Psychiat.*, **113**, 1237–1264.

COPPEN, A., JULIAN, T., FRY, D. E. AND MARKS, V. (1967) Body build and urinary steroid excretion in mental illness. *Brit. J. Psychiat.*, **113**, 269–276.

CRISP, A. H. AND ROBERTS, F. J. (1963) The response of an adrenalectomised patient to ECT. *Amer. J. Psychiat.*, **119**, 784–785.

FAWCETT, J. A. AND BUNNEY, W. E. (1967) Pituitary adrenal function and depression. *Arch. Gen. Psychiat.*, **16**, 517–535.

FERGUSON, H. C., BARTRAM, A. C. G., FOWLIE, H. C., CATHRO, D. M., BIRCHALL, K. AND MITCHELL, F.L. (1964) A preliminary investigation of steroid excretion in depressed patients before and after electroconvulsive therapy. *Acta Endocrinol.*, **47**, 58–68.

GIBBONS, J. L. AND McHUGH, P. R. (1962) Plasma cortisol in depressive illness. *J. Psychiat. Res.*, **1**, 162–171.

GIBBONS, J. L. (1966) The secretion rate of corticosterone in depressive illness. *J. Psychosomat. Res.*, **10**, 263–266.

GIBBONS, J. L. AND FAHY, T. J. (1966) Effect of dexamethasone on plasma corticosteroids in depressive illness. *Neuroendocrinology*, **1**, 358–363.

GIBBONS, J. L. (1968) The adrenal cortex and psychological distress. In: *Endocrinology and Human Behaviour*, R. MICHAEL (Ed.), Oxford University Press, London, pp. 220–236.

GOODWIN, F. K., MURPHY, D. L. AND BUNNEY, W. E. (1968) *Amer. Psychiat. Assoc. Meeting in Boston.*

HODGES, J. R., JONES, M., ELITHORN, A. AND BRIDGES, P. (1964) Effect of electroconvulsive therapy on plasma cortisol levels. *Nature*, **204**, 754–755.

KURLAND, H. D. (1964) Steroid excretion in depressive disorders. *Arch. Gen. Psychiat.*, **10**, 554–560.

LINDQVIST, B. E. R. AND LINDQVIST, G. (1964) The antidepressant effect of amitriptyline in an adrenalectomised patient. *Amer. J. Psychiat.*, **120**, 912–913.

MICHAEL, R. P. AND GIBBONS, J. L. (1963) Interrelationships between the endocrine system and neuropsychiatry. *Intern. Rev. Neurobiol.*, **5**, 243–302.

SACHAR, E. J. (1967) Corticosteroids in depressive illness. *Arch. Gen. Psychiat.*, **17**, 544–567.

STENBÄCK, A., JAKOBSON, T. AND RIMON, R. (1966) Depression and anxiety ratings in relation to the excretion of urinary total 17-OHCS in depressive subjects. *J. Psychosomat. Res.*, **9**, 355–362.

DISCUSSION

KLEIN: In children admitted to hospital for random problems, morning cortisol levels fall to normal after only 3–4 days, according to studies we and others have done. Is the slower decrease you have shown due to the fact that you study adults, or due to the underlying disease?

COPPEN: The adaptation of depressed adult patients to the hospital environment parallels the adaptation which is found in mentally normal subjects, given similar circumstances.

SACHAR: In reference to Dr. Gibbons' studies reported by Dr. Coppen, I learned on visiting Dr. Gibbons that virtually all the cases showing large changes in cortisol production rate were in fact patients undergoing psychotic disorganization with beginning delusion formation. His sample of depressed patients was therefore highly selective; in fact he had been specially looking for these patients. I think that the data Dr. Coppen has reported and put together with some of the other data available really begins to make a consistent picture of adreno-cortical activity in depressions.

NIJDAM: I would like to ask if you have any experience with manic depressive patients and whether you have investigated in the same patients manic and depressive states. Commenting on the observation that E.C.T. is working in mania and in depression as well, it is still intriguing that sith drugs we have to use different treatments, ant-depressants for depression and neuroleptics for mania.

COPPEN: I think that the chemical pathology of mania and depression are markedly similar. I think they show the same changes in indolamines and electrolyte distribution. Looked from this point of view manies are disturbed depressives. E.C.T. is certainly used both in mania and depression.

NIJDAM: Have you any experience with manic and depressive states in the same patient as far as levels of cortisol are concerned.

COPPEN: Plasma cortisol levels show a decline with recovery from depression, but little change is observed when they swing to mania.

McCLURE: Do you think there is any correlation between your indolamine and your corticosteroid findings?

COPPEN: We have no direct evidence on this point.

JONES: Do you know of any abnormality of the circadian rhythm of plasma cortisol in depression?

COPPEN: We measured 8 AM and 9 PM plasma cortisol levels in 29 depressed patients before and after recovery and could detect no change in the diurnal variation.

Summing–up of session IV

ACTH, corticosteroids and the Brain: Clinical studies

R. A. CLEGHORN

Department of Psychiatry, Allan Memorial Institute, McGill University,
1025 Pine Avenue West, Montreal 112, P. Quebec. (Canada)

The rapid expansion of research in endocrinology, about which we have been hearing, emphasizes an interrelationship with the central nervous system. This was long ago suspected but only proven in recent years. Much of what we have been hearing at this conference recapitulates and recalls major events of the last 70 years. I have tried to capture in a thumbnail sketch a few of those events which highlight critical developments in endocrinology by itemizing in terms of decades a few outstanding advances.

In *1901*, there was the isolation of adrenalin.

In *1910*, there appeared that monumental landmark, Biedl's "die innere Sekretion." A short two years later, Cushing's "Pituitary Body and Its Disorders" was published.

By *1922*, arguments raged about the responsibility of pituitary and hypothalamus for the disabilities following ablation of the gland. This issue was clarified five years later by P. E. Smith's new technique for hypophysectomy in the rat.

1932 was noteworthy because of Edgar Allen's timely monograph on "Sex and Internal Secretions" which provided a clear summary of a field that was about to flower so abundantly. So the next decade was bursting with significant discoveries and developments. Many steroid hormones were isolated, while Selye enunciated his theory of stress and the adrenals.

By *1942*, critical evidence of the action of corticosteroids on the central nervous system appeared in the reports of Engel and Margolin, and Thorn and his colleagues, on the altered EEG in Addison's disease and the psychological changes in that condition.

By *1952*, ACTH and cortisone stirred therapeutic hopes and renewed interest in the influence of hormones on the central nervous system because of the mental symptoms evoked. The following year, Mirsky reported on effects of ACTH on conditioned responses, thereby initiating a whole new area of study.

By *1961*, when Young's classical edition of "Sex and Internal Secretions" was published, so much more data on the influence of hormones on behaviour had been recorded that it hardly seemed like the same discipline described 30 years earlier by Allen. Since then, still more facts have accumulated on the inter-relationships of the endocrinological and central nervous systems, and our debt now is to Dr. de Wied and his staff of the Rudolf Magnus Institute for organizing this conference which deals with recent investigations and carries us to the periphery of knowledge in that field.

We have heard papers describing details of the reciprocal action of the nervous and hormonal systems. We have heard accounts of scientific studies demonstrating clearly the mutual interdependence of these two systems. Now, the degree of inter-relatedness and interdependence is so well established that these new data, and points of view, must be incorporated in the current knowledge of the informed clinician. In the achievement of these advances, one must recognize not only the painstaking skill of the investigators, but also their dependence on those elaborate and sensitive chemical and electronic methods developed in the last two or three decades. By combining these with conditioning techniques, there has been opened up a new and more subtle appreciation of central nervous system activity. The finding of an action of ACTH directly on the brain provided exciting results — while seeming at first like heresy to older students like myself who were schooled in a fixed view of a limited trophic action on a target gland. The extension of this research to demonstrate that a fraction of the ACTH molecule, itself no longer active on the adrenal, has a pro-found influence on brain functioning, is a revelation of the first order. This was demonstrated on human subjects in this 4th section in experiments where the ACTH fraction was described as having a disintegrating action on EEG conditioned syn-chrony. It remains to be seen in what way this is significantly related to previously reported experiments on animals in which the ACTH delayed extinction of a con-ditioned response.

The pertinence of physiological studies on lower animals for an understanding of the comparable but more complicated activity in man was repeatedly in evidence during this last session. Concepts, such as arousal, homeostasis and stress, were recurring themes. Growth, development, performance and emotions, were topics of major concern. It was shown that physiological parameters can be correlated to body build. This raises the hope that further studies of this order may clarify that tantali-zingly conflicting topic of physique and character, about which so much has been written and from which so little of significance has emerged.

The effect of corticosteroids (CS) on sensory systems has long been known from work on rats and, indeed, from some clinical observations. Now this has been expertly studied in untreated Addison's disease in which both taste and hearing are exquisitely sensitive. Restoration to normal occurs only with the carbohydrate-active steroids. Apparently word recognition also declines in adrenal insufficiency, so that it seems that processing of information to and in the brain is badly integrated. Here is a rich area ripe for study by neurologists and psychiatrists.

The influence of hormonal deficiency was further demonstrated in this session in the accounts of dwarfs and the identification of their metabolic faults. The contrary influence of hormonal excess on growth and development may be a higher I.Q. in either the naturally occurring syndrome or those iatrogenically induced by progester-one treatment of women with treatened abortion. Female issue of such prenatal exposure behave in rough male ways, rather like Harlow's testosterone-induced hermaphroditic monkeys. Our concepts of character traits seem to be shifting from an excessively environmentally-oriented point of view, emphasizing social influences, to the probability of greater biological control.

Psychological control of endocrine activity is also a very live issue as shown by studies on the emotional disturbances associated with depressive and psychotic states and adrenocortical activity. The high blood or urinary level of CS, earlier reported as charasteristic of depression, now seems to be more probably dependent upon the degree of emotional turmoil associated with the upset of admission to hospital or the occurrence of panic or anxiety attacks. This is an area where psychodynamic thinking, derived from Freudian psychoanalysis, integrates profitably in the interpretation of findings. This is so because it has been found that denial, delusional or paranoid thinking may protect the emotional core of the subject from distressing arousal. By this inappropriate type of mental reorganization, bodily homeostasis is maintained.

In closing, I cannot refrain from a quotation which seems to say a lot in a gracious, literary way about the concepts and psychobiological events we have been considering. It is from Samuel Butler's "The Way of All Flesh." He says:

"All our lives long, every day and every hour, we are engaged in the process of accommodating our changed and unchanged selves to changed and unchanged surroundings; living, in fact, is nothing else than this process of accommodation; when we fail in it a little we are stupid, when we fail flagrantly, we are mad, when we suspend it temporarily, we sleep, when we give up the attempt altogether, we die. In quiet, uneventful lives the changes internal and external are so small that there is little or no strain in the process of fusion and accomodation; in other lives there is great strain, but there is also great fusing and accommodating power. A life will be successful or not, according as the power of accommodation is equal to or unequal to the strain of fusing and adjusting internal and external things."

From this paragraph, I would like to use the words *accommodation, change, surroundings, strain* and *success* in another context. We have been accommodated in this beautiful place, Vierhouten. We have listened in gracious surroundings to great changes taking place in our science; it has been no strain but a great success because of the hospitality, perspicacity and the magnificent organization of the conference by our hosts of the Rudolf Magnus Institute for Pharmacology. To them and to the Rector-Magnificus Professor Lanjouw, we offer our heartfelt thanks for so much food for the mind and the body.

Author Index

Subject Index

International Conference on the Pituitary-Adrenal Axis and the Nervous System, Vierhouten, Netherlands, 1969.

Pituitary, adrenal and the brain. Ed. by D. de Wied and J. A. W. M. Weijnen. Amsterdam, New York, Elsevier Publishing Co., 1970.

xv, 357 p. with illus. 27 cm. (Progress in brain research, v. 32)

fl 78.00   Ne 70–42

"Organized by the Rudolf Magnus Institute for Pharmacology, University of Utrecht, and held at Vierhouten, The Netherlands, 22–24 July, 1969."

Includes bibliographies.

1. Pituitary body—Congresses. 2. Adrenal glands—Congresses. 3. Brain — Congresses.   I. Wied, David de, ed.   II. Weijnen, J. A. W. M., ed. III. Utrecht. Rijksuniversiteit. Rudolf Magnus Instituut voor   Farmacologie. IV. Title. (Series)

QP376.P7 vol. 32   612'.8   70–110965

ISBN 90–444–40854–1

Library of Congress   71 (4)